Traumatic Brain Injury: Clinical Characteristics and Outcomes

Traumatic Brain Injury: Clinical Characteristics and Outcomes

Editor

Rafael Badenes

MDPI • Basel • Beijing • Wuhan • Barcelona • Belgrade • Manchester • Tokyo • Cluj • Tianjin

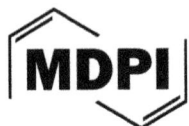

Editor
Rafael Badenes
University of Valencia
Spain

Editorial Office
MDPI
St. Alban-Anlage 66
4052 Basel, Switzerland

This is a reprint of articles from the Special Issue published online in the open access journal *Journal of Clinical Medicine* (ISSN 2077-0383) (available at: https://www.mdpi.com/journal/jcm/special_issues/Traumatic_Brain_Injury_Characteristics_Outcomes).

For citation purposes, cite each article independently as indicated on the article page online and as indicated below:

LastName, A.A.; LastName, B.B.; LastName, C.C. Article Title. *Journal Name* **Year**, *Volume Number*, Page Range.

ISBN 978-3-0365-5527-0 (Hbk)
ISBN 978-3-0365-5528-7 (PDF)

© 2022 by the authors. Articles in this book are Open Access and distributed under the Creative Commons Attribution (CC BY) license, which allows users to download, copy and build upon published articles, as long as the author and publisher are properly credited, which ensures maximum dissemination and a wider impact of our publications.

The book as a whole is distributed by MDPI under the terms and conditions of the Creative Commons license CC BY-NC-ND.

Contents

About the Editor vii

Małgorzata Barud, Wojciech Dabrowski, Dorota Siwicka-Gieroba, Chiara Robba, Magdalena Bielacz and Rafael Badenes
Usefulness of Cerebral Oximetry in TBI by NIRS
Reprinted from: *J. Clin. Med.* **2021**, *10*, 2938, doi:10.3390/jcm10132938 1

Annachiara Marra, Maria Vargas, Pasquale Buonanno, Carmine Iacovazzo, Antonio Coviello and Giuseppe Servillo
Early vs. Late Tracheostomy in Patients with Traumatic Brain Injury: Systematic Review and Meta-Analysis
Reprinted from: *J. Clin. Med.* **2021**, *10*, 3319, doi:10.3390/jcm10153319 11

Wojciech Dabrowski, Dorota Siwicka-Gieroba, Chiara Robba, Magdalena Bielacz, Joanna Sołek-Pastuszka, Katarzyna Kotfis, Romuald Bohatyrewicz, Andrzej Jaroszyński, Manu L. N. G. Malbrain and Rafael Badenes
Potentially Detrimental Effects of Hyperosmolality in Patients Treated for Traumatic Brain Injury
Reprinted from: *J. Clin. Med.* **2021**, *10*, 4141, doi:10.3390/jcm10184141 21

Dong-Ki Kim, Dong-Hun Lee, Byung-Kook Lee, Yong-Soo Cho, Seok-Jin Ryu, Yong-Hun Jung, Ji-Ho Lee and Jun-Ho Han
Performance of Modified Early Warning Score (MEWS) for Predicting In-Hospital Mortality in Traumatic Brain Injury Patients
Reprinted from: *J. Clin. Med.* **2021**, *10*, 1915, doi:10.3390/jcm10091915 33

Nicole von Steinbuechel, Katrin Rauen, Fabian Bockhop, Amra Covic, Ugne Krenz, Anne Marie Plass, Katrin Cunitz, Suzanne Polinder, Lindsay Wilson, Ewout W. Steyerberg, Andrew I. R. Maas, David Menon, Yi-Jhen Wu, Marina Zeldovich and the CENTER-TBI Participants and Investigators
Psychometric Characteristics of the Patient-Reported Outcome Measures Applied in the CENTER-TBI Study
Reprinted from: *J. Clin. Med.* **2021**, *10*, 2396, doi:10.3390/jcm10112396 43

Nicole von Steinbuechel, Katrin Rauen, Ugne Krenz, Yi-Jhen Wu, Amra Covic, Anne Marie Plass, Katrin Cunitz, Isabelle Mueller, Fabian Bockhop, Suzanne Polinder, Lindsay Wilson, Ewout W. Steyerberg, Andrew I. R. Maas, David Menon, Marina Zeldovich and The Linguistic Validation Group of CENTER-TBI
Translation and Linguistic Validation of Outcome Instruments for Traumatic Brain Injury Research and Clinical Practice: A Step-by-Step Approach within the Observational CENTER-TBI Study
Reprinted from: *J. Clin. Med.* **2021**, *10*, 2863, doi:10.3390/jcm10132863 77

Won Pyo Hong, Ki Jeong Hong, Sang Do Shin, Kyoung Jun Song, Tae Han Kim, Jeong Ho Park, Young Sun Ro, Seung Chul Lee, Chu Hyun Kim and Joo Jeong
Association of Flow Rate of Prehospital Oxygen Administration and Clinical Outcomes in Severe Traumatic Brain Injury
Reprinted from: *J. Clin. Med.* **2021**, *10*, 4097, doi:10.3390/jcm10184097 109

Romuald Bohatyrewicz, Joanna Pastuszka, Wojciech Walas, Katarzyna Chamier-Cieminska, Wojciech Poncyljusz, Wojciech Dabrowski, Joanna Wojczal, Piotr Luchowski, Maciej Guzinski, Elzbieta Jurkiewicz, Monika Bekiesinska-Figatowska, Radoslaw Owczuk, Jerzy Walecki, Olgierd Rowinski, Maciej Zukowski, Krzysztof Kusza, Mariusz Piechota, Andrzej Piotrowski, Marek Migdal, Marzena Zielinska and Marcin Sawicki
Implementation of Computed Tomography Angiography (CTA) and Computed Tomography Perfusion (CTP) in Polish Guidelines for Determination of Cerebral Circulatory Arrest (CCA) during Brain Death/Death by Neurological Criteria (BD/DNC) Diagnosis Procedure
Reprinted from: *J. Clin. Med.* **2021**, *10*, 4237, doi:10.3390/jcm10184237 . . . . **119**

Carlos Lam, Ju-Chuan Yen, Chia-Chieh Wu, Heng-Yu Lin and Min-Huei Hsu
Effects of the COVID-19 Pandemic on Treatment Efficiency for Traumatic Brain Injury in the Emergency Department: A Multicenter Study in Taiwan
Reprinted from: *J. Clin. Med.* **2021**, *10*, 5314, doi:10.3390/jcm10225314 . . . . **133**

Wojciech Dabrowski, Dorota Siwicka-Gieroba, Todd T. Schlegel, Chiara Robba, Sami Zaid, Magdalena Bielacz, Andrzej Jaroszyński and Rafael Badenes
Suppression of Electrographic Seizures Is Associated with Amelioration of QTc Interval Prolongation in Patients with Traumatic Brain Injury
Reprinted from: *J. Clin. Med.* **2021**, *10*, 5374, doi:10.3390/jcm10225374 . . . . **145**

Francesco Corallo, Viviana Lo Buono, Rocco Salvatore Calabrò and Maria Cristina De Cola
Can Cranioplasty Be Considered a Tool to Improve Cognitive Recovery Following Traumatic Brain Injury? A 5-Years Retrospective Study
Reprinted from: *J. Clin. Med.* **2021**, *10*, 5437, doi:10.3390/jcm10225437 . . . . **157**

About the Editor

Rafael Badenes

Rafael Badenes is a Medical Doctor, PhD, specialist in Anesthesiology and Intensive Care. Head of Department of Anesthesiology and Surgical-Trauma Intensive Care, Hospital Clínic Universitari de Valencia, Valencia, Spain. Full Professor at Department of Surgery, Anesthesia & Critical Care Unit, University of Valencia. Spain. Scientist of INCLIVA Research Health Intitute, Valencia, Spain. His primary research interests are currently neuroscience related to intensive care medicine.

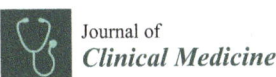

Review

Usefulness of Cerebral Oximetry in TBI by NIRS

Małgorzata Barud [1,*], Wojciech Dabrowski [1], Dorota Siwicka-Gieroba [1], Chiara Robba [2], Magdalena Bielacz [3] and Rafael Badenes [4]

1 Department of Anaesthesiology and Intensive Therapy, Medical University of Lublin, 20-954 Lublin, Poland; w.dabrowski5@yahoo.com (W.D.); dsiw@wp.pl (D.S.-G.)
2 Department of Anaesthesia and Intensive Care, Policlinico San Martino, 16100 Genova, Italy; kiarobba@gmail.com
3 Institute of Tourism and Recreation, State Vocational College of Szymon Szymonowicz, 22-400 Zamosc, Poland; magda.bielacz@gmail.com
4 Department of Anaesthesiology and Intensive Care, Hospital Clínico Universitario de Valencia, University of Valencia, 46010 Valencia, Spain; rafaelbadenes@gmail.com
* Correspondence: gosiekbar@wp.pl

Abstract: Measurement of cerebral oximetry by near-infrared spectroscopy provides continuous and non-invasive information about the oxygen saturation of haemoglobin in the central nervous system. This is especially important in the case of patients with traumatic brain injuries. Monitoring of cerebral oximetry in these patients could allow for the diagnosis of inadequate cerebral oxygenation caused by disturbances in cerebral blood flow. It could enable identification of episodes of hypoxia and cerebral ischemia. Continuous bedside measurement could facilitate the rapid diagnosis of intracranial bleeding or cerebrovascular autoregulation disorders and accelerate the implementation of treatment. However, it should be remembered that the method of monitoring cerebral oximetry by means of near-infrared spectroscopy also has its numerous limitations, resulting mainly from its physical properties. This paper summarizes the usefulness of monitoring cerebral oximetry by near-infrared spectroscopy in patients with traumatic brain injury, taking into account the advantages and the disadvantages of this technique.

Keywords: cerebral oximetry; near-infrared spectroscopy; traumatic brain injury; cerebrovascular autoregulation; intracranial pressure

1. Introduction

Traumatic brain injuries (TBIs) are some of the main causes of mortality in patients injured as a result of traffic accidents, falls from a height, battery, or firearm assault. TBIs are classified in various ways. Depending on the severity of the injury, they are divided into mild, moderate, and severe injuries. Depending on the mechanism of injury, they are classified into focal injuries and primary diffuse brain injuries. They can be isolated or part of a multi-organ trauma. TBI leads to primary brain injury.

Treatment of patients with TBI is primarily focused on preventing secondary brain injury. For many years, the standard of care for patients with TBI has been the monitoring of intracranial pressure (ICP) and cerebral perfusion pressure (CPP), estimated as the difference between ICP and mean arterial pressure (MAP) [1]. Continuous EEG monitoring is also increasingly used. However, these methods do not provide direct information on hypoxia and ischemia or the metabolic needs of the brain tissue. Hence, there is a need to use a method that would allow the assessment of cerebral oxygenation.

For almost 30 years now, a method of non-invasive monitoring of cerebral oximetry using near-infrared spectroscopy (NIRS) has been available. This technique was initially used in neonatal intensive care [2] and cardiac surgery [3], and has since been increasingly employed in adult intensive care.

2. Near-Infrared Spectroscopy (NIRS)

Cerebral oximetry measurements are performed using near-infrared spectroscopy (NIRS). It is a continuous, non-invasive method that enables monitoring of regional cerebral oxygen saturation. Normal NIRS readings represent a balance between oxygen supply and consumption in peripheral tissues.

The technique was first described by Jobsis in 1977 [4]. Under physiological conditions, tissues are relatively translucent to near-infrared light with wavelengths of 700–1000 nm, and the absorption of light by tissues is low. As a result, light can penetrate to a depth of up to 8 cm and still be completely detectable. [5]. Near-infrared light beams can penetrate bones, which is essential for transcranial monitoring of cerebral oximetry.

Cerebral oximetry measurements are cheap and easy to take. Special sensors are applied to the scalp which allow one to obtain measurements mainly from the external parts of the brain. For practical reasons, the sensors are commonly attached to the scalp overlying the frontal lobe, but measurements can be made from above any brain lobe. Each probe has a near-infrared light generator (diode or laser) and a proximal and distal light detector. Mixed arterial and venous blood in the brain and external tissues is measured. The arterial to venous blood ratio in the brain is 15:85 [6]. Hemoglobin oxygenation in brain vessels is estimated using percutaneous measurements of the amount of light absorbed by hemoglobin in the cerebral cortex.

The light transmitted through biological tissues is reflected, absorbed and scattered. Light reflection is determined by the angle between the light beam and the tissue surface. The absorption of light by tissues, causing the attenuation of light, depends on the chromophores—oxyhemoglobin, deoxyhaemoglobin and cytochrome oxidase. NIRS uses the different absorption properties of oxyhemoglobin, deoxyhaemoglobin and cytochrome oxidase to quantify their concentrations in tissues [7]. The relationship between the concentration of chromophore (c), its extinction coefficient (α), distance traveled by light in tissues (d), and the ratio of the incident light intensity (I_0) to the intensity of transmitted light (I) is determined by the Beer-Lambert equation [5,8]:

$$A = \log(I_0/I) = \alpha \times c \times d \tag{1}$$

Most photons in tissues are scattered, so the path traveled by photons can be much longer than the direct distance between the optodes. Most of the total attenuation of an infrared light beam is due to scattering, and only a small portion is absorbed. That is why the differential pathlength factor (DPF) and factor G, which depends on light losses other than attenuation, need to be added to the above equation [5,9]:

$$A = \log(I_0/I) = \alpha \times c \times d \times DPF + G \tag{2}$$

NIRS measurements in adults can be performed with the emitter and detectors placed on the same side of the head, providing "regional" information on brain oxygenation as only a small volume of brain tissue between the optodes is examined. In this method, the light travels along an arc with a tissue penetration depth of approximately half the distance between the emitter and the detectors. It is recommended that the distance between the optodes be not less than 2.5 to 3 cm, because the shorter the distance between the optodes, the more strongly the extracerebral tissues attenuate the light [5].

The first NIRS devices used two or three wavelengths and were mainly trend monitors. Nowadays, a four-wavelength generation of NIRS monitors are available, which provide reliable real-time regional cerebral oxygen saturation readings. NIRS devices can use three different detection modes: continuous wave (CW), frequency domain (FD), and time domain (TD). CW monitors are the most popular and the simplest devices. They measure the attenuation of incident light. FD monitors use high-frequency modulation to measure the phase and intensity of the signals generated. This technique allows a more quantitative assessment of the optical properties of tissues. TD monitors measure the time of flight of photons and are the most expensive of all NIRS devices [10].

3. Usefulness of Monitoring Cerebral Oximetry in TBI Patients by NIRS

3.1. Identification of Episodes of Impaired Cerebral Oxygenation

Adequate cerebral oxygenation is essential in treating patients with TBI. There exist invasive measurement methods, such as the measurement of jugular bulb oxygen saturation (SjvO2) or the measurement of brain tissue oxygen pressure (PbtO2). However, cerebral oximeters using NIRS are more and more frequently employed to obtain non-invasive measurements of cerebral oxygenation.

In a study by Esnault et al., cerebral oximetry (rScO2) values obtained by NIRS were compared with the results of an invasive measurement of brain tissue oxygen pressure. A PbtO2 probe was inserted into the frontal lobe of the cerebral hemisphere with more severe tissue injury/damage. The rScO2 sensor, on the other hand, was placed on the skin in the frontal area ipsilateral to the PbtO2 probe. The authors found no correlation between the readings obtained with NIRS and the tissue oxygen pressure probe. Cerebral oximetry allowed one to identify only about 15% of the ischemic episodes detected by the PbtO2 measurement. When one of the subjects developed brain death, NIRS continued to show normal rScO2 values, while PbtO2 dropped to 0 mmHg. Esnault et al. concluded that rScO2 measurement could not be used interchangeably with PbtO2 as a monitor of cerebral oxygenation in patients with TBI [11].

The correlation between rScO2 and PbtO2 in TBI patients was also investigated by Leal-Noval et al. In their study, involving 56 patients, a weak correlation was observed between rScO2 and PbtO2 measurements. Moreover, rScO2 was shown to have poor accuracy in detecting moderate cerebral hypoxia [12], which is in agreement with the observations made by Esnault et al. [11]. Detectability improved when hypoxia reached PbtO2 values <12 mmHg [12].

Entirely different observations have been reported by Brawanski et al. Over 90% of their rScO2 readings from the frontal area and PbtO2 measurements from the white matter of the frontal lobe showed a significant correlation. An analysis of their data indicated that the PbrO2 and the rScO2 signals contained similar information despite the fact that they were obtained using completely different technologies [13]. A significant correlation between PbtO2 and rScO2 readings has also been demonstrated in patients with TBI in other research [14].

In a study comparing two types of NIRS monitors—NIRO 200, which measures the cerebral tissue oxygenation index (TOI), and INVOS 5100, which monitors rScO2, jugular bulb oxygen saturation (SjvO2) and central venous saturation (ScvO2) were also measured. Thirty one pediatric patients with congenital heart defects were examined. A significant correlation was demonstrated between the rScO2 and SjvO2 measurements, and an even higher correlation between rScO2 and ScvO2. Similarly, a high correlation between readings was observed for TOI [15].

Monitoring of cerebral oximetry using NIRS in septic shock patients allowed investigation of the relationship between rScO2 and ScvO2. rScO2 and ScvO2 values increased with the progressing stabilization of the patients' condition and the decrease in lactic acidosis. The study demonstrated that there was a significant negative correlation between lactic acid levels and rScO2 values. On the other hand, a significant positive correlation between rScO2 and ScvO2 readings was observed at 8, 24, 48, and 72 h after admission to the ICU [16].

Many authors believe that cerebral oximetry monitoring using NIRS is an unreliable technique for monitoring oxygen metabolism in the brain tissue compared to measurements of brain tissue oxygen pressure. However, it should be noted that rScO2 and PbtO2 measure different parameters using different techniques. Moreover, PbtO2 is not acknowledged as a gold standard for monitoring oxygen metabolism in the brain. PbtO2 measurements are representative of a small area of tissue in the immediate vicinity of the probe. On the other hand, monitoring of rScO2 could prove very useful in patients in whom an invasive technique cannot or should not be used for various reasons. Both of these parameters could be monitored simultaneously to obtain a more complete picture of changes in cerebral oxygen metabolism [17]. Of note, jugular bulb oxygen saturation measurement, commonly used in TBI patients, gives a more global picture of cerebral oxygenation, and so local tissue hypoxia may go unnoticed when using this technique [18].

3.2. Monitoring of Cerebrovascular Autoregulation

Autoregulation of cerebral blood flow (CBF) is one of the most important mechanisms for maintaining intracranial homeostasis. It keeps CBF at a constant level in the face of changing cerebral perfusion pressure (CPP). This prevents disturbances in CBF during significant changes in arterial blood pressure. Autoregulation is extremely important in TBI patients in the context of the development of secondary injuries. As a result of impaired autoregulation, the balance between the cerebral metabolic rate of oxygen (CMRO2), cerebral blood volume (CBV) and CBF can be disturbed. This may lead to ischemic or hyperemic brain lesions, hypoxia or increased intracranial pressure. There is ample scientific evidence that abnormal autoregulation of CBF is associated with poorer treatment outcomes in patients with TBI [19,20]. Monitoring of CBF autoregulation may allow to individualize CPP targets in patients with TBI, which is associated with improved treatment outcomes [21,22].

Currently, different methods are available for assessing CBF autoregulation. The most widely used invasive techniques include measurement of intracranial pressure (ICP) and direct measurement of oxygen content in the brain tissue (parenchymal PbtO2 monitoring). Among non-invasive methods, transcranial Doppler (TCD) ultrasonography, which measures CBF velocity [23], and NIRS cerebral oximetry are commonly employed.

The values of cerebral oximetry are mainly influenced by CBF, cerebral metabolic rate of oxygen and arterial blood oxygen content. Owing to the fact that the factors affecting oxygen metabolism are relatively stable over short periods of time, NIRS can be used in place of invasive methods of bedside monitoring of changes in CBF [24,25].

Depending on the manufacturer and the technology used, NIRS devices generate various measurements, such as regional cerebral oxygen saturation (rScO2), cerebral blood flow index (rCBFi), tissue oxygenation index (TOI), and relative total tissue hemoglobin concentration (rTHb) [26].

Analyses of cerebrovascular autoregulation include computing correlations of CBF or CBV with CPP using mathematical models (e.g., COx for rScO2 or TOx for TOI) [27]. Brady et al. monitored cerebral autoregulation with a NIRS monitor in piglets using the cerebral oximetry index (COx) as an indicator of autoregulatory vascular reactivity. By correlating rScO2 values measured using NIRS with mean arterial pressure (MAP) readings, one can calculate COx. If COx is close to zero, there is no correlation between rScO2 and MAP because blood pressure is in the autoregulation range. On the other hand, COx values close to one, point to a strong correlation between cerebral oximetry and MAP, which is interpreted as impaired CBF autoregulation or as a MAP beyond the limit of autoregulation [25]. In Brady et al.'s study, COx values were compared with invasive measurements using the laser-Doppler index (LDx). Those authors demonstrated that COx displayed high sensitivity and specificity in detecting cerebrovascular autoregulation disorders caused by hypotension in piglets. The COx readings correlated with those obtained using LDx. Brady et al. showed that COx was sensitive to the loss of cerebrovascular autoregulation and could be a valuable non-invasive method for continuous monitoring of autoregulation in patients with TBI.

Monitoring of CBF autoregulation using NIRS has also been studied in patients with sepsis. NIRS readings were consistent with measurements of changes in autoregulation performed using TCD [27]. Similar results, showing the compatibility of NIRS with TCD measurements, were obtained by Zheng et al. [28].

Currently, the market offers a CBF monitoring device called c-FLOW Ornim Medical LTD device, which uses low-power ultrasound and near-infrared laser light to continuously monitor blood flow in tissue microcirculation. It tracks CBF trends, continuously measures blood pressure, and correlates the measurements to provide a real-time autoregulation index. This allows to identify the limits of cerebrovascular autoregulation and detect impairments in autoregulation [29].

3.3. Monitoring of Cerebral Blood Flow

In a study of non-invasive CBF measurement using NIRS and indocyanine green, Gora et al. obtained CBF values that were low compared to those obtained with conventional positron emission tomography (PET) [30]. Similarly, NIRS measurements of CBV yielded low results, which appeared to be related to contamination of the path near-infrared light travels from the emitter to the detector by extracerebral tissues. It is difficult to assess the volume and density of these tissues and their optical properties [31]. It seems that in order for NIRS to be used for the measurement of CBF and CBV in clinical settings, the contribution of extracerebral signals to NIRS readings must be further investigated [30]. Also, the influence of indocyanine green on the values of cerebral oximetry measured with NIRS does not seem to be entirely clear. Yoo et al. obtained falsely elevated cerebral oximetry readings after an intravenous bolus of indocyanine green. This marker mainly absorbs light in the near-infrared range of 600–900 nm. Therefore, one should expect that, similarly to indigo carmine or methylene blue, the use of indocyanine green would dampen cerebral oximetry readings. In Yoo et al.'s study, a several-minute increase in rScO2 co-occurred with a significantly shorter-lasting decrease in blood saturation (SpO2). The authors lean towards the theory that indocyanine green reduces the amount of light detected by NIRS devices at a wavelength of 810 nm, which is interpreted as an increase in the concentration of oxyhemoglobin and results in falsely elevated cerebral oximetry readings [32].

In contrast to these observations are the results of a study by Keller et al., in which measurements obtained by NIRS and indocyanine green were consistent with those obtained by MRI [33]. Also in the study by Milej et al. a significant correlation of the CBF values obtained with the NIRS and indocyanine green was demonstrated with the CBF measurements obtained by MRI [34].

3.4. Detection of Increased Intracranial Pressure

In patients with TBI, monitoring of ICP is extremely important in preventing secondary injuries. An increase in ICP is associated with a decrease in CPP, and thus a decline in CBF, which can lead, among others, to a secondary ischemic phenomenon. Moreover, elevated ICP values in patients with TBI are associated with a higher risk of death [35].

Typically, ICP is measured invasively using a probe placed inside the brain. However, attempts are being made at using NIRS cerebral oximetry measurements as a non-invasive ICP monitor.

Kampfl et al. used NIRS to monitor cerebral oximetry in two groups of patients with TBI—with ICP higher or lower than 25 mmHg. They observed significantly lower values of rScO2 in patients with increased ICP compared to the group of patients with ICP below 25 mmHg. Moreover, no differences were observed between CPP, TCD or blood gas values between these two groups. It seems that cerebral oximetry monitoring using NIRS may be of help in detecting CBF abnormalities in patients with elevated ICP [36].

Similar observations were made by Dias et al. in a study of the characteristics of plateau waves of intracranial pressure. They observed that an increase in ICP was associated with the detection of brain hypoxia by NIRS [37].

By contrast, Zuluaga et al. observed different trends in rScO2 in a pediatric population depending on the underlying disease causing intracranial hypertension. rScO2 decreased with increasing ICP in children with brain tumors and hydrocephalus, but increased when ICP was caused by intracranial hemorrhage. The authors clearly demonstrated that changes in rScO2 were not significantly related to CPP or ICP. Accordingly, NIRS does not seem to be an appropriate method for monitoring and predicting changes in ICP [38].

It should be noted that in all the studies reviewed here, authors observed changes in cerebral oximetry readings in response to an increase in ICP, thus confirming the usefulness of NIRS in detecting hypoxic episodes. However, these studies do not confirm that NIRS allows to directly diagnose changes in ICP. Nonetheless, it seems that monitoring of rScO2 in patients with TBI may be used as an auxiliary method to signal a possible increase in ICP and the need to initiate more invasive monitoring.

3.5. NIRS and Diffuse Correlation Spectroscopy

A newer method of monitoring CBF that uses infrared light is diffuse correlation spectroscopy (DCS), which is based on the use of the intensity fluctuations of near-infrared light.

In a study carried out on neonatal piglets with closed head injury simulating TBI, CBF was monitored with DCS and cerebral blood oxygenation using NIRS. A significant correlation of the results obtained with the DCS with the values obtained with the fluorescent microsphere technique was demonstrated. Measurements made with DCS correlated with the values of arterial oxygen saturation, mean arterial pressure and heart rate. DCS was also sensitive to changing physiological conditions such as cardiac arrest [39].

Baker et al. monitored CBF and oxidative metabolism in brain-injured adults. In the research, they used both invasive methods such as ICP monitor or cerebral microdialysis, as well as non-invasive measurement of NIRS and DCS. Conducted observations confirmed the usefulness of non-invasive methods in monitoring patients with brain injury. There were no significant correlations between the absolute values of the parameters measured with invasive and non-invasive methods. However, the NIRS and DCS measurements allowed the detection of disproportions between cerebral perfusion and oxygen metabolism during specific clinical events, which were also observed by invasive methods. The possibility of longitudinal assessment of cerebral autoregulation, based on non-invasive measurements, has also been demonstrated [40].

Due to the use of hybrid monitors, using both the NIRS and DCS techniques, it is also possible to estimate CMRO2 [41]. The combination of both monitoring techniques has also been successfully used in studies among patients undergoing elective cardiac surgery with use of circulatory arrest by measuring cerebral oximetry, CBF and CMRO2. DCS allows the identification of periods of brain hyperperfusion and hypoperfusion during circulatory arrest [42].

4. Limitations of the Use of Cerebral Oximetry Measurements with NIRS

Although monitoring of cerebral oximetry using NIRS has been refined over the years, it still has some limitations.

An unquestionable disadvantage of this monitoring technique is the multitude of devices available on the market, which differ in the technical aspects of making measurements, and therefore cannot be used interchangeably [43].

The results obtained with the use of NIRS are influenced by extracerebral blood flow, cerebrospinal fluid, thickness of skull bones, and myelin sheaths [44]. Interference from the lighting used in the room in which oximetry is performed, which is often overlooked in practice, is important as well. Oximetry readings can also be affected by skin pigmentation. Another problem is the falsification of measurements by myoglobin, as hemoglobin and myoglobin have similar optical properties. This may cause an overestimation of hemoglobin saturation readings [45]. Hirasawa et al. demonstrated that extracranial blood flow had an effect on cerebral oximetry readings regardless of the distance between the emitter and the detector [46].

The range of normal cerebral oximetry values is also still being discussed. The most commonly used lower and upper limits are 60% and 75%, respectively, with deviations from these baseline values as high as 10%. These limits are individually variable and depend on comorbidities [47].

In patients with TBI, there are also other issues. These patients very often have multiple wounds or postoperative sutures on the scalp, as well as subcutaneous hematomas accompanied by swelling of the soft tissues. These lesions make it impossible to properly attach NIRS electrodes, or cause disturbances in signal reception and falsify readings.

The influence of the presence of hematomas and brain edema on the absorption and scattering of near-infrared light in TBI patients has also been debated [48].

Importantly, there have been reports of measuring devices registering normal cerebral oximetry values in patients with confirmed absence of cerebral perfusion [49]. These reports seem to call into question all the other observations and the knowledge gained from them.

5. Conclusions

Cerebral oximetry monitoring using NIRS is increasingly employed in the therapy of TBI patients, not only to register cerebral oximetry. The greatest advantage of this method is that it enables continuous and non-invasive measurement of rScO2. Despite technical imperfections, cerebral oximetry measurements can be an important complement to other parameters monitored, providing a more holistic picture of intracranial pathologies. However, attention should be paid to the still present technical imperfections of the method, which significantly affect the obtained, often inconclusive results.

Author Contributions: Conceptualization, M.B. (Małgorzata Barud) and W.D.; methodology, M.B. (Małgorzata Barud); formal analysis, M.B. (Małgorzata Barud), W.D.; writing—original draft preparation, M.B., W.D., D.S.-G.; writing—review and editing, M.B. (Małgorzata Barud), W.D., D.S.-G., C.R., M.B. (Magdalena Bielacz), R.B.; visualization, M.B. (Małgorzata Barud), W.D., D. S-G., C.R., M.B. (Magdalena Bielacz), R.B.; supervision, M.B. (Małgorzata Barud), W.D., D.S-G., C.R., M.B. (Magdalena Bielacz), R.B.; project administration, M.B. (Małgorzata Barud), W.D., D.S.-G., C.R., M.B. (Magdalena Bielacz), R.B. All authors have read and agreed to the published version of the manuscript.

Funding: This manuscript received no external funding.

Institutional Review Board Statement: Not applicable.

Informed Consent Statement: Not applicable.

Data Availability Statement: Not applicable.

Conflicts of Interest: The authors declare no conflict of interest.

References

1. Carney, N.; Totten, A.M.; O'Reilly, C.; Ullman, J.S.; Hawryluk, G.W.; Bell, M.J.; Bratton, S.L.; Chesnut, R.; Harris, O.A.; Kissoon, N.; et al. Guidelines for the Management of Severe Traumatic Brain Injury, Fourth Edition. *Neurosurgery* **2017**, *80*, 6–15. [CrossRef]
2. Brazy, J.E.; Lewis, D.V.; Mitnick, M.H.; Jöbsis vander Vliet, F.F. Noninvasive monitoring of cerebral oxygenation in preterm infants: Preliminary observations. *Pediatrics* **1985**, *75*, 217–225. [PubMed]
3. Murkin, J.M.; Adams, S.J.; Novick, R.J.; Quantz, M.; Bainbridge, D.; Iglesias, I.; Cleland, A.; Schaefer, B.; Irwin, B.; Fox, S. Monitoring brain oxygen saturation during coronary bypass surgery: A randomized, prospective study. *Anesth. Analg.* **2007**, *104*, 51–58. [CrossRef] [PubMed]
4. Jobsis, F.F. Noninvasive infrared monitoring of cerebral and myocardial oxygen sufficiency and circulatory parameters. *Science* **1977**, *23*, 1264–1267. [CrossRef] [PubMed]
5. Pellicer, A.; Bravo, M.C. Near-infrared spectroscopy: A methodology-focused review. *Semin. Fetal Neonatal Med.* **2011**, *16*, 42–49. [CrossRef]
6. Casati, A.; Spreafico, E.; Putzu, M.; Fanelli, G. New technology for noninvasive brain monitoring: Continuous cerebral oximetry. *Minerva Anestesiol.* **2006**, *72*, 605–625. [PubMed]
7. Murkin, J.M.; Arango, M. Near-infrared spectroscopy as an index of brain and tissue oxygenation. *Br. J. Anaesth.* **2009**, *103*, i3–i13. [CrossRef]
8. Owen-Reece, H.; Smith, M.; Elwell, C.E.; Goldstone, J.C. Near infrared spectroscopy. *Br. J. Anaesth.* **1999**, *82*, 418–444. [CrossRef]
9. Madsen, P.L.; Secher, N.H. Near-infrared oximetry of the brain. *Prog. Neurobiol.* **1999**, *58*, 541–560. [CrossRef]
10. Davies, D.J.; Su, Z.; Clancy, M.T.; Lucas, S.J.E.; Dehghani, H.; Logan, A.; Belli, A. Near-Infrared Spectroscopy in the Monitoring of Adult Traumatic Brain Injury: A Review. *J. Neurotrauma* **2015**, *32*, 933–941. [CrossRef]
11. Esnault, P.; Boret, H.; Montcriol, A.; Carre, E.; Prunet, B.; Bordes, J.; Simon, P.; Joubert, C.; Dagain, A.; Kaiser, E.; et al. Assessment of cerebral oxygenation in neurocritical care patients: Comparison of a new four wavelengths forehead regional saturation in oxygen sensor (EQUANOX®) with brain tissue oxygenation. A prospective observational study. *Minerva Anestesiol.* **2015**, *81*, 876–884.

12. Leal-Noval, S.R.; Cayuela, A.; Arellano-Orden, V.; Marín-Caballos, A.; Padilla, V.; Ferrándiz-Millón, C.; Corcia, Y.; García-Alfaro, C.; Amaya-Villar, R.; Murillo-Cabezas, F. Invasive and noninvasive assessment of cerebral oxygenation in patients with severe traumatic brain injury. *Intensive Care Med.* **2010**, *36*, 1309–1317. [CrossRef]
13. Brawanski, A.; Faltermeier, R.; Rothoerl, R.D.; Woertgen, C. Comparison of near-infrared spectroscopy and tissue P(O2) time series in patients after severe head injury and aneurysmal subarachnoid hemorrhage. *J. Cereb. Blood Flow Metab.* **2002**, *22*, 605–611. [CrossRef]
14. Holzschuh, M.; Woertgen, C.; Metz, C.; Brawanski, A. Dynamic changes of cerebral oxygenation measured by brain tissue oxygen pressure and near infrared spectroscopy. *Neurol. Res.* **1997**, *19*, 246–248. [CrossRef]
15. Nagdyman, N.; Ewert, P.; Peters, B.; Miera, O.; Fleck, T.; Berger, F. Comparison of different near-infrared spectroscopic cerebral oxygenation indices with central venous and jugular venous oxygenation saturation in children. *Paediatr. Anaesth.* **2008**, *18*, 160–166. [CrossRef]
16. Al Tayar, A.; Abouelela, A.; Mohiuddeen, K. Can the cerebral regional oxygen saturation be a perfusion parameter in shock? *J. Crit. Care* **2017**, *38*, 164–167. [CrossRef]
17. Forcione, M.; Ganau, M.; Prisco, L.; Chiarelli, A.M.; Bellelli, A.; Belli, A.; Davies, D.J. Mismatch between Tissue Partial Oxygen Pressure and Near-Infrared Spectroscopy Neuromonitoring of Tissue Respiration in Acute Brain Trauma: The Rationale for Implementing a Multimodal Monitoring Strategy. *Int. J. Mol. Sci.* **2021**, *22*, 1122. [CrossRef] [PubMed]
18. Gupta, A.K.; Hutchinson, P.J.; Al-Rawi, P.; Gupta, S.; Swart, M.; Kirkpatrick, P.J.; Menon, D.K.; Datta, A.K. Measuring brain tissue oxygenation compared with jugular venous oxygen saturation for monitoring cerebral oxygenation after traumatic brain injury. *Anesth. Analg.* **1999**, *88*, 549–553. [CrossRef] [PubMed]
19. Lam, J.M.; Hsiang, J.N.; Poon, W.S. Monitoring of autoregulation using laser Doppler flowmetry in patients with head injury. *J. Neurosurg.* **1997**, *86*, 438–445. [CrossRef] [PubMed]
20. Rivera-Lara, L.; Zorrilla-Vaca, A.; Geocadin, R.G.; Healy, R.J.; Ziai, W.; Mirski, M.A. Cerebral Autoregulation-oriented Therapy at the Bedside: A Comprehensive Review. *Anesthesiology* **2017**, *126*, 1187–1199. [CrossRef] [PubMed]
21. Budohoski, K.P.; Czosnyka, M.; Smielewski, P.; Varsos, G.V.; Kasprowicz, M.; Brady, K.M.; Pickard, J.D.; Kirkpatrick, P.J. Cerebral autoregulation after subarachnoid hemorrhage: Comparison of three methods. *J. Cereb. Blood Flow Metab.* **2013**, *33*, 449–456. [CrossRef]
22. Aries, M.J.; Czosnyka, M.; Budohoski, K.P.; Steiner, L.A.; Lavinio, A.; Kolias, A.G.; Hutchinson, P.J.; Brady, K.M.; Menon, D.K.; Pickard, J.D.; et al. Continuous determination of optimal cerebral perfusion pressure in traumatic brain injury. *Crit. Care Med.* **2012**, *40*, 2456–2463. [CrossRef]
23. Joshi, B.; Ono, M.; Brown, C.; Brady, K.; Easley, R.B.; Yenokyan, G.; Gottesman, R.F.; Hogue, C.W. Predicting the limits of cerebral autoregulation during cardiopulmonary bypass. *Anesth. Analg.* **2012**, *114*, 503–510. [CrossRef]
24. Smielewski, P.; Kirkpatrick, P.; Minhas, P.; Pickard, J.D.; Czosnyka, M. Can cerebrovascular reactivity be measured with near-infrared spectroscopy? *Stroke* **1995**, *26*, 2285–2292. [CrossRef] [PubMed]
25. Brady, K.M.; Lee, J.K.; Kibler, K.K.; Smielewski, P.; Czosnyka, M.; Easley, R.B.; Koehler, R.C.; Shaffner, D.H. Continuous time-domain analysis of cerebrovascular autoregulation using near-infrared spectroscopy. *Stroke* **2007**, *38*, 2818–2825. [CrossRef]
26. Bush, B.; Sam, K.; Rosenblatt, K. The Role of Near-infrared Spectroscopy in Cerebral Autoregulation Monitoring. *J. Neurosurg. Anesthesiol.* **2019**, *31*, 269–270. [CrossRef]
27. Steiner, L.A.; Pfister, D.; Strebel, S.P.; Radolovich, D.; Smielewski, P.; Czosnyka, M. Near-infrared spectroscopy can monitor dynamic cerebral autoregulation in adults. *Neurocrit. Care* **2009**, *10*, 122–128. [CrossRef]
28. Zheng, Y.; Villamayor, A.J.; Merritt, W.; Pustavoitau, A.; Latif, A.; Bhambhani, R.; Frank, S.; Gurakar, A.; Singer, A.; Cameron, A.; et al. Continuous cerebral blood flow autoregulation monitoring in patients undergoing liver transplantation. *Neurocrit. Care* **2012**, *17*, 77–84. [CrossRef] [PubMed]
29. Tsalach, A.; Ratner, E.; Lokshin, S.; Silman, Z.; Breskin, I.; Budin, N.; Kamar, M. Cerebral Autoregulation Real-Time Monitoring. *PLoS ONE* **2016**, *11*, e0161907. [CrossRef]
30. Gora, F.; Shinde, S.; Elwell, C.E.; Goldstone, J.C.; Cope, M.; Delpy, D.T.; Smith, M. Noninvasive measurement of cerebral blood flow in adults using near-infrared spectroscopy and indocyanine green: A pilot study. *J. Neurosurg. Anesthesiol.* **2002**, *14*, 218–222. [CrossRef]
31. Hopton, P.; Walsh, T.S.; Lee, A. Measurement of cerebral blood volume using near-infrared spectroscopy and indocyanine green elimination. *J. Appl. Physiol.* **1999**, *87*, 1981–1987. [CrossRef]
32. Yoo, K.Y.; Baek, H.Y.; Jeong, S.; Hallacoglu, B.; Lee, J. Intravenously administered indocyanine green may cause falsely high near-infrared cerebral oximetry readings. *J. Neurosurg. Anesthesiol.* **2015**, *27*, 57–60. [CrossRef]
33. Keller, E.; Nadler, A.; Alkadhi, H.; Kollias, S.S.; Yonekawa, Y.; Niederer, P. Noninvasive measurement of regional cerebral blood flow and regional cerebral blood volume by near-infrared spectroscopy and indocyanine green dye dilution. *NeuroImage* **2003**, *20*, 828–839. [CrossRef]
34. Milej, D.; He, L.; Abdalmalak, A.; Baker, W.B.; Anazodo, U.C.; Diop, M.; Dolui, S.; Kavuri, V.C.; Pavlosky, W.; Wang, L.; et al. Quantification of cerebral blood flow in adults by contrast-enhanced near-infrared spectroscopy: Validation against MRI. *J. Cereb. Blood Flow Metab.* **2020**, *40*, 1672–1684. [CrossRef] [PubMed]
35. Balestreri, M.; Czosnyka, M.; Hutchinson, P.; Steiner, L.A.; Hiler, M.; Smielewski, P.; Pickard, J.D. Impact of intracranial pressure and cerebral perfusion pressure on severe disability and mortality after head injury. *Neurocrit. Care* **2006**, *4*, 8–13. [CrossRef]

36. Kampfl, A.; Pfausler, B.; Denchev, D.; Jaring, H.P.; Schmutzhard, E. Near infrared spectroscopy (NIRS) in patients with severe brain injury and elevated intracranial pressure. A pilot study. *Acta Neurochir. Suppl.* **1997**, *70*, 112–114. [CrossRef]
37. Dias, C.; Maia, I.; Cerejo, A.; Smielewski, P.; Paiva, J.A.; Czosnyka, M. Plateau Waves of Intracranial Pressure and Multimodal Brain Monitoring. *Acta Neurochir. Suppl.* **2016**, *122*, 143–146. [CrossRef]
38. Zuluaga, M.T.; Esch, M.E.; Cvijanovich, N.Z.; Gupta, N.; McQuillen, P.S. Diagnosis influences response of cerebral near infrared spectroscopy to intracranial hypertension in children. *Pediatr. Crit. Care Med.* **2010**, *11*, 514–522. [CrossRef] [PubMed]
39. Zhou, C.; Eucker, S.A.; Durduran, T.; Yu, G.; Ralston, J.; Friess, S.H.; Ichord, R.N.; Margulies, S.S.; Yodh, A.G. Diffuse optical monitoring of hemodynamic changes in piglet brain with closed head injury. *J. Biomed. Opt.* **2009**, *14*, e034015. [CrossRef]
40. Baker, W.B.; Balu, R.; He, L.; Kavuri, V.C.; Busch, D.R.; Amendolia, O.; Francis Quattrone, F.; Suzanne Frangos, S.; Maloney-Wilensky, E.; Abramson, K.; et al. Continuous non-invasive optical monitoring of cerebral blood flow and oxidative metabolism after acute brain injury. *J. Cereb. Blood Flow Metab.* **2019**, *39*, 1469–1485. [CrossRef] [PubMed]
41. Boas, D.A.; Franceschini, M.A. Haemoglobin oxygen saturation as a biomarker: The problem and a solution. *Philos. Trans. A Math. Phys. Eng. Sci.* **2011**, *369*, 4407–4424. [CrossRef]
42. Zavriyev, A.I.; Kaya, K.; Farzam, P.; Farzam, P.Y.; Sunwoo, J.; Jassar, A.S.; Sundt, T.M.; Carp, S.A.; Franceschini, M.A.; Qu, J.Z. The role of diffuse correlation spectroscopy and frequency-domain near-infrared spectroscopy in monitoring cerebral hemodynamics during hypothermic circulatory arrests. *JTCVS Tech.* **2021**, *7*, 161–177. [CrossRef]
43. Fellahi, J.L.; Butin, G.; Fischer, M.O.; Zamparini, G.; Gérard, J.L.; Hanouz, J.L. Dynamic evaluation of near-infrared peripheral oximetry in healthy volunteers: A comparison between INVOS and EQUANOX. *J. Crit. Care* **2013**, *28*, 881. [CrossRef]
44. Yoshitani, K.; Kawaguchi, M.; Miura, N.; Okuno, T.; Kanoda, T.; Ohnishi, Y.; Kuro, M. Effects of hemoglobin concentration, skull thickness, and the area of the cerebrospinal fluid layer on near-infrared spectroscopy measurements. *Anesthesiology* **2007**, *106*, 458–462. [CrossRef] [PubMed]
45. Scheeren, T.W.; Schober, P.; Schwarte, L.A. Monitoring tissue oxygenation by near infrared spectroscopy (NIRS): Background and current applications. *J. Clin. Monit. Comput.* **2012**, *26*, 279–287. [CrossRef]
46. Hirasawa, A.; Yanagisawa, S.; Tanaka, N.; Funane, T.; Kiguchi, M.; Sørensen, H.; Secher, N.H.; Ogoh, S. Influence of skin blood flow and source-detector distance on near-infrared spectroscopy-determined cerebral oxygenation in humans. *Clin. Physiol. Funct. Imaging* **2015**, *35*, 237–244. [CrossRef] [PubMed]
47. Thavasothy, M.; Broadhead, M.; Elwell, C.; Peters, M.; Smith, M. A comparison of cerebral oxygenation as measured by the NIRO 300 and the INVOS 5100 Near-Infrared Spectrophotometers. *Anaesthesia* **2002**, *57*, 999–1006. [CrossRef]
48. Calderon-Arnulphi, M.; Alaraj, A.; Slavin, K.V. Near infrared technology in neuroscience: Past, present and future. *Neurol. Res.* **2009**, *31*, 605–614. [CrossRef]
49. Gomersall, C.D.; Joynt, G.M.; Gin, T.; Freebairn, R.C.; Stewart, I.E. Failure of the INVOS 3100 cerebral oximeter to detect complete absence of cerebral blood flow. *Crit. Care Med.* **1997**, *25*, 1252–1254. [CrossRef]

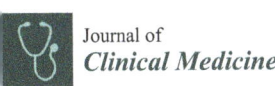

Journal of Clinical Medicine

Review

Early vs. Late Tracheostomy in Patients with Traumatic Brain Injury: Systematic Review and Meta-Analysis

Annachiara Marra, Maria Vargas *, Pasquale Buonanno, Carmine Iacovazzo, Antonio Coviello and Giuseppe Servillo

Department of Neurosciences, Reproductive and Odontostomatological Sciences, University of Naples "Federico II", 80100 Naples, Italy; dottmarraannachiara@gmail.com (A.M.); pasqual3.buonanno@gmail.com (P.B.); dott.iacovazzo@gmail.com (C.I.); antonio_coviello@live.it (A.C.); maria.vargas@unina.it (G.S.)
* Correspondence: vargas.maria82@gmail.com; Tel.: +39-081746-3708

Abstract: Introduction. Tracheostomy can help weaning in long-term ventilated patients, reducing the duration of mechanical ventilation and intensive care unit length of stay, and decreasing complications from prolonged tracheal intubation. In traumatic brain injury (TBI), ideal timing for tracheostomy is still debated. We performed a systematic review and meta-analysis to evaluate the effects of timing (early vs. late) of tracheostomy on mortality and incidence of VAP in traumatic brain-injured patients. **Methods.** This study was conducted in conformity with the Preferred Reporting Items for Systematic Reviews and Meta-Analyses (PRISMA) guideline. We performed a search in PubMed, using an association between heading terms: early, tracheostomy, TBI, prognosis, recovery, impact, mortality, morbidity, and brain trauma OR brain injury. Two reviewers independently assessed the methodological quality of eligible studies using the Newcastle–Ottawa Scale (NOS). Comparative analyses were made among Early Tracheostomy (ET) and late tracheostomy (LT) groups. Our primary outcome was the odds ratio of mortality and incidence of VAP between the ET and LT groups in acute brain injury patients. Secondary outcomes included the standardized mean difference (MD) of the duration of mechanical ventilation, ICU length of stay (LOS), and hospital LOS. **Results.** We included two randomized controlled trials, three observational trials, one cross-sectional study, and three retrospective cohort studies. The total number of participants in the ET group was 2509, while in the LT group it was 2597. Early tracheostomy reduced risk for incidence of pneumonia, ICU length of stay, hospital length of stay and duration of mechanical ventilation, but not mortality. **Conclusions.** In TBI patients, early tracheostomy compared with late tracheostomy might reduce risk for VAP, ICU and hospital LOS, and duration of mechanical ventilation, but increase the risk of mortality.

Keywords: acute brain injury; early tracheostomy; late tracheostomy; tracheostomy timing; mortality; ventilatory acquired pneumonia

Citation: Marra, A.; Vargas, M.; Buonanno, P.; Iacovazzo, C.; Coviello, A.; Servillo, G. Early vs. Late Tracheostomy in Patients with Traumatic Brain Injury: Systematic Review and Meta-Analysis. *J. Clin. Med.* **2021**, *10*, 3319. https://doi.org/10.3390/jcm10153319

Academic Editor: Rafael Badenes

Received: 3 July 2021
Accepted: 26 July 2021
Published: 28 July 2021

Publisher's Note: MDPI stays neutral with regard to jurisdictional claims in published maps and institutional affiliations.

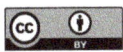

Copyright: © 2021 by the authors. Licensee MDPI, Basel, Switzerland. This article is an open access article distributed under the terms and conditions of the Creative Commons Attribution (CC BY) license (https://creativecommons.org/licenses/by/4.0/).

1. Introduction

Traumatic brain injury (TBI) is a complex disorder which can affect the central nervous system, leading to temporary or permanent physical, cognitive, and psychosocial impairments [1]. The worldwide incidence of TBI is estimated at 939 cases per 100,000 people with the highest peak of incidence in North America and Europe [2].

In patients with TBI, endotracheal intubation is often necessary to maintain airway patency and prevent hypoxia [3]. Tracheostomy may facilitate weaning in long-term mechanical ventilated patients, reduce duration of intensive care unit (ICU) length of stay (LOS), and decrease complications from prolonged tracheal intubation [4,5].

In TBI patients, the main indications for tracheostomy include weaning failure, absence of protective airway reflexes, impairment of respiratory drive, and difficulties in managing secretions [6]. However, the beneficial effects, timing and indications of tracheostomy in TBI are still debating [7,8].

In ICU patients, the use of tracheostomy may improve the comfort of patients, allow more effective secretions suctioning and a more secure airway, decrease airway resistance, enhance patient mobility, opportunities for speech and eating orally. Early and late complications after tracheotomy include bleeding, wound infection, subcutaneous emphysema, laryngeal nerve or esophageal injury, and tracheal stenosis.

Tracheostomies performed during the first week of mechanical ventilation are classified as early, while tracheostomies performed later than seven days are defined as late [9]. Evidence on the advantages of early over late tracheostomy is conflicting [5], and there are limited robust data to guide the ideal timing to perform a tracheostomy.

Systematic reviews of randomized controlled trials (RCTs) in general critical care populations have generally not found benefit from early tracheostomy [8–10], but these results cannot be generalized to traumatic brain-injured patients, who typically require tracheostomy for airway protection for depressed airway reflexes rather than respiratory failure.

Observational studies in traumatic brain-injured patients suggest that tracheostomy performed earlier may be associated with lower in-hospital morbidity and improved clinical outcomes [11–14], but the best timing for tracheostomy continues to be debated.

To address these gaps in knowledge, we performed a systematic review and meta-analysis to evaluate the effects of early vs. late tracheostomy on mortality and VAP incidence in acutely brain-injured patients.

2. Materials and Methods

Our study was conducted according to the Preferred Reporting Items for Systematic Reviews and Meta-Analyses (PRISMA) guideline [15]. The following terms were used to perform a PubMed search: early, tracheostomy, TBI, prognosis, recovery, impact, mortality, morbidity, and brain trauma OR brain injury. Inclusion criteria were (1) English language; (2) TBI as the main cause of trauma; (3) clear outcome; (4) reliable patient's admission assessment; (5) late tracheostomy (LT) clearly defined and not confused with prolonged intubation; and (6) a minimum of two outcomes: ICU stay, hospital stay, mortality rates, or ventilator-associated pneumonia (VAP) diagnosis. We included randomized controlled studies, retrospective and prospective studies. We excluded studies without full reports or abstracts, commentaries, editorials, and reviews.

3. Data Extraction

Two reviewers (A.M. and M.V.) independently screened studies for inclusion, retrieved potentially relevant studies, and decided on study eligibility using a standardized data extraction form, checked by the other authors. Any disagreement was solved by discussion or by the judgment of a third author (P.B.). We collected the following data from every study included in our analysis: study design, year, patient's demographics, mean time between admission and tracheostomy, neurologic assessment at admission, confirmed VAP, median ICU stay, median hospital stay, mortality rates, and ICU or hospital costs. Two investigators (P.B. and C.I.) independently screened the citations to identify other potentially eligible studies not included in the previous PubMed search.

4. Risk of Bias

Two reviewers (M.V. and P.B.) independently assessed the methodological quality of eligible studies using the Newcastle–Ottawa Scale (NOS) for assessing the quality of nonrandomized studies in a meta-analysis [16] for each included trial. Any disagreement was resolved asking for the opinion of a third reviewer (G.S.).

5. Data Synthesis and Analysis

The primary outcome were the odds ratio of mortality and the incidence of VAP between the early tracheostomy (ET) and LT groups. The secondary outcomes were the duration of mechanical ventilation, ICU length of stay (LOS), and hospital LOS. A standardized mean difference was used as effect size to compare the two groups. Consequently, random effects model was used [17]. This model is more conservative and reduces the likelihood of type II errors. Heterogeneity was assessed by I^2 calculation, and it was considered low, moderate, or high if I^2 values were 25%, 50%, and 75%, respectively. Results expressed with median and range were converted in mean and standard deviation according to Hozo et al. [18]. Trial sequential analysis (TSA) was performed to determine the required information size (RIS), i.e., the number of subjects to enroll in order to confirm or reject the supposed effect of an intervention. TSA was undertaken using TSA 0.9 beta software if the number of included trials was more than five. The RIS was estimated using relative risk reduction and heterogeneity-adjusted information size for dichotomous outcomes. Results are considered conclusive if the cumulative Z-curve crosses the conventional significance boundary (Z = 1.96) or the trial sequential boundary (i.e., significance or futility boundaries) or if the RIS is reached. TSA-adjusted 95% CIs were also presented.

6. Results

A total of nine studies [5,11,13,19–24] were selected for the systematic review (Figure 1) (Table 1). According to the NOS [16], the quality scores of the included studies ranged from 5 to 8. Most of them (7/9) were greater than or equal to seven stars, as listed. We included two randomized controlled trials [19,24], three observational trials [5,13,21], one cross-sectional study [20], and three retrospective cohort studies [11,22,23]. Great heterogeneity was observed in the definition of the early tracheostomy. Shibahashi et al. [22] performed tracheostomy within 72 h after admission, in two studies [19,24] early tracheostomy was performed on post-injury day 3–5, while, in Khalili et al. [21], ET was performed before or at the sixth day of admission, in 2 other studies [5,23] early tracheostomy was performed ≤7 days from admission, Alali et al. [11] classified as early tracheostomy a procedure executed ≤8 days, and in 2 other studies [13,20] ET was defined as the performance of the procedure within the first 10 days of mechanical ventilation or after decompressive craniectomy. The total number of participants in the ET group was 2509, while in the LT group it was 2597. Reduced risk for incidence of pneumonia was found in the ET group (OR = 0.63, 95% CI = 0.52, 0.76, I^2 = 0%, p = 0.89) (Figure 2), but this result was confirmed only by the analysis including the prospective and retrospective studies but not the RCTs (OR = 0.62, 95% CI = 0.51, 0.75, I^2 = 0%, p = 0.71) (Supplemental Figure S1). ET was significantly associated to reduced ICU length of stay (MD = −5.96, 95% CI = −7,99, −3.92, I^2 = 88%, p < 0.001) (Figure 3), hospital length of stay (MD = −6.97, 95% CI= −8.25, −5.68, I^2 = 0%, p = 0.59) (Figure 4), and duration of mechanical ventilation (MD = −4.86.56, 95% CI= −6.98, −2.75, I^2 = 93%, p < 0.001) (Figure 5). Increased risk of mortality was found in the ET group (OR = 1.56, 95%CI = 1.06, 2.3, I^2 = 38.3%, p = 0.11) (Figure 6; Supplemental Figure S2). The TSA adjusted 95% CI was ranged from 0.57 to 46.86. The cumulative z-curve crossed neither the conventional boundary for benefit nor the trial sequential futility boundary for benefit, suggesting that the current evidence was inconclusive (Supplemental Figure S3). Furthermore, we need 151 from randomized controlled trials to assess the impact of ET on mortality.

PRISMA 2009 Flow Diagram

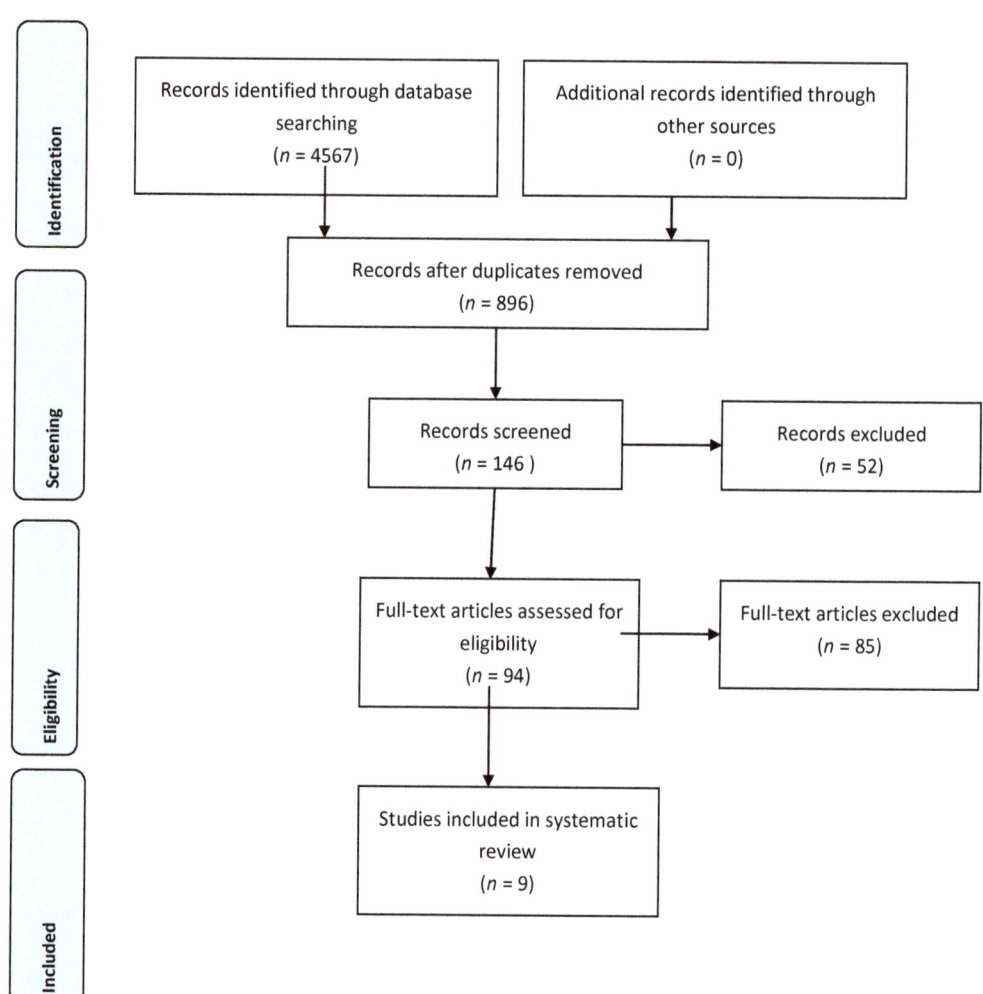

Figure 1. PRISMA 2009 Flow Diagram.

Table 1. Characteristics of the studies included in this meta-analysis. NA = not available.

Authors	Study Design	Age (Years) in ET vs. LT Groups	Sex (Male) in ET vs. LT Groups	GCS Score Information ET vs. LT Groups	How Early Tracheostomy Was Defined by the Studies
Alali et al. [12]	Retrospective cohort	49 (30–64) vs. 53 (35–68)	75.6% vs. 73%	4 (3–7) vs. 7 (3–13)	≤8 days
Bouderka et al. [23]	Retrospective cohort	NA	NA	NA	<7 days
Dunham et al. [19]	Randomized controlled trial	NA	NA	NA	3–5 days of endotracheal tube
Huang et al. [20]	Cross-sectional study	NA	NA	NA	≤10 days after decompressive tracheotomy
Khalili et al. [21]	Observational cohort	41.6 vs. 37.8	50% vs. 86%	6.15 vs. 5.70	≤6 days
Robba et al. [6]	Prospective observational	48.5 (31–67) vs. 44 (28–59	77.2% vs. 76.7%	5.5 (3–10 vs. 5 (3–9)	≤7 days
Shibahashi et al. [22]	Retrospective cohort	68 (62–74) vs. 68 (53–74)	33 vs. 33	6 (3–7) vs. 6 (6–9)	≤3 days
Surgeman et al. [24]	Randomized controlled trial	NA	NA	NA	3–5 days
Wang et al. [14]	Observational cohort	55.3 (19–80) vs. 57.5 (18–85)	87.5% vs. 66%	5.9 (3–8) vs. 5.7 83–8)	≤10 days

(A)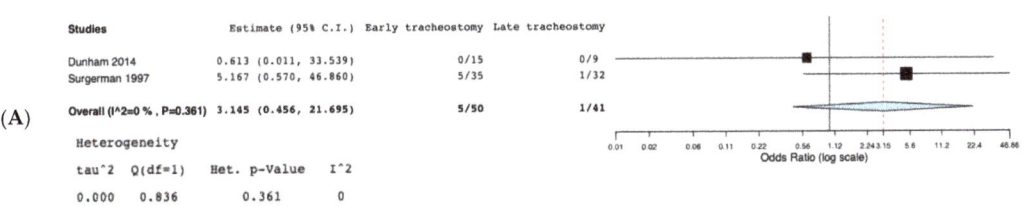

(B)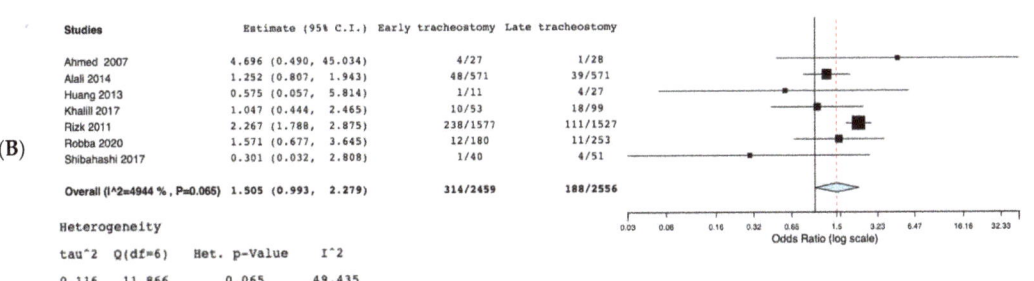

Figure 2. (A): Forest plot for incidence of pneumonia; (B): Forest plot for incidence of pneumonia in RCTs.

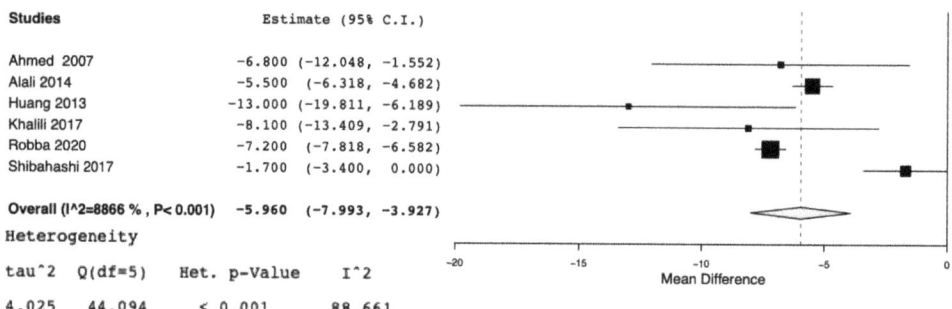

Figure 3. Forest plot for ICU length of stay.

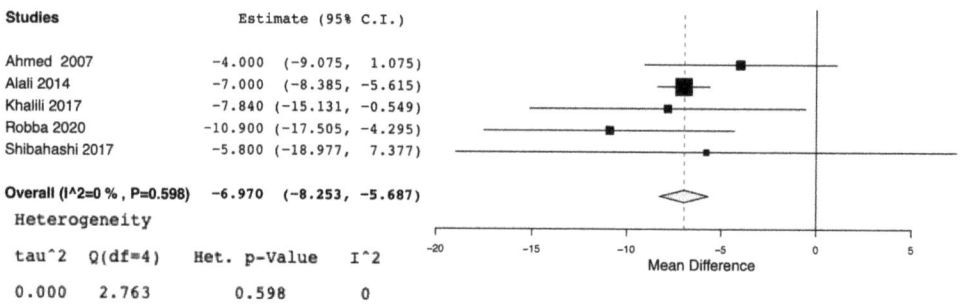

Figure 4. Forest plot for hospital length of stay.

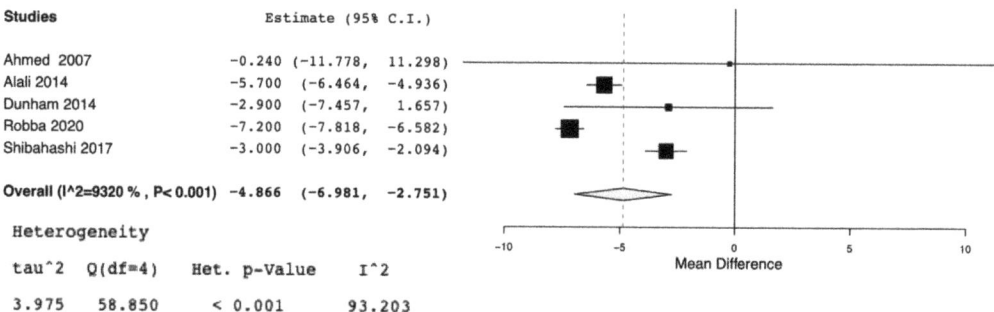

Figure 5. Forest plot for duration of mechanical ventilation.

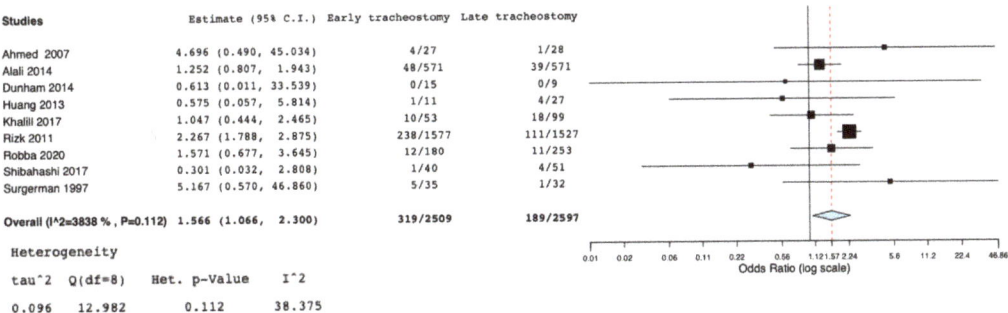

Figure 6. Forest plot for mortality in included studies.

7. Discussion

In this systematic review involving 9 studies and 5106 patients, we found that early tracheostomy, compared with late tracheostomy, might reduce risk for VAP, ICU and hospital LOS, and duration of mechanical ventilation, while an increased risk of mortality was found in the LT group.

Tracheostomy is a common procedure performed in critically ill patients. Patients with severe TBI may need prolonged MV to avoid complications such as hypoxemia and hypercapnia [13]. Robba et al. [5] found that TBI patients underwent tracheostomy more frequently than the general ICU population (31.8% vs. 10%, respectively) [25,26]; this could be due to a higher risk of extubation failure, and the impairment of airways protection reflexes secondary to the neurological injury.

In ICU patients, tracheostomy is most commonly performed after 14 days from admission [27,28], and only a quarter of tracheostomies are accomplished in the first week [25]. In TBI patients, multiple factors, related to severity of neurological injury, pre- and post-hospitalization management, evolution of trauma, local medical practices, ethical and legal implications, and costs [5,25,29,30], play a role in the decision-making process of whether and when to perform the tracheotomy. Literature reported a median time to tracheostomy of 9 days post-admission, probably reflecting a change in treatment goals [5] no longer aimed to manage acute intracranial emergencies, but focused on weaning from ventilator support and rehabilitation [5]. Moreover, this timing of tracheostomy also prevents the use of the procedure in patients with lesser or higher severities of injury; in the former case, patients have enough time to recover spontaneous breathing and an adequate level of consciousness, in the latter case they succumb early because of the rapid progression of the lesions [5].

This process still leads to performing tracheostomy at an earlier stage than in patients without TBI, but allows for the identification of patients who are most likely to benefit from the procedure [21,31–35].

Pneumonia, especially VAP, is one of the major complications of TBI that adversely affects outcome, and its risk showed a 10% increase per day of mechanical ventilation [36,37]. Similarly to De Franca et al., our results show that ET, compared with LT, might reduce the risk for VAP, probably due to the reduction of ventilation days of ET compared to LT [1,3,8,38].

Like other literature reports, we found that early tracheostomy may potentially reduce hospital stay, duration of mechanical ventilation and mortality rates [1,3,23,24,31,39]. In a propensity-matched cohort study on TBI patients, early tracheostomy (≤7 days) was associated with shorter ICU and hospital LOS but did not affect mortality [11]. Khalili et al. [21], in a cohort of 152 TBI patients, showed similar results on ICU and hospital LOS and mortality. A meta-analysis by McCredie et al. [39] found that ET might reduce the long-term mortality, duration of mechanical ventilation, and LOS. Robba et al. [5] found that each delay of 1 day to perform a tracheostomy was associated with a 4% increase in the risk of an unfavorable outcome and with a 6% increase in the hazard of death. While this association may suggest a benefit from an ET, patients with more severe injury may need more time to control the intracranial damage evolution and stabilize their condition, thus delaying tracheostomy, or may have a worse expected outcome, restraining the decision for the tracheostomy. The same study showed that patients who received LT had a significant longer ICU and hospital LOS; for every 2 days of deferral in tracheostomy, ICU and hospital LOS increase of about 1 and 2 days, respectively [5]. De Franca et al. [1] demonstrated that patients undergoing ET had a shorter ICU and hospital stay, which can reflect the impact of tracheostomy in patient recovery from hemodynamic instability and in a faster weaning from mechanical ventilation.

We found that the LT group had an increased risk of mortality. Conversely, Lu et al. [3], as in other previous finding [8,40–43], found no differences in mortality between the ET and not-ET groups. These studies showed improved outcomes for the ET groups with no survival benefit. The high mortality rate in tracheostomy patients could be related to the complications of tracheostomy (e.g., wound infection, esophageal injury, pneumothorax, and tracheal stenosis) [44]; moreover, the majority of patients undergoing tracheostomy are in severe clinical conditions with a probable high risk of death [45], which can influence the statistical significance of mortality rates. Our results could depend on the fact that mortality in ICU is a complex outcome, taking into account different variables including age, sex, comorbidities, and the length of follow-up time. According to this, mortality could be not driven by a single parameter like timing of tracheostomy, that is, a procedure that may allow a better management of critically ill patients. In addition, results of TSA suggested that current evidence is inconclusive and that more randomized controlled trials are necessary to assess the real impact of ET on mortality.

Despite the known advantages, there are still some controversies regarding tracheotomy in TBI. According to Cox et al., tracheostomy increases the proportion of patients with chronic burden, contributing to raising the costs outside the hospital [44,46].

This systematic review and meta-analysis added several novelties compared to the current literature. We included the huge study of Robba et al. [5] that selected TBI patients from CENTER-TBI, a prospective observational longitudinal cohort study, including 1358 patients, of which 433 (31.8%) had a tracheostomy. Moreover, in our systematic review and meta-analysis, we carried out a sub-group analysis according to the type of the included studies (RCT vs. non RCT) and performed a trial sequential analysis on RCTs.

Of note, this meta-analysis has some limitations. First, there is the ambiguous definition of timing to differentiate an early and a late tracheostomy. Second, heterogeneity more than 50% was found in 2 out of 5 considered outcomes like ICU LOS and duration of mechanical ventilation. Third, only published articles were reviewed, which might have contributed to a publication bias.

8. Conclusions and Future Perspectives

Our meta-analysis suggests that ET in TBI patients could help in reducing duration of mechanical ventilation, ICU and hospital LOS, contribute to a lower exposure to secondary injuries and nosocomial adverse events, increasing the opportunity of patients' early rehabilitation and discharge.

Further studies, especially multicenter RCTs, are needed to collect more data about the different outcomes of TBI patients undergoing ET compared to those treated with LT in order to confirm the superiority of the former airway management in such a challenging clinical condition.

Supplementary Materials: The following are available online at https://www.mdpi.com/article/10.3390/jcm10153319/s1, Figure S1: Forest plot for incidence of pneumonia in non RCTs, Figure S2: A: Forest plot for mortality in RCTs; B: forest plot for mortality in non RCTs, Figure S3: Trial Sequential Analysis on mortality.

Author Contributions: A.M. and M.V. had full access to all study data, take responsibility for the integrity of the data and the accuracy of the data analysis; design and conduct of the study: A.M.,

M.V. and P.B.; data acquisition, analysis and interpretation of the data: All authors; statistical analysis: M.V., P.B. and A.C.; drafting of the manuscript: A.M., M.V., P.B., C.I. and G.S.; critical revision of the article for important intellectual content: All authors. All authors have read and agreed to the published version of the manuscript.

Funding: This research received no external funding.

Institutional Review Board Statement: Not applicable.

Informed Consent Statement: Not applicable.

Data Availability Statement: Not applicable.

Conflicts of Interest: The authors declare no conflict of interest.

References

1. De Franca, S.A.; Tavares, W.M.; Salinet, A.S.M.; Paiva, W.; Teixeira, M.J. Early Tracheostomy in Severe Traumatic Brain Injury Patients: A meta-analysis and comparison with late tracheostomy. *Crit. Care Med.* **2020**, *48*, e325–e331. [CrossRef]
2. Dewan, M.C.; Rattani, A.; Gupta, S.; Baticulon, R.; Hung, Y.-C.; Punchak, M.; Agrawal, A.; Adeleye, A.O.; Shrime, M.G.; Rubiano, A.M.; et al. Estimating the global incidence of traumatic brain injury. *J. Neurosurg.* **2019**, *130*, 1080–1097. [CrossRef]
3. Lu, Q.; Xie, Y.; Qi, X.; Li, X.; Yang, S.; Wang, Y. Is Early Tracheostomy Better for Severe Traumatic Brain Injury? A Meta-Analysis. *World Neurosurg.* **2018**, *112*, e324–e330. [CrossRef]
4. Rumbak, M.J.; Newton, M.; Truncale, T.; Schwartz, S.W.; Adams, J.W.; Hazard, P.B. A prospective, randomized, study comparing early percutaneous dilational tracheotomy to prolonged translaryngeal intubation (delayed tracheotomy) in critically ill medical patients. *Crit. Care Med.* **2004**, *32*, 1689–1694. [CrossRef]
5. Robba, C.; The CENTER-TBI ICU Participants and Investigators; Galimberti, S.; Graziano, F.; Wiegers, E.J.A.; Lingsma, H.F.; Iaquaniello, C.; Stocchetti, N.; Menon, D.; Citerio, G. Tracheostomy practice and timing in traumatic brain-injured patients: A CENTER-TBI study. *Intensiv. Care Med.* **2020**, *46*, 983–994. [CrossRef] [PubMed]
6. Raimondi, N.; Vial, M.R.; Calleja, J.; Quintero, A.; Cortés, A.; Celis, E.; Pacheco, C.; Ugarte, S.; Añón, J.M.; Hernández, G.; et al. Evidence-based guidelines for the use of tracheostomy in critically ill patients. *J. Crit. Care* **2017**, *38*, 304–318. [CrossRef] [PubMed]
7. Lazaridis, C.; DeSantis, S.M.; McLawhorn, M.; Krishna, V. Liberation of neurosurgical patients from mechanical ventilation and tracheostomy in neurocritical care. *J. Crit. Care* **2012**, *27*, 417.e1–417.e8. [CrossRef] [PubMed]
8. Siempos, I.I.; Ntaidou, T.K.; Filippidis, F.; Choi, A.M.K. Effect of early versus late or no tracheostomy on mortality and pneumonia of critically ill patients receiving mechanical ventilation: A systematic review and meta-analysis. *Lancet Respir. Med.* **2015**, *3*, 150–158. [CrossRef]
9. Andriolo, B.N.G.; Andriolo, R.B.; Saconato, H.; Atallah, Á.N.; Valente, O. Early versus late tracheostomy for critically ill patients. *Cochrane Database Syst. Rev.* **2015**. [CrossRef] [PubMed]
10. Szakmany, T.; Russell, P.; Wilkes, A.R.; Hall, J.E. Effect of early tracheostomy on resource utilization and clinical outcomes in critically ill patients: Meta-analysis of randomized controlled trials. *Br. J. Anaesth.* **2015**, *114*, 396–405. [CrossRef]
11. Alali, A.S.; Scales, D.C.; Fowler, R.A.; Mainprize, T.G.; Ray, J.G.; Kiss, A.; de Mestral, C.; Nathens, A.B. Tracheostomy timing in traumatic brain injury. *J. Trauma Acute Care Surg.* **2014**, *76*, 70–78. [CrossRef]
12. Pinheiro, B.D.V.; Tostes, R.D.O.; Brum, C.I.; Carvalho, E.V.; Pinto, S.P.S.; De Oliveira, J.C.A. Early versus late tracheostomy in patients with acute severe brain injury. *J. Bras. Pneumol.* **2010**, *36*, 84–91. [CrossRef]
13. Wang, H.-K.; Lu, K.; Liliang, P.-C.; Wang, K.-W.; Chen, H.-J.; Chen, T.-B.; Liang, C.-L. The impact of tracheostomy timing in patients with severe head injury: An observational cohort study. *Injury* **2012**, *43*, 1432–1436. [CrossRef]
14. Rizk, E.B.; Patel, A.S.; Stetter, C.M.; Chinchilli, V.M.; Cockroft, K.M. Impact of Tracheostomy Timing on Outcome After Severe Head Injury. *Neurocritical Care* **2011**, *15*, 481–489. [CrossRef]
15. Moher, D.; Shamseer, L.; Clarke, M.; Ghersi, D.; Liberati, A.; Petticrew, M.; Shekelle, P.; Stewart, L.A.; PRISMA-P Group. Preferred reporting items for systematic review and meta-analysis protocols (PRISMA-P) 2015 statement. *Syst. Rev.* **2015**, *4*, 1. [CrossRef] [PubMed]
16. Wells, G.A.; Shea, B.; O'Connell, D.; Peterson, J.; Welch, V.; Losos, M.; Tugwell, P. *The Newcastle-Ottawa Scale (NOS) for Assessing the Quality of Nonrandom-Ised Studies in Meta-Analyses*; Ottawa Hospital Research Institute: Ottawa, ON, USA, 2000.
17. DerSimonian, R.; Laird, N. Meta-analysis in clinical trials revisited. *Contemp. Clin. Trials* **2015**, *45*, 139–145. [CrossRef] [PubMed]
18. Hozo, S.P.; Djulbegovic, B.; Hozo, I. Estimating the mean and variance from the median, range, and the size of a sample. *BMC Med. Res. Methodol.* **2005**, *5*, 13. [CrossRef]
19. Dunham, C.M.; Cutrona, A.F.; Gruber, B.S.; Calderon, J.E.; Ransom, K.J.; Flowers, L.L. Early tracheostomy in severe traumatic brain injury: Evidence for decreased mechanical ventilation and increased hospital mortality. *Int. J. Burn. Trauma* **2014**, *4*, 14–24.
20. Huang, Y.-H.; Lee, T.-C.; Liao, C.-C.; Deng, Y.-H.; Kwan, A.-L. Tracheostomy in craniectomised survivors after traumatic brain injury: A cross-sectional analytical study. *Injury* **2013**, *44*, 1226–1231. [CrossRef]
21. Khalili, H.; Paydar, S.; Safari, R.; Arasteh, P.; Niakan, A.; Foroughi, A.A. Experience with Traumatic Brain Injury: Is Early Tracheostomy Associated with Better Prognosis? *World Neurosurg.* **2017**, *103*, 88–93. [CrossRef] [PubMed]

22. Shibahashi, K.; Sugiyama, K.; Houda, H.; Takasu, Y.; Hamabe, Y.; Morita, A. The effect of tracheostomy performed within 72 h after traumatic brain injury. *Br. J. Neurosurg.* **2017**, *31*, 564–568. [CrossRef]
23. Bouderka, M.A.; Fakhir, B.; Bouaggad, A.; Hmamouchi, B.; Hamoudi, D.; Harti, A. Early Tracheostomy versus Prolonged Endotracheal Intubation in Severe Head Injury. *J. Trauma Inj. Infect. Crit. Care* **2004**, *57*, 251–254. [CrossRef] [PubMed]
24. Sugerman, H.J.; Wolfe, L.; Pasquale, M.D.; Rogers, F.B.; O'Malley, K.F.; Knudson, M.; Dinardo, L.; Gordon, M.; Schaffer, S. Multicenter, Randomized, Prospective Trial of Early Tracheostomy. *J. Trauma Inj. Infect. Crit. Care* **1997**, *43*, 741–747. [CrossRef] [PubMed]
25. Sabelnikovs, O.; The LUNG-SAFE Investigators and the ESICM Trials Group; Madotto, F.; Pham, T.; Nagata, I.; Uchida, M.; Tamiya, N.; Kurahashi, K.; Bellani, G.; Laffey, J.G. Epidemiology and patterns of tracheostomy practice in patients with acute respiratory distress syndrome in ICUs across 50 countries. *Crit. Care* **2018**, *22*, 195. [CrossRef]
26. Mehta, A.B.; Syeda, S.N.; Bajpayee, L.; Cooke, C.R.; Walkey, A.; Wiener, R. Trends in Tracheostomy for Mechanically Ventilated Patients in the United States, 1993–2012. *Am. J. Respir. Crit. Care Med.* **2015**, *192*, 446–454. [CrossRef]
27. Vargas, M.; Pelosi, P.; Servillo, G. Percutaneous tracheostomy: It's time for a shared approach! *Crit. Care* **2014**, *18*, 448. [CrossRef]
28. Vargas, M.; Sutherasan, Y.; Antonelli, M.; Brunetti, I.; Corcione, A.; Laffey, J.G.; Putensen, C.; Servillo, G.; Pelosi, P. Tracheostomy procedures in the intensive care unit: An international survey. *Crit. Care* **2015**, *19*, 362. [CrossRef] [PubMed]
29. Durbin, C.G. Indications for and timing of tracheostomy. *Respir. Care* **2005**, *50*, 483–487.
30. Vargas, M.; Servillo, G.; Antonelli, M.; Brunetti, I.; De Stefano, F.; Putensen, C.; Pelosi, P. Informed consent for tracheostomy procedures in Intensive Care Unit: An Italian national survey. *Minerva Anestesiol* **2013**, *79*, 741–749.
31. Frutos-Vivar, F.; Esteban, A.; Apezteguía, C.; Anzueto, A.; Nightingale, P.; González, M.; Soto, L.; Rodrigo, C.; Raad, J.; David, C.M.; et al. Outcome of mechanically ventilated patients who require a tracheostomy. *Crit. Care Med.* **2005**, *33*, 290–298. [CrossRef]
32. Wang, Y.; Guo, Z.; Fan, D.; Lu, H.; Xie, D.; Zhang, D.; Jiang, Y.; Li, P.; Teng, H. A Meta-Analysis of the Influencing Factors for Tracheostomy after Cervical Spinal Cord Injury. *BioMed Res. Int.* **2018**, *2018*, 5895830. [CrossRef]
33. Bösel, J.; Schiller, P.; Hook, Y.; Andes, M.; Neumann, J.-O.; Poli, S.; Amiri, H.; Schönenberger, S.; Peng, Z.; Unterberg, A.; et al. Stroke-Related Early Tracheostomy Versus Prolonged Orotracheal Intubation in Neurocritical Care Trial (SETPOINT). *Stroke* **2013**, *44*, 21–28. [CrossRef] [PubMed]
34. MacIntyre, N. Discontinuing Mechanical Ventilatory Support. *Chest* **2007**, *132*, 1049–1056. [CrossRef] [PubMed]
35. Blot, F.; Similowski, T.; Trouillet, J.-L.; Chardon, P.; Korach, J.-M.; Costa, M.-A.; Journois, D.; Thiéry, G.; Fartoukh, M.; Pipien, I.; et al. Early tracheotomy versus prolonged endotracheal intubation in unselected severely ill ICU patients. *Intensive care Med.* **2008**, *34*, 1779–1787. [CrossRef] [PubMed]
36. Chastre, J.; Fagon, J. State of the Art Ventilator-associated Pneumonia. *Am. J. Respir. Crit. Care Med.* **2002**. [CrossRef] [PubMed]
37. Combes, A.; Figliolini, C.; Trouillet, J.-L.; Kassis, N.; Wolff, M.; Gibert, C.; Chastre, J. Incidence and outcome of polymicrobial ventilator-associated pneumonia. *Chest* **2002**, *121*, 1618–1623. [CrossRef]
38. Hui, X.; Haider, A.H.; Hashmi, Z.G.; Rushing, A.P.; Dhiman, N.; Scott, V.K.; Selvarajah, S.; Haut, E.; Efron, D.T.; Schneider, E.B. Increased risk of pneumonia among ventilated patients with traumatic brain injury: Every day counts! *J. Surg. Res.* **2013**, *184*, 438–443. [CrossRef]
39. McCredie, V.A.; Alali, A.S.; Scales, D.C.; Adhikari, N.K.J.; Rubenfeld, G.D.; Cuthbertson, B.H.; Nathens, A.B. Effect of Early versus Late Tracheostomy or Prolonged Intubation in Critically Ill Patients with Acute Brain Injury: A Systematic Review and Meta-Analysis. *Neurocritical Care* **2017**, *26*, 14–25. [CrossRef]
40. Romero, J.; Vari, A.; Gambarrutta, C.; Oliviero, A. Tracheostomy timing in traumatic spinal cord injury. *Eur. Spine J.* **2009**, *18*, 1452–1457. [CrossRef]
41. Brook, A.; Sherman, G.; Malen, J.; Kollef, M. Early versus late tracheostomy in patients who require prolonged mechanical ventilation. *Am. J. Crit. Care* **2000**, *9*, 352–359. [CrossRef]
42. Jeon, Y.-T.; Hwang, J.-W.; Lim, Y.-J.; Lee, S.-Y.; Woo, K.-I.; Park, H.-P. Effect of Tracheostomy Timing on Clinical Outcome in Neurosurgical Patients. *J. Neurosurg. Anesthesiol.* **2014**, *26*, 22–26. [CrossRef] [PubMed]
43. Griffiths, J.; Barber, V.S.; Morgan, L.; Young, J.D. Systematic review and meta-analysis of studies of the timing of tracheostomy in adult patients undergoing artificial ventilation. *BMJ* **2005**, *330*, 1243. [CrossRef]
44. Vargas, M.; Sutherasan, Y.; Brunetti, I.; Micalizzi, C.; Insorsi, A.; Ball, L.; Folentino, M.; Sileo, R.; De Lucia, A.; Cerana, M.; et al. Mortality and long-term quality of life after percutaneous tracheotomy in Intensive Care Unit: A prospective observational study. *Minerva Anestesiol.* **2018**, *84*, 1024–1031. [CrossRef] [PubMed]
45. Cheung, N.H.; Napolitano, L.M. Tracheostomy: Epidemiology, Indications, Timing, Technique, and Outcomes. *Respir. Care* **2014**, *59*, 895–919. [CrossRef] [PubMed]
46. Cox, C.E.; Carson, S.S.; Holmes, G.M.; Howard, A.; Carey, T.S. Increase in tracheostomy for prolonged mechanical ventilation in North Carolina, 1993–2002. *Crit. Care Med.* **2004**, *32*, 2219–2226. [CrossRef]

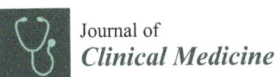

Review

Potentially Detrimental Effects of Hyperosmolality in Patients Treated for Traumatic Brain Injury

Wojciech Dabrowski [1,*,†], Dorota Siwicka-Gieroba [1,*,†], Chiara Robba [2], Magdalena Bielacz [3], Joanna Sołek-Pastuszka [4], Katarzyna Kotfis [5], Romuald Bohatyrewicz [4], Andrzej Jaroszyński [6], Manu L. N. G. Malbrain [1,7,8] and Rafael Badenes [9]

1. Department of Anaesthesiology and Intensive Care, Medical University of Lublin, 20-954 Lublin, Poland; manu.malbrain@umlub.pl
2. Department of Anaesthesia and Intensive Care, Policlinico San Martino, 16100 Genova, Italy; kiarobba@gmail.com
3. Institute of Tourism and Recreation, State Vocational College of Szymon Szymonowicz, 22-400 Zamosc, Poland; magda.bielacz@gmail.com
4. Department of Anaesthesiology and Intensive Care, Pomeranian Medical University, 71-252 Szczecin, Poland; pastuszka@mp.pl (J.S.-P.); romuald.bohatyrewicz@pum.edu.pl (R.B.)
5. Department of Anaesthesiology, Intensive Therapy and Acute Intoxications, Pomeranian Medical University, 70-111 Szczecin, Poland; katarzyna.kotfis@pum.edu.pl
6. Department of Nephrology, Institute of Medical Science, Jan Kochanowski University of Kielce, 25-736 Kielce, Poland; jaroszynskiaj@interia.pl
7. International Fluid Academy, Dreef 3, 3360 Lovenjoel, Belgium
8. Medical Department, AZ Jan Palfjin Hospital, Watersportlaan 5, 9000 Gent, Belgium
9. Department of Anaesthesiology and Intensive Care, Hospital Clínico Universitario de Valencia, University of Valencia, 46010 Valencia, Spain; rafaelbadenes@gmail.com
* Correspondence: w.dabrowski5@yahoo.com (W.D.); dsiw@wp.pl (D.S.-G.)
† Wojciech Dabrowski and Dorota Siwicka-Gieroba contributed equally to this article.

Abstract: Hyperosmotic therapy is commonly used to treat intracranial hypertension in traumatic brain injury patients. Unfortunately, hyperosmolality also affects other organs. An increase in plasma osmolality may impair kidney, cardiac, and immune function, and increase blood–brain barrier permeability. These effects are related not only to the type of hyperosmotic agents, but also to the level of hyperosmolality. The commonly recommended osmolality of 320 mOsm/kg H_2O seems to be the maximum level, although an increase in plasma osmolality above 310 mOsm/kg H_2O may already induce cardiac and immune system disorders. The present review focuses on the adverse effects of hyperosmolality on the function of various organs.

Keywords: osmolality; traumatic brain injury (TBI); hypertonic saline; mannitol; osmolar gap

1. Introduction

Hyperosmotic therapy has been recommended for treatment of cerebral edema (CE) and increased intracranial pressure (ICP) in patients with traumatic brain injury (TBI) and other cerebral diseases [1,2]. The main purpose of increasing the plasma osmolality is to force the shift of water from the brain to the vascular space through the blood–brain barrier (BBB) [2]. According to the Monroe–Kellie doctrine, the sum of the volumes of intracerebral blood, cerebrospinal fluid (CSF), and brain is constant, therefore a decrease of water from the interstitial space of the brain reduces cerebral volume and cerebral edema, which may improve cerebral perfusion [3,4]. Experimental studies have also documented that hyperosmolar therapy attenuates trauma-related inflammatory response by reducing neutrophil activation and neutrophil-endothelium binding [5,6]. Currently, mannitol and hypertonic saline (HTS) have only been recommended for the treatment of intracranial hypertension (ICH) and cerebral edema, and the final goal of hyperosmotic therapy is the achievement of plasma osmolality not higher than 320 mOsm/kg H_2O [1,2,7]. The choice

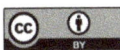

of agents depends on clinical experience and local protocol, however HTS is frequently used to reduce ICH as well as tissue edema, whereas mannitol is used only to reduce ICH [8,9].

2. The Most Popular Hyperosmotic Agents

The main problem for choosing hyperosmotic agents is their different osmotic activity. The reflection coefficient (a number which reflects the difficulty for the molecule to pass through the endothelium: 0 = fully permeable and 1.0 = completely impermeable) is 0.9 in the normal brain and a little less in the injured brain [10]. It means that mannitol practically did not pass through the BBB, but it penetrates the injured BBB and the intact BBB. Mannitol at a daily dose of 0.5–1.5 g/kg body weight is commonly used as an osmotically active medication in patients with TBI. Chemically, it is a metabolically inert sugar alcohol ($C_6H_{14}O_6$), which is similar to xylitol or sorbitol. It elevates plasma osmolality, which enhances flow from the extravascular to the intravascular space. Interestingly, inhaled mannitol was also indicated by the Food and Drug Administration (FDA) in the treatment of cystic fibrosis in the lung [11,12].

HTS elevates plasma osmolality via plasma increase in osmotically active ions, such as sodium. Additionally, HTS also reduces single erythrocyte volume, improving their passage through the capillaries. Its reflection coefficient is 1 [13,14]. It seems to reduce ICH and improve cerebral perfusion pressure more effectively than mannitol [15–17]. Some studies also documented better outcomes in patients treated with HTS compared to mannitol, however the osmotherapy-related electrolyte disequilibrium appears to be an independent predictor of poor outcome, regardless of the type of osmotically active medication [18–20]. This improves the rheological properties of the blood and the osmotic activity of aquaporin receptors in the BBB [21,22]. Clinicians commonly use HTS with different 3%, 7.5%, or 23.4% solutions, and each of those presents a different osmotic activity (Table 1) [21,22]. Regardless of the type of the osmotically active agents, the main target of osmotherapy is to maintain plasma osmolality around 300–320 mOsm/kg H_2O [1,2].

Table 1. Theoretical osmolality of the most popular osmotically active agents [17–25].

Solution	0.9% NaCl	3% NaCl	7.5% NaCl	23.4% NaCl	10% Mannitol	15% Mannitol	20% Mannitol	1‰ Ethanol
Osmolality (mOsm/kg H_2O)	308	1026	2567	8008	550	825	1100	22

3. Basic Knowledge

Hyperosmotic therapy is based on osmosis—a phenomenon in which the water molecules migrate through a semi-permeable barrier from a solution rich in osmotically active molecules to a solution poor in the concentration of these agents. The difference in solutes, which cannot pass across the semi-permeable membrane, causes a chemical potential. According to the Gibbs–Duhen equation, the chemical potential and activity of water molecules is higher in a solvent in which the activity of saluted agents is lower, and the movement of water is forced from the solvent to the solution [26]. Osmolarity is defined as the number of solutes per liter of solution, however the concentration of solutes is very low in human body fluids. Therefore, the plasma osmolarity is calculated in milliosmoles (mOsm/L). Osmolality is defined as the number of milliosmoles of solutes per one kilogram of water (mOsm/kg H_2O). Physiologically, Na^+, K^+, Cl^-, HCO_3^-, glucose, and urea are the main osmotically active substances in the human body, however a lot of medicaments exhibit osmotic properties. Some of them, such as urea and ethanol, freely cross the cell membranes and are called "ineffective osmoles", whereas others such as Na^+, K^+, Cl^-, HCO_3^-, and glucose are called effective osmoles because they do not cross the cell membranes, forcing water shifts through the cellular membranes (tonicity). Chemically, osmolarity is strongly related to osmolality in solutions with the same composition but different concentrations of osmotically active agents. These relationship changes occur in the blood because the blood contains lipids, proteins, and others small solutes contributing to plasma osmolality, thus sodium solutions are not completely dissociated in the aqueous medium. Additionally, the plasma contains only 93% of water [27]. Therefore, plasma osmolality can be calculated by multiplying the plasma osmolarity by 0.93. Hence, osmotic pressure is more closely related to plasma osmolality than osmolarity. Plasma osmolality should be measured by a cryoscopy technique, which is considered as the reference method for osmolality measurement [28]. However, several clinicians have calculated plasma osmolality using a different equation. The most popular, the simplest, and the best is known as the Worthley equation [25,27]:

$$Plasma\ osmolality = 2xNa^+ + \frac{Glucose\ (mg/dL)}{18} + \frac{BUN\ (mg/dL)}{2.8} = 275 - 295\ mOsm/kg\ H_2O$$

The difference between the measured and the calculated plasma osmolality is called the osmolal gap. Physiologically, its value ranges between −10 and +10 mOsm/L. An osmolal gap higher than 10 mOsm/L documents the presence of osmotically active agents in the blood, while its values above 20 mOsm/L suggest blood intoxication with strong osmotic substances [29–31]. Despite the beneficial effect of elevated plasma osmolality on cerebral water content in TBI patients with cerebral edema, hyperosmolality per se or associated with high osmolal gap may affect organ function, increase the risk of multiorgan dysfunction, and worsen the outcome in critically ill patients (Figure 1) [30–34]. The aim of this article was to provide a narrative review regarding the effect of recommended plasma hyperosmolality on organ function in patients treated for TBI.

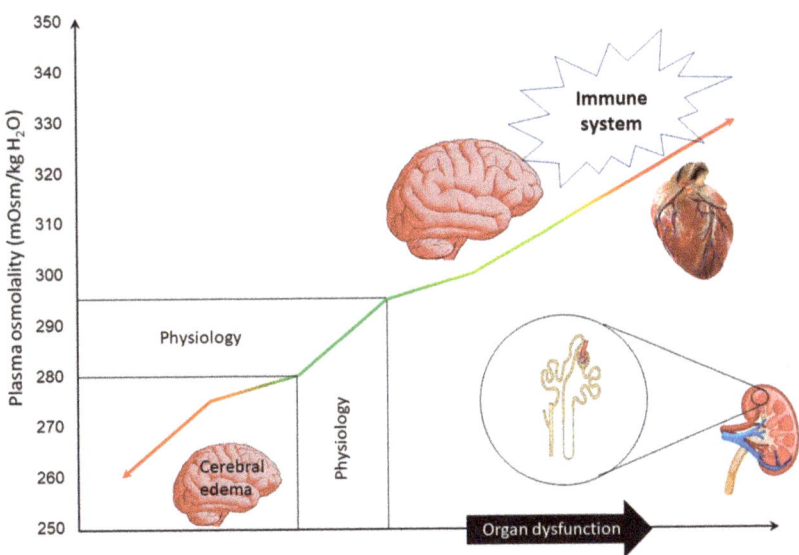

Figure 1. General scheme showing the organs that can be damaged as a result of increased plasma osmolality.

4. Plasma Hyperosmolality and the Heart

The disorders of plasma osmolality can impair cardiac function and increase the risk of life-threatening cardiac arrhythmias and sudden cardiac death [32,35–38]. An analysis of relationships between plasma osmolality, and the 30-day and 1-year outcomes in 985 patients diagnosed with acute coronary syndrome, showed a significantly higher mortality rate in patients with hyperosmolal plasma [38]. Another clinical analysis of 3748 patients treated for acute coronary diseases also documented an increase in short and long mortality in patients with hyperosmolality [36]. Interestingly, the rate of ventricular arrhythmias, cardiogenic shock, and major adverse cardiac events was two-fold higher in those patients. Indeed, an increase in plasma osmolality following mannitol administration above 313 mOsm/kg H_2O significantly increased the risk for prolongation of corrected QT interval above 500 ms, which is associated with the incidence of atrial fibrillation in patients without any cardiac history treated for TBI [32]. An experimental study has shown that HTS-induced hyperosmolality per se may exert potentially deleterious effects on myocardial contractility, leading to systolic and diastolic dysfunction, cytosolic Ca^{2+} accumulation with diastolic contracture, and increased susceptibility to life-threatening arrhythmias [27]. Additionally, HTS-related hyperosmotic stress is associated with an increase in the intracellular Ca^{2+} concentration and generation of reactive oxygen species, which promotes stress in the endoplasmic reticulum, leading to apoptosis and death of adult and neonatal cardiomyocytes [39,40]. Plasma osmolality plays a crucial role in the function of cardiac aquaporins. Hyperosmolality increases the mRNA of aquaporin-1, mRNA of upregulated aquaporin-7, protein glycosylation, and intracellular translocation, which may modulate water transport in cardiac myocytes [41–43]. A rapid increase in plasma osmolality following hypertonic saline administration depresses the sensitivity of the cardiac baroreflex independently of changes in blood pressure, causing an increase in heart rate [44]. Accumulating data have shown that a rapid increase in plasma osmolality activates sympathetic nerve activity, both in humans and animals [45–47]. Moreover, prolonged hyperosmolality also increases sympathetic nerve activity through activation of osmoreceptors and raised excitatory amino acid release in the forebrain [47,48]. A dysregulation of sympathetic/parasympathetic activity as well as dysfunction of cardiac myocytes following an increase in plasma osmolality may depress cardiac function, leading to acute cardiac failure. Thus, it can be speculated that hyperosmolality may play an important role in cardiac dysfunction that develops in patients treated for TBI, which is commonly known as the brain–heart interaction.

In some clinical situations, hyperosmolality may also have a beneficial effect on cardiac function. Experimental studies documented that hyperosmotic perfusion significantly reduced total and intracellular myocardial water content, reduced sarcolemmal rupture, and increased coronary flow in ischemia/reperfusion-induced cellular edema [49,50]. Another study documented that hyperosmotic pretreatment also reduced the infarct size following regional-induced ischemia in a rat heart model [51]. The beneficial effect of hyperosmotic perfusion after cardiac ischemia may be explained by the relatively small osmotic gradient between the intra- and extra-cellular spaces during reperfusion. An increase of the level of intracellular lactate following ischemia-induced anaerobic glycolysis results in a relative hyperosmotic condition within the ischemic area. Hence, the normo- or hypo-osmotic reperfusion increases the water shift from the vascular into the intracellular space, leading to cellular edema, whereas hyperosmotic reperfusion does not induce water extravasation (Figure 2). It is also worth stressing that a lot of research analyzing the beneficial effect of hyperosmolal reperfusion in ischemic heart with swollen cardiomyocytes showed that the increased osmolality of the perfusate (with mannitol) had cardioprotective properties [52]. Taken together, we can suggest that hyperosmolality may impair cardiac function in TBI patients without any previous history of cardiac diseases. Hence, osmotherapy requires strict control of plasma osmolality (not osmolarity).

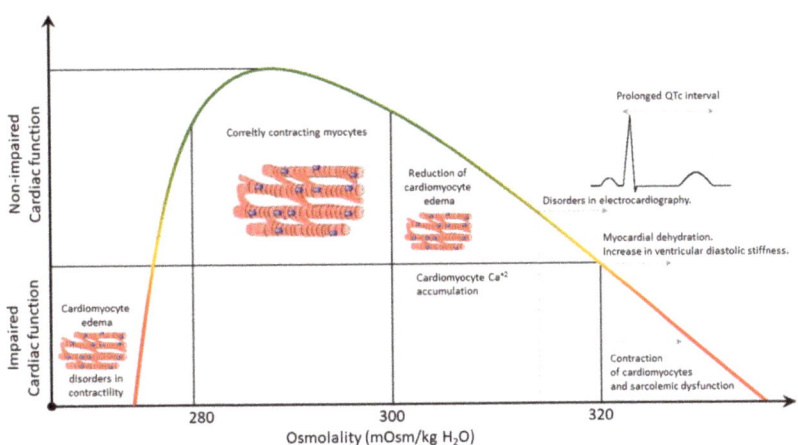

Figure 2. General scheme showing the effect of hyperosmolality on the heart.

5. Plasma Hyperosmolality and the Kidney

Kidneys are especially vulnerable to disorders in plasma osmolality because they play a crucial role in plasma osmolality regulation. The kidney is responsible for regulation of salt and water excretion. Under physiological conditions, sodium is the predominant cation affecting fluid osmolality in mammals, and the osmoregulation and the control of total body sodium operate independently to its plasma concentration, at least to some extent [53]. Several factors play a role in the regulation of kidney excretory function, and inner medullary cells are especially vulnerable to elevation of plasma osmolality. Hyperosmolality induces salt excretion, increasing its concentration in urea and inner medullary cells. This process forces increased urea removal. It is noteworthy that Na^+ and Cl^- exert different effects on cells due to their different permeability of the cell membranes, whereas urea penetrates the cell membrane similarly to water. Extracellular hypertonicity following elevated extracellular salt content increases passive water shift from the intracellular into the extracellular space, leading to cellular shrinkage. On the other hand, elevated urea concentration in the extracellular space forces its shift to the inner medullary cells due to osmosis. Accumulated intracellular urea is a trigger for uncontrolled protein denaturation. Additionally, the non-specific effect of hyperosmolality may result from osmolar-forced diuresis with activation of tubulo-glomerular feedback associated with an increase in hydrostatic pressure in the tubules and a decrease in intrarenal microcirculation flow, which ultimately reduces the glomerular filtration rate. An impairment of renal blood flow disturbs oxygen delivery to the renal cells, inducing hypoxia-related cell damage [54]. Hence, hyperosmolality itself affects cell volume, cell metabolism, intracellular ion homeostasis, and stability of nucleic acids, which can induce an apoptotic process and upregulate several genes in the renal inner medullary cells [55–58]. A lot of osmotically active agents may also induce or intensify hyperosmosis-related acute kidney injury (AKI). This pathology is commonly known as "osmotic nephrosis" or "sucrose nephrosis" (Figure 3). Several studies showed that intravenous administration of immune globulin, mannitol, contrast media, hydroxyethyl starch solutions, or glucose can induce AKI injury via osmotic cell destruction [59–65]. It was well-documented that osmotically active agents entered the tubular cells by means of pinocytosis, leading to cellular edema with increased lysosomes and endocytotic vacuoles. Interestingly, the use of iso-osmolar contrast media also results in nephrotoxicity, similar to the effect of the hyperosmolar media, which cannot be explained by hyperosmolality itself, but rather the increased viscosity of the iso-osmolar agents [65,66]. However, plasma osmolality plays an important role for renal function. Clinical observations documented a significant relationship between plasma osmolality and a higher incidence of AKI noted in patients with diabetic ketoacidosis when osmolality exceeded 320 mOsm/kg [67,68]. The osmotic nephrosis is usually reversible after discontinuation of osmotically active agents; however, some patients require temporary renal replacement therapy [63,68–71].

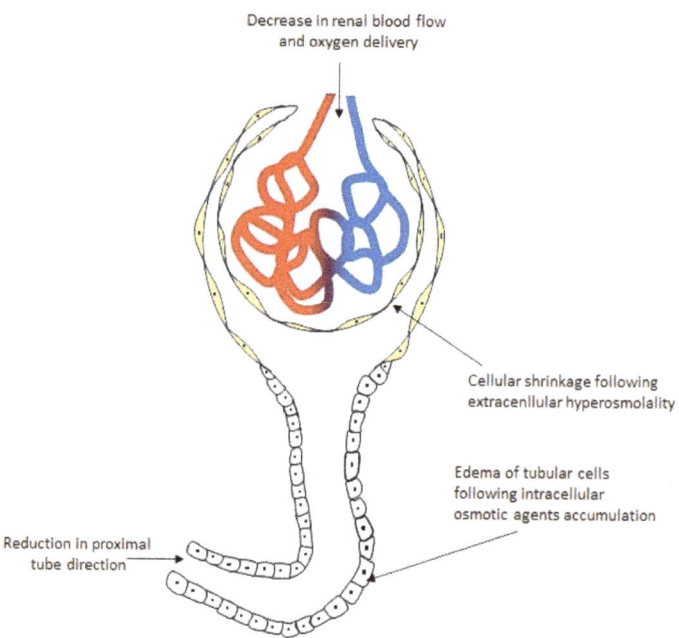

Figure 3. General scheme presenting an effect of hyperosmosis on glomerulus and tubular cells [54–57,66].

Mannitol is not recommended for use in the management of severe TBI when ICP and brain tissue oxygen are monitored [2]. Several studies documented AKI following mannitol administration [62,69–71]. Mannitol-induced osmotic nephrosis has been well-documented, as it exerts nephrotoxic activity [61–63,65,72]. There is a dose–response relationship between the use of mannitol and the incidence and severity of AKI, with a cut-off of the daily dose at 1.34 g/kg body weight [73]. Interestingly, the combined therapy of ICH with mannitol and HTS did not increase the risk of AKI more than HTS alone, however several authors suggested to use HTS, demonstrating its superiority over mannitol [13,14,16,18,74]. In conclusion, it can be postulated that an increase in plasma hyperosmolality per se, as well as the use of osmotically active medications, may impair renal function, and that maintaining adequate renal perfusion may reduce the risk of AKI.

6. Plasma Hyperosmolality and Immune System

The effects of hyperosmolality on the immune system are still controversial and not very well-recognized, however several in vitro studies have attributed an important role to hypertonicity in the inflammatory response [75–80]. Elevated plasma osmolality is especially associated with stimulation of macrophages and dendric cells [5,75]. An increase in plasma osmolality by 10 to 20 mOsm/kg suppresses neutrophil function by modulating cellular signaling, fosters B cell activation and differentiation, and reduces macrophage activation [5,76–78]. Several experimental studies have documented that increasing tonicity inhibits the production of proinflammatory cytokines in pulmonary epithelial cells [78,79]. The inhibitory effect of hypertonicity on inflammatory responses is especially important after brain injury. An increase in plasma osmolality following mannitol or HTS administration reduces microglial activation and promotes the anti-inflammatory phagocytic M2-like microglial phenotype in an experimental model of intracerebral hemorrhage [5]. Such relationships between hyperosmolality and the inflammatory response may result from direct regulation of nuclear factor in the T cells, which affect TNF-α and lymphotoxin-β [80]. Additionally, hyperosmotic stress leads to cell apoptosis that involves changes in the apoptotic signaling molecules such as mitogen-activated protein kinase, c-Jun amino terminal kinase, mitogen-activated kinase, and p38 mitogen-activated kinase in a primary cultured nucleus pulpous cells [81]. Hyperosmolarity following mannitol administration at the dose of 1.0–1.5 g/kg body weight induces programmed cell death in a dose-dependent manner in both endothelial and smooth muscle cells [82]. The cell loss within the endothelial monolayers was the most pronounced, with serum osmolarity above 320 mOsm/L. Quite the opposite, it has been documented that hyperosmotic stress is associated with pro-inflammatory cytokine secretion, such as: TNF, IL1-β, IL-6, and IL-8, and that hyperosmolality may be an important factor for survival of macrophages at the inflammatory site after injection of the Bacille Calmette-Guerin (BCG) vaccine [83]. Additionally, prolonged dietary sodium administration increases activation of stress-sensitive neurons of the hypothalamic paraventricular nucleus and basolateral amygdala, leading to stress coping behaviors in mice [84]. In a clinical study including 44 healthy volunteers who received a 250 mL intravenous bolus of 3% saline solution to increase plasma osmolality to 315 mOsm/L, the authors showed that both hyponatremia and plasma hyperosmolality did not induce an increase in circulating markers of inflammation and led to a decrease in the level of TNFα and IL-8 at an unchanged level of IL-6 plasma concentration [85]. Another study documented that the increase in plasma osmolality following mannitol at a dose of 0.5 g/kg body weight significantly limited cardiopulmonary bypass-related inflammatory response, with a reduction of pro-inflammatory and an increase of anti-inflammatory cytokines [86]. It is noteworthy that the majority of studies analyzing the effects of hyperosmolality on the immune system are based on experimental observations. Therefore, one can only speculate that hyperosmolality seems to have a beneficial effect on the immune system, and this hypothesis should be confirmed in further studies.

7. Plasma Hyperosmolality and the Blood–Brain Barrier

Hyperosmolar therapy is the cornerstone treatment of ICH. Administration of hyperosmolar agents increases the osmotic gradient between blood and brain, forcing the water flux from the brain to blood through the BBB. In the central nervous system of mammals, the BBB is created at the level of the endothelial brain cells, where multiple protein complexes accumulate at the cell-junctions, restricting the paracellular diffusion of ions and other polar solutes, hence effectively blocking the penetration of macromolecules. Unfortunately, therapeutic hyperosmolar agents can reversibly open thigh junctions in the cerebrovascular endothelium, and their conductivity depends on the degree of plasma hyperosmolality [87–90]. An experimental study has shown a temporal induction of neuroinflammatory response following intracarotid infusion of mannitol [89]. Elevation of cytokines, chemokines, trophic factors, and cell adhesion molecules was noted within 5 min after mannitol administration that persisted for 4 days. It is noteworthy that the BBB's susceptibility to increase plasma osmolality decreases with age and is the greatest in fetuses and premature infants [90].

Currently, the effect of a rapid increase of plasma osmolality on the function of the BBB is used to increase delivery of poorly penetrating medications to the brain (Figure 4). This type of treatment may be especially attractive for treating malignant brain tumors [91,92]. Administration of a small volume of chemotherapeutics after mannitol into the tumor circulation increases their therapeutic properties without the need for increased systemic doses and without adverse effects [91]. A lot of preclinical and clinical studies have convincingly documented the high potency of this approach to elevate the delivery of chemotherapy and other medications to the brain. Experimental studies have also presented a better brain delivery of other drugs, such as antiepileptic drugs or docosahexaenoic acid (DHA), in hypertonicity-related hyperpermeability of the BBB [93,94]. Interestingly, an increase of DHA attenuates BBB disruption, and reduces cerebral edema and TBI-induced neuroinflammation [94,95].

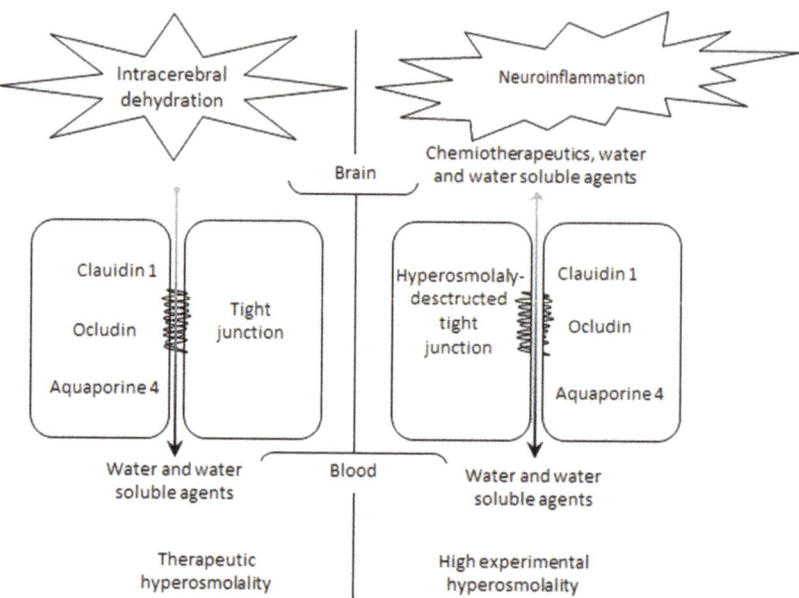

Figure 4. General scheme showing the effect of hyperosmolality on the blood–brain barrier. Therapeutic increase in plasma osmolality intense water removal from the brain. Experimentally raised osmolality to the high value disrupts the blood–brain barrier from opening the tight junction for intracerebral shifts of chemotherapeutics, water, and other water-soluble and insoluble agents.

It is difficult to show a destructive effect of plasma hyperosmolality on the BBB in patients treated for TBI. An experimental and therapeutic decrease in BBB permeability is induced by intra-arterial administration of mannitol. Hence, many clinicians prefer HTS over mannitol to increase plasma osmolality, because HTS does not affect the BBB permeability. However, a decrease in BBB permeability following hypertonicity seems to be useful in treating secondary brain damage from different antioxidants and anti-inflammatory agents. This hypothesis needs confirmation in future studies.

8. Conclusions

Osmotherapy is the cornerstone treatment of ICH. An increase in plasma osmolality to the recommended 320 mOsm/kg H_2O is commonly achieved by mannitol or HTS. The choice of osmotic agents is still the subject of debate, and HTS seems to be preferred over mannitol. An increase in plasma osmolality may impair cardiac, kidney, immune, and BBB function, however a deleterious effect of mannitol-induced hyperosmolality has only been clinically documented with respect to kidney and cardiac function. An increase in plasma osmolality per se above 313 mOsm/kg H_2O may by itself impair cardiac function. Future trials are awaited to bring more answers and solutions.

Author Contributions: W.D., A.J., C.R. and R.B. (Romuald Bohatyrewicz) reviewed the concept; D.S.-G., W.D., K.K., M.B., J.S.-P., C.R. and R.B. (Rafael Badenes) performed literature collection and analysis; W.D., M.L.N.G.M. and A.J. drafted the first version; K.K. reviewed the initial draft. All authors have read and agreed to the published version of the manuscript.

Funding: This research received no external funding.

Data Availability Statement: Not applicable—not original data.

Conflicts of Interest: The authors declare no conflict of interest.

References

1. Raslan, A.; Bhardwaj, A. Medical management of cerebral edema. *Neurosurg. Focus* **2007**, *22*, E12. [CrossRef]
2. Chesnut, R.; Aguilera, S.; Buki, A.; Bulger, E.; Citerio, G.; Cooper, D.J.; Arradtia, R.D.; Diringer, M.; Figaji, A.; Gao, G.; et al. A management algorithm for patients with intracranial pressure monitoring: The Seattle International Severe Traumatic Brain Injury Consensus Conference (SIBICC). *Intensive Care Med.* **2020**, *46*, 1783–1794. [CrossRef]
3. Macintyre, I. A hotbed of medical innovation: George Kellie (1770–1829), his colleagues at Leith and the Monro-Kellie doctrine. *J. Med. Biogr.* **2014**, *22*, 93–100. [CrossRef] [PubMed]
4. Mokri, B. The Monro-Kellie hypothesis: Applications in CSF volume depletion. *Neurology* **2001**, *56*, 1746–1748. [CrossRef] [PubMed]
5. Schreibman, D.L.; Hong, C.M.; Keledjian, K.; Ivanowa, S.; Tsymbalyuk, S.; Gerzanich, V.; Simard, J.M. Mannitol and hypertonic saline reduce swelling and modulate inflammatory markers in a rat model of intracerebral haemorrhage. *Neurocrit. Care* **2018**, *29*, 253–263. [CrossRef] [PubMed]
6. Pascual, J.L.; Ferri, L.E.; Seely, A.J.E.; Campisi, G.; Chaudhury, P.; Giannias, B.; Evans, D.C.; Razek, T.; Michel, R.P.; Cgristou, N.V. Hypertonic saline resuscitation of hemorrhagic shock diminishes neutrophil rolling and adherence to endothelium and reduces in vivo vascular leakage. *Ann. Surg.* **2002**, *236*, 634–642. [CrossRef] [PubMed]
7. Oddo, M.; Poole, D.; Helbok, R.; Meyfroidt, G.; Stocchetti, N.; Bouzat, P.; Cecconi, M.; Geeraets, T.; Martin-Loeches, I.; Quintard, H.; et al. Fluid therapy in neurointensive care patients: ESCIM consensus and clinical practice recommendations. *Intenvive Care Med.* **2018**, *44*, 449–463. [CrossRef] [PubMed]
8. Toung, T.J.; Chen, C.H.; Lin, C.; Bhardwaj, A. Osmotherapy with hypertonic saline attenuates water content in brain and extracerebral organs. *Crit. Care Med.* **2007**, *35*, 526–531. [CrossRef]
9. Hays, A.N.; Lazaridis, C.; Neyens, R.; Nicholas, J.; Gay, S.; Chalela, J.A. Osmotherapy: Use among neurointensivists. *Neurocrit Care* **2011**, *14*, 222–228. [CrossRef]
10. Bhardwaj, A. Osmotherapy in neurocritical care. *Curr. Neurol. Neurosci. Rep.* **2007**, *7*, 513–521. [CrossRef]
11. FDA Approved Drug Products: BRONCHITOL (mannitol) Oral Inhalation Power. Available online: https://www.accessdata.fda.gov/drugsatfda_docs/label/2020/202049s000lbl.pdf (accessed on 30 October 2020).
12. Southern, K.W.; Clancy, J.P.; Ranganathan, S. Aerosolized agents for airway clearance in cystic fibrosis. *Pediatr. Pulmonol.* **2019**, *54*, 858–864. [CrossRef]
13. Georgidis, A.L.; Suarez, J.I. Hypertonic saline for cerebral edema. *Curr. Neurol. Neurosci. Rep.* **2003**, *6*, 524–530. [CrossRef]
14. Kheirbek, T.; Pascual, J.L. Hypertonic saline for the treatment of intracranial hypertension. *Curr. Neurol. Neurosci. Rep.* **2014**, *14*, 482. [CrossRef] [PubMed]
15. Badaut, J.; Ashwal, S.; Obenaus, A. Aquaporins in cerebrovascular disease: A target for treatment of brain edema? *Cerebrovasc Dis.* **2011**, *31*, 521–531. [CrossRef] [PubMed]
16. Badenes, R.; Hutton, B.; Citerio, G.; Robba, C.; Aguilar, G.; Alonso-Arroyo, A.; Taccone, F.S.; Tornero, C.; Catala-Lopez, F. Hyperosmolar therapy for acute brain injury: Study protocol for an umbrella rewie of meta-analyses and evidence mapping. *BMJ Open* **2020**, *10*, e033913. [CrossRef] [PubMed]
17. Himmelsehr, S. Hypertonic saline solutions for treatment of intracranial hypertension. *Curr. Opin. Anaesthesiol.* **2007**, *20*, 414–426. [CrossRef] [PubMed]
18. Garrard, A.; Sollee, D.R.; Butterfields, R.C.; Johannsen, L.; Wood, A.; Bertholf, R.L. Validation of pre-existing formula to calculate the contribution of ethanol to the osmolar gap. *Clin. Toxicol.* **2012**, *50*, 562–566. [CrossRef]
19. Cochrane, T.T. Improvements in the equation for calculating the contribution to osmotic potential of the separate solutes of water solutions. *Med. Phys.* **1984**, *11*, 338–340. [CrossRef] [PubMed]
20. Moucka, F.; Nezbeda, I.; Smith, W.R. Molecular simulation of aqueous electrolytes: Water chemical potential results and Gibbs-Duhem equation consistency tests. *J. Chem. Phys.* **2013**, *139*, 124505. [CrossRef]
21. Rasouli, M.; Kalantari, K.R. Comparison of methods for calculating serum osmolality: Multivariate linear regression analysis. *Clin. Chem. Lab. Med.* **2005**, *43*, 635–640. [CrossRef]
22. Sweeney, T.E.; Beuchat, C.A. Limitation of methods of osmometry: Measuring the osmolality of biological FLUIDS. *Am. J. Physiol.* **1993**, *264*, R469–R480. [CrossRef] [PubMed]
23. Kruse, J.A.; Cadnapaphornachai, P. The serum osmole gap. *J. Crit. Care* **1994**, *9*, 185–197. [CrossRef]
24. Skaaland, H.; Larstorp, A.C.K.; Lindberg, M.; Jacobsen, D. Reference values for osmolal gap in healthy subject and in medical inpatients. *Scand. J. Clin. Lab. Investig.* **2020**, *80*, 1–5. [CrossRef] [PubMed]
25. Liams, G.; Fillppatos, T.D.; Liontos, A.; Elisaf, M.S. Serum osmolal gap in clinical practice: Usefulness and limitations. *Postgrad. Med.* **2017**, *129*, 456–459. [CrossRef]
26. Dabrowski, W.; Siwicka-Gieroba, D.; Robba, C.; Badenes, R.; Bialy, M.; Iwaniuk, P.; Schlegel, T.T.; Jaroszynski, A. Plasma hyperosmolality prolongs QTc interval and increases rosk for atrial fibrillation in traumatic brain injury patients. *J. Clin. Med.* **2020**, *9*, 1293. [CrossRef]
27. Bealer, S.L. Peripheral hyperosmolality reduces cardiac baroreflex sensitivity. *Auton. Neurosci.* **2003**, *104*, 24–31. [CrossRef]

28. Kultz, D. Hyperosmolality triggers oxidative damage in kidney cells. *Proc. Nat. Acad. Sci. USA* **2004**, *101*, 9177–9178. [CrossRef]
29. Steinberg, C. Diagnosis and clinical management of long-QT syndrome. *Curr. Opin. Cardiol.* **2018**, *33*, 31–41. [CrossRef]
30. Tatlisu, M.A.; Kaya, A.; Keskin, M.; Uzman, O.; Borklu, E.B.; Cinier, G.; Hayiroglu, M.I.; Tatlisu, K.; Eren, M. Can we use plasma hyperosmolality as a predictor of mortality for ST-segment elevation myocardial infarction? *Coron. Artery Dis.* **2017**, *28*, 70–76. [CrossRef]
31. Kaya, H.; Yücel, O.; Ege, M.R.; Zorlu, A.; Yücel, H.; Günes, H.; Ekmekci, A.; Yilmaz, M.B. Plasma osmolality predicts mortality in patients with heart failure with reduced ejection fraction. *Kardiol. Pol.* **2017**, *75*, 316–322. [CrossRef]
32. Rohla, M.; Freynhofer, M.K.; Tentzeris, I.; Farhan, S.; Wojte, J.; Huber, K.; Weiss, T.W. Plasma osmolality predicts clinical outcome in patients with acute coronary syndrome undergoing percutaneous coronary intervention. *Eur. Heart J. Acuta Cardiovasc. Care* **2014**, *3*, 84–92. [CrossRef] [PubMed]
33. Ricardo, R.A.; Bassani, R.A.; Bassani, J.W.M. Osmolality- and Na+-dependent effect of hyperosmotic NaCl solution on contractile activity and Ca2+ cycling in rat ventricular myocytes. *Pflugers Arch.* **2008**, *455*, 617–626. [CrossRef] [PubMed]
34. Burgos, J.I.; Morell, M.; Mariangelo, J.I.E.; Petroff, M.V. Hyperosmotic stress promotes endoplasmic reticulum stress-dependent apoptosis in adult rat cardiac myocytes. *Apoptosis* **2019**, *24*, 785–797. [CrossRef]
35. Galvez, A.; Morales, M.P.; Eltit, J.M.; Ocaranza, P.; Carrasco, L.; Campos, X.; Sapag-Hagar, M.; Díaz-Araya, G.; Lavandero, S. A rapid and strong apoptotic process is triggering by hyperosmotic stress in cultured rat cardiac myocytes. *Cell Tissue Res.* **2001**, *304*, 279–285. [CrossRef]
36. Page, E.; Winterfield, J.; Goings, G.; Bastawrous, A.; Upshaw-Early, J. Water channel proteins in rat cardiac myocyte caveolae: Osmolarity-dependent reversible internalization. *Am. J. Physiol.* **1998**, *274*, H1988–H2000. [CrossRef]
37. Rutkovskiy, A.; Mariero, L.H.; Nygard, S.; Stenslokken, K.O.; Valen, G.; Vaage, J. Transient hyperosmolality modulates expression of cardiac aquaporins. *Biochem. Biophys. Res. Commun.* **2012**, *425*, 70–75. [CrossRef]
38. Aggeli, I.K.; Kapogiannatou, A.; Paraskevopoulou, F.; Gaitanaki, C. Differential response of cardiac aquaporins of hyperosmotic stress; salutary role of AQ1 against the induced apoptosis. *Eur. Rev. Med. Pharmacol. Sci.* **2021**, *25*, 313–325.
39. Farquhar, W.B.; Wenner, M.M.; Delaney, E.P.; Prettyman, A.V.; Stillabower, M.E. Sympathetic neural response to increased osmolality in humans. *Am. J. Physiol. Heart Circ. Physiol.* **2006**, *291*, H2181–H2186. [CrossRef] [PubMed]
40. Kinsman, B.J.; Browning, K.N.; Stocker, S.D. NaCl and osmolarity produce different responses in organum vasculosum if the lamina terminalis neurons, sympathetic nerve activity and blood pressure. *J. Physiol.* **2017**, *595*, 6187–6201. [CrossRef]
41. Brooks, V.L.; Freeman, K.L.; O'Donaughy, T.L. Acute and chronic increase in osmolality increase excitatory amino acid drive of the rostral ventrolateral medulla in rats. *Am. J. Physiol. Regul. Integr. Comp. Physiol.* **2004**, *287*, R1359–R1368. [CrossRef] [PubMed]
42. Kamijo, Y.I.; Okazaki, K.; Ikegawa, S.; Okada, Y.; Nose, H. Rapid saline infusion and/or drinking enhance skin sympathetic nerve activity components reduced by hypovolaemia and hyperosmolality in hyperthermia. *J. Physiol.* **2018**, *596*, 544–5459. [CrossRef]
43. Andreas-Villarreal, M.; Barba, I.; Poncelas, M.; Inserte, J.; Rodriguea-Palomares, J.; Pineda, V.; Gracia-Dorado, D. Measuring water distribution in the heart: Preventing edema reducas ischemia-reperfusion injury. *J. Am. Hert. Assoc.* **2016**, *5*, e003843. [CrossRef]
44. Cao, Y.; Wang, L.; Chen, H.; Lv, Z. Beneficial effect of hyperosmotic perfusion in the myocardium after ischemia/reperfusion injury in isolated rat hearts. *Rev. Bras. Cir. Cardiovasc.* **2013**, *28*, 545–560. [CrossRef]
45. Falck, G.; Schjott, J.; Jynge, P. Hyperosmotic pretreatment reduces infarct size in the rat heart. *Physiol. Rev.* **1999**, *48*, 331–340.
46. Feige, K.; Rubbert, J.; Raupach, A.; Stroethoff, M.; Heinen, J.; Hollmann, M.W.; Huhn, R.; Torregroza, C. Cardioprotective properties of mannitol-involvement of mitochondrial potassium channels. *Int. J. Mol. Sci.* **2021**, *22*, 2395. [CrossRef]
47. Bie, P.; Damkjaer, M. Renin secretion and total body sodium: Pathways of integrative control. *Clin. Exp. Pharmacol. Physiol.* **2010**, *37*, e34–e42. [CrossRef] [PubMed]
48. Bansal, S.; Patel, R.N. Pathophysiology of contrast-induced acute kidney injury. *Interv. Cardiol. Clin.* **2020**, *9*, 293–298. [CrossRef] [PubMed]
49. Berl, T. How do kidney cells adopt to survive in hypertonic inner medulla? *Trans. Am. Clin. Climatol. Assoc.* **2009**, *120*, 389–401.
50. Blasum, B.S.; Schröter, R.; Neugebauer, U.; Hofchsröer, V.; Pavenstädt, H.; Ciarimboli, G.; Schlatter, E.; Edemir, B. The kidney-sepcific expression of genes can be modulated by the extracellular osmolality. *FASEB J.* **2016**, *30*, 3588–3597. [CrossRef]
51. Orbach, H.; Tishler, M.; Shoenfeld, Y. Intravenous immunoglobulin and the kidney—A two-edged sword. *Semin. Arthritis Rheum.* **2004**, *34*, 593–601. [CrossRef]
52. Kwan, T.H.; Tong, M.K.; Siu, Y.P.; Leung, K.T.; Lee, H.K.; Young, C.Y.; Au, T.C. Acute renal failure related to intravenous immunoglobulin infusion in an elderly woman. *Hong Kong Med. J.* **2005**, *11*, 45–49. [PubMed]
53. Gaut, J.P.; Liapis, H. Acute kidney injury pathology and pathophysiology: A retrospective review. *Clin. Kidney J.* **2020**, *14*, 526–536. [CrossRef] [PubMed]
54. Shi, J.; Qian, J.; Li, H.; Luo, H.; Luo, W.; Lin, Z. Renal tubular epithelial cells injury induced by mannitol and its potential mechanism. *Ren. Fail.* **2018**, *40*, 85–91. [CrossRef] [PubMed]
55. Dickenmann, M.; Oettl, T.; Mihatsch, M.J. Osmotic nephrosis: Acute kidney injury with accumulation of proximal tubular lysosomes due to administration of exogenous solutes. *Am. J. Kidney Dis.* **2008**, *51*, 491–503. [CrossRef] [PubMed]
56. Visweswaran, P.; Massin, E.K.; Dubose, T.D., Jr. Mannitol-induced acute renal failure. *J. Am. Soc. Nephrol.* **1997**, *8*, 1028–1033. [CrossRef] [PubMed]
57. Lin, S.Y.; Tang, S.C.; Tsai, L.K.; Yeh, S.J.; Shen, L.J.; Wu, F.L.; Jeng, J.S. Incidence and risk factors for acute kidney injury following mannitol infusion in patients with acute stroke: A retrospective cohort study. *Medicine* **2015**, *94*, e2032. [CrossRef] [PubMed]

58. Asif, A.; Preston, R.A.; Roth, D. Radiocontrast-induced nephropathy. *Am. J. Ther.* **2003**, *10*, 137–147. [CrossRef] [PubMed]
59. Seeliger, E.; Lenhard, D.C.; Persson, P.B. Contrast media velocity versus osmolality in kidney injury: Lesson from animal studies. *BioMed Res. Int.* **2014**, *2014*, 358136. [CrossRef]
60. Lancelot, E.; Idee, J.P.; Lacledere, C.; Santus, R.; Corot, C. Effects of two dimetric iodinated contrast media on renal medullary blood perfusion and oxygenation in dogs. *Invest. Radiol.* **2002**, *37*, 368–375. [CrossRef]
61. Skrifvars, M.B.; Bailey, M.; Moore, E.; Martensson, J.; French, C.; Presneill, J.; Nichol, A.; Little, L.; Duranteau, J.; Huet, O.; et al. A post hoc analysis of osmotherapy use in the erythropoietin in traumatic brain injury study—Associations with acute kidney injury and mortality. *Crit. Care Med.* **2021**, *49*, e394–e403. [CrossRef]
62. Dorman, H.R.; Sondheimer, J.H.; Cadnapaphornchai, P. Mannitol-induced acute renal failure. *Medicine* **1990**, *69*, 153–159. [CrossRef]
63. Moustafa, H.; Schoene, D.; Altarsha, E.; Rahmig, J.; Schneider, H.; Pallesen, L.P.; Prakapenia, A.; Siepmann, T.; Barlinn, J.; Paussauer, J.; et al. Acute kidney injury in patients with malignant middle cerebral artery infarction undergoing hyperosmolar therapy with mannitol. *J. Crit. Care* **2021**, *64*, 22–28. [CrossRef]
64. Schmitt, J.; Rahman, A.F.; Ashraf, A. Concurrent diabetic ketoacidosis with hyperosmolality and/or severe hyperglycemia in youth with type 2 diabetes. *Endocrinol. Diab. Metab.* **2020**, *3*, e00160. [CrossRef] [PubMed]
65. Royal Australian College of General Practitioners. General Practice Management of Type 2 Diabetes 2016–2018. Available online: www.racgp.org.au/clinical-resources/clinical-guidelines/key-racgp-guidelines/view-all-racgp-guidelines/management-of-type-2-diabetes (accessed on 5 May 2021).
66. Nomani, A.Z.; Nabi, Z.; Rashid, H.; Janjua, J.; Nomani, H.; Majeed, A.; Chaudry, S.R.; Mazhar, A.S. Osmotic nephrosis with mannitol: A review article. *Ren. Fail.* **2014**, *36*, 1169–1176. [CrossRef]
67. Kim, M.Y.; Park, J.H.; Kang, N.R.; Jang, H.R.; Lee, J.E.; Huh, W.; Kim, Y.G.; Kim, D.J.; Hong, S.C.; Kim, J.S.; et al. Intreased risk of acute kidney injury associated with higher infusion rate of mannitol in patients with intracranial haemorrhage. *J. Neurosurg.* **2014**, *120*, 1340–1348. [CrossRef] [PubMed]
68. Narayan, S.W.; Castelino, R.; Hammond, N.; Patanwala, A.E. Effect of mannitol plus hypertonic saline combination versus hypertonic saline monotherapy on acute kidney injury after traumatic brain injury. *J. Crit. Care* **2020**, *57*, 220–224. [CrossRef] [PubMed]
69. Gu, J.; Huang, H.; Huang, Y.; Sun, H.; Xu, H. Hypertonic saline or mannitol for treating elevated intracranial pressure in traumatic brain injury: A meta-analysis of randomized controlled trials. *Neurosurg. Rev.* **2019**, *42*, 499–509. [CrossRef]
70. Huang, X.; Yang, L.; Ye, J.; He, S.; Wang, B. Equimolar doses of hypertonic agents (saline or mannitol) in the treatment of intracranial hypertension after severe traumatic brain injury. *Medicine* **2020**, *99*, e22004. [CrossRef] [PubMed]
71. Shi, J.; Tan, L.; Ye, J.; Hu, L. Hypertonic saline and mannitol in patients with traumatic brain injury: A systematic and meta-analysis. *Medicine* **2020**, *99*, e21655. [CrossRef]
72. Patil, H.; Gupta, R. A comparative study of bolus dose of hypertonic saline, mannitol, and mannitol plus glycerol combination in patients with severe traumatic brain injury. *World Neurosurg.* **2019**, *125*, e221–e228. [CrossRef]
73. DeNett, T.; Feltner, C. Hypertonic saline versus mannitol for the treatment of increased intracranial pressure in traumatic brain injury. *J. Am. Assoc. Nurse Pract.* **2019**, *33*, 283–293. [CrossRef]
74. Wiorek, A.; Jaworski, T.; Krzych, Ł.J. Hyperosmolar threatment for patients at risk for increased intracranial pressure: A single-center cohort study. *Int. J. Environ. Res. Public Health* **2020**, *17*, 4573. [CrossRef]
75. Popovic, Z.V.; Embgenbroich, M.; Chessa, F.; Nordström, V.; Bonrouhy, M.; Hielscher, T.; Gretz, N.; Wang, S.; Mathow, D.; Quast, T.; et al. Hyperosmolarity impedes the cross-priming competence of dendric cells in a TRIF-dependent manner. *Sci. Rep.* **2017**, *7*, 311. [CrossRef] [PubMed]
76. Junger, W.T.; Hoyt, D.B.; Davis, R.E.; Herdon-Remelius, C.; Namiki, S.; Junger, H.; Loomis, W.; Altman, A. Hypertonicity regulates the function of human neutrophils by modulating chemoattractant receptor signalling and activating mitogen-activated protein kinase p38. *J. Clin. Investig.* **1998**, *101*, 2768–2779. [CrossRef]
77. Cvetkovic, L.; Perisic, S.; Titze, J.; Jäck, H.M.; Schuh, W. The impact of hyperosmolality on activation and differentiation of B lymphoid cells. *Front. Immunol.* **2019**, *10*, 808. [CrossRef] [PubMed]
78. Powers, K.A.; Zurawska, J.; Szaszi, K.; Khadaroo, R.G.; Kapus, A.; Rotstein, O.D. Hypertonic resuscitation of hemorrhagic shock prevents alveolar macrophage activation by preventing systemic oxidative stress due to gut ischemia/reperfusion. *Surgery* **2005**, *137*, 66–74. [CrossRef] [PubMed]
79. Wright, F.L.; Gamboni, F.; Moore, E.E.; Nydam, T.L.; Mitra, S.; Silliman, C.C.; Banerjee, A. Hyperosmolarity invokes distinct anti-inflammatory mechanisms in pulmonary epithelial cells: Evidence from signalling and transcription layers. *PLoS ONE* **2014**, *9*, e114129. [CrossRef]
80. Lopez-Rodríguez, C.; Aramburu, J.; Jin, L.; Rakeman, A.S.; Michino, M.; Rao, A. Bridging the NFAT and NF-κB families: NFAT5 dimerization regulates cytokine gene transcription in response to osmotic stress. *Immunity* **2001**, *15*, 47–58. [CrossRef]
81. Dong, Z.H.; Wang, D.C.; Liu, T.T.; Li, F.H.; Liu, R.L.; Wei, J.W.; Zhou, C.L. The roles of MAPKs in rabbit nucleus pulposus cell apoptosis induced by high osmolality. *Eur. Rev. Med. Pharmacol. Sci.* **2014**, *18*, 2835–2845.
82. Malek, A.M.; Goss, G.G.; Jiang, L.; Izumo, S.; Alper, S.L. Mannitol at clinical concentrations activated multiple signaling pathways and induces apoptosis in endothelial cells. *Stroke* **1998**, *29*, 2631–2640. [CrossRef]

83. Schwartz, L.; Guais, A.; Pooya, M.; Abolhassani, M. Is inflammation a concequence of extracellular hyperosmolarity? *J. Inflamm.* **2009**, *6*, 21. [CrossRef] [PubMed]
84. Mitchell, N.C.; Gilman, T.L.; Daws, L.C.; Toney, G.M. High salt intake enhances swim stress-induced PVN vasopressin cell activation and active stress coping. *Psychoneuroendocrinology* **2018**, *93*, 29–38. [CrossRef]
85. Sailer, C.O.; Wiedemann, S.J.; Strauss, K.; Schnyder, I.; Fenske, W.K.; Christ-Crain, M. Markers of systemic inflammation in response to osmotic stimuli in healthy volunteers. *Endocr. Connect.* **2019**, *8*, 1282–1287. [CrossRef]
86. Ziegeler, S.; Raddatz, A.; Schneider, S.O.; Sandman, I.; Sasse, H.; Bauer, I.; Kubulus, D.; Mathes, A.; Lausberg, H.F.; Rensing, H. Effect of haemofiltration and mannitol treatment on cardiopulmonary-bypass induced immunosuppression. *Scand. J. Immunol.* **2009**, *69*, 234–241. [CrossRef] [PubMed]
87. Al-Sarraf, H.; Ghaaedi, F.; Redic, Z. Time course of hyperosmolar opening of the blood-brain and blood-CSF barriers in spontaneously hypertensive rats. *J. Vasc. Res.* **2007**, *44*, 99–109. [CrossRef]
88. Huang, K.; Zhou, L.; Alanis, K.; Hou, J.; Baker, L.A. Imaging effect of hyperosmolality on individual tricellular junctions. *Chem. Sci.* **2020**, *11*, 1307–1315. [CrossRef]
89. Burks, S.R.; Kersch, C.N.; Witko, J.A.; Pagel, M.A.; Sundby, M.; Muldoon, L.L.; Neuwelt, E.A.; Frank, J.A. Blood-brain barrier opening by intracarotid artery hyperosmolar mannitol induces sterile inflammatory and innate immune responses. *Proc. Natl. Acad. Sci. USA* **2021**, *118*, e2021915118. [CrossRef] [PubMed]
90. Stonestreet, B.S.; Sadowska, G.B.; Leeman, J.; Hanumara, R.C.; Petersson, K.H.; Patlak, C.S. Effects of acute hyperosmolality on blood-brain barrier function in ovine foetuses and lambs. *Am. J. Physiol. Regul. Integr. Comp. Physiol.* **2006**, *291*, R1031–R1039. [CrossRef]
91. Joshi, S.; Ellis, J.A.; Ornstein, E.; Bruce, J.N. Intraarterial drug delivery for glioblastoma multiforme: Will the phoenix rise again? *J. Neurooncol.* **2015**, *124*, 333–343. [CrossRef]
92. Fortin, D.; Desjardins, A.; Benko, A.; Niyonsega, T.; Boudrias, M. Enhanced chemotherapy delivery by intraarterial infusion and blood-brain barrier disruption in malignant brain tumors: The Sherbrooke experience. *Cancer* **2005**, *103*, 2606–2615. [CrossRef]
93. Marchi, N.; Betto, G.; Fazio, V.; Fan, Q.; Ghosh, C.; Machado, A.; Janigro, D. Blood-brain barrier damage and brain penetration of antiepileptic drugs: Role of serum proteins and brain edema. *Epilepsia* **2009**, *50*, 664–677. [CrossRef] [PubMed]
94. Godinho, B.M.D.C.; Henninger, N.; Bouley, J.; Alterman, J.F.; Haraszti, R.A.; Gilbert, J.W.; Sapp, E.; Coles, A.H.; Biscans, A.; Nikan, M.; et al. Transvascular delivery of hydrophobically modified siRNAs: Gene silencing in the rat brain upon disruption of the blood-brain barrier. *Mol. Ther.* **2018**, *26*, 2580–2591. [CrossRef] [PubMed]
95. Liu, A.H.; Chen, N.Y.; Tu, P.H.; Wu, C.T.; Chiu, S.C.; Huang, Y.C.; Lim, S.N.; Yip, P.K. DHA attenuates cerebral edema following traumatic brain injury via the reduction in blood-brain barrier permeability. *Int. J. Mol. Sci.* **2020**, *21*, 6291. [CrossRef] [PubMed]

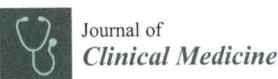

Article

Performance of Modified Early Warning Score (MEWS) for Predicting In-Hospital Mortality in Traumatic Brain Injury Patients

Dong-Ki Kim, Dong-Hun Lee *, Byung-Kook Lee, Yong-Soo Cho, Seok-Jin Ryu, Yong-Hun Jung, Ji-Ho Lee and Jun-Ho Han

Department of Emergency Medicine, Chonnam National University Medical School, 160 Baekseo-ro, Dong-gu, Gwangju 61469, Korea; lifelorddg@naver.com (D.-K.K.); bbukkuk@hanmail.net (B.-K.L.); semi-moon@hanmail.net (Y.-S.C.); samahalak@naver.com (S.-J.R.); xnxn77@hanmail.net (Y.-H.J.); rake21c@naver.com (J.-H.L.); ckris12345@naver.com (J.-H.H.)
* Correspondence: ggodhkekf@hanmail.com; Tel.: +82-62-220-6809

Abstract: The present study aimed to analyze and compare the prognostic performances of the Revised Trauma Score (RTS), Injury Severity Score (ISS), Shock Index (SI), and Modified Early Warning Score (MEWS) for in-hospital mortality in patients with traumatic brain injury (TBI). This retrospective observational study included severe trauma patients with TBI who visited the emergency department between January 2018 and December 2020. TBI was considered when the Abbreviated Injury Scale was 3 or higher. The primary outcome was in-hospital mortality. In total, 1108 patients were included, and the in-hospital mortality was 183 patients (16.3% of the cohort). Receiver operating characteristic curve analyses were performed for the ISS, RTS, SI, and MEWS with respect to the prediction of in-hospital mortality. The area under the curves (AUCs) of the ISS, RTS, SI, and MEWS were 0.638 (95% confidence interval (CI), 0.603–0.672), 0.742 (95% CI, 0.709–0.772), 0.524 (95% CI, 0.489–0.560), and 0.799 (95% CI, 0.769–0.827), respectively. The AUC of MEWS was significantly different from the AUCs of ISS, RTS, and SI. In multivariate analysis, age (odds ratio (OR), 1.012; 95% CI, 1.000–1.023), the ISS (OR, 1.040; 95% CI, 1.013–1.069), the Glasgow Coma Scale (GCS) score (OR, 0.793; 95% CI, 0.761–0.826), and body temperature (BT) (OR, 0.465; 95% CI, 0.329–0.655) were independently associated with in-hospital mortality after adjustment for confounders. In the present study, the MEWS showed fair performance for predicting in-hospital mortality in patients with TBI. The GCS score and BT seemed to have a significant role in the discrimination ability of the MEWS. The MEWS may be a useful tool for predicting in-hospital mortality in patients with TBI.

Keywords: traumatic brain injury; scoring system; modified early warning score; mortality

Citation: Kim, D.-K.; Lee, D.-H.; Lee, B.-K.; Cho, Y.-S.; Ryu, S.-J.; Jung, Y.-H.; Lee, J.-H.; Han, J.-H. Performance of Modified Early Warning Score (MEWS) for Predicting In-Hospital Mortality in Traumatic Brain Injury Patients. *J. Clin. Med.* **2021**, *10*, 1915. https://doi.org/10.3390/jcm10091915

Academic Editor: Rafael Badenes

Received: 23 March 2021
Accepted: 22 April 2021
Published: 28 April 2021

Publisher's Note: MDPI stays neutral with regard to jurisdictional claims in published maps and institutional affiliations.

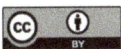

Copyright: © 2021 by the authors. Licensee MDPI, Basel, Switzerland. This article is an open access article distributed under the terms and conditions of the Creative Commons Attribution (CC BY) license (https:// creativecommons.org/licenses/by/ 4.0/).

1. Introduction

Trauma is the leading cause of death in people aged below 46 years [1]. Although the mortality of trauma patients has declined over the last decades, the cause of trauma-related death has gradually shifted from multiple organ dysfunction syndrome to central nervous injury [2]. Therefore, it is important to identify risk factors early and provide intensive care for patients with traumatic brain injury (TBI).

Several triage tools for TBI have been developed, and studies have reported the efficacies of these tools for predicting prognosis [3–8]. Among these, the Injury Severity Score (ISS) and Revised Trauma Score (RTS) are the most commonly used tools in severe trauma patients, including those with TBI [3,4]. However, the relationship between these tools and the prognosis of patients with TBI is not well understood, and some studies have even questioned these relationships [9–11]. The Shock Index (SI), the ratio of heart rate to systolic blood pressure (SBP), was related to hypovolemic shock in patients with severe trauma, including TBI [5,6], and may be related to the mortality of patients with TBI [7]. In addition, previous studies have reported that early warning scores, such as the Modified Early Warning Score (MEWS), are related to adverse events, including hypotension and the need for advanced airway management, need for intensive care, and early mortality in patients with TBI [8]. However, few studies have shown the association between various triage tools and outcomes in patients with TBI.

Therefore, this study aimed to analyze and compare the prognostic performances of the RTS, ISS, SI, and MEWS for in-hospital mortality in patients with TBI. We also investigated the risk factors associated with in-hospital mortality in patients with TBI.

2. Materials and Methods

2.1. Study Design and Population

We performed a retrospective observational study involving patients with TBI at Chonnam National University Hospital, Gwangju, South Korea, who were admitted between January 2018 and December 2020. Severe trauma was defined as an ISS greater than 15 [12]. TBI was considered when the head Abbreviated Injury Scale (AIS) score was 3 or higher [13]. Isolated TBI was defined as a head AIS score of ≥3 and any other AIS score of <3 [14]. Combined TBI was defined as a head AIS score of ≥3 and at least one other AIS score of ≥3 [14]. The following exclusion criteria were applied: age below 18 years; cardiac arrest following trauma before arrival at the emergency department (ED); specific trauma mechanisms, such as drowning, burns, or hanging; and missing data. This study was approved by the institutional review board of Chonnam National University Hospital (CNUH-2021-064).

Vital sign and Glasgow Coma Scale (GCS) scores were measured by triage nurses who have received in-hospital education and training in the triage room at ED visits. All the triage nurses have been working in the ED for at least 2 years before performing triage. The AIS and ISS scores were calculated by physicians who have received training in Korean Trauma Assessment and Treatment (KTAT).

2.2. Data Collection

Data on the following variables were obtained for each patient: age, sex, mechanism of trauma, SBP (mmHg) on admission, respiratory rate on admission, pulse rate on admission, body temperature (BT, °C) on admission, initial Glasgow Coma Scale (GCS) score, amount of transfused packed red blood cells (PRC), fresh frozen plasma (FFP), and platelet concentrates (PC) within 24 h after arrival at the ED, and in-hospital mortality.

The RTS was calculated based on vital signs and the GCS score (Table 1) [15]. The SI was calculated as the heart rate divided by SBP [5]. The AIS score and ISS were calculated on ED arrival. The MEWS was calculated based on vital signs and AVPU (Alert, Voice, Pain, Unresponsive) scale data on ED arrival (Table 2) [16]. The primary outcome was in-hospital mortality.

Table 1. Revised Trauma Score.

The Revised Trauma Score (RTS)			
Glasgow Coma Scale (GCS)	Systolic Blood Pressure (SBP)	Respiratory Rate (RR)	Coded Value
13–15	>89	10–29	4
9–12	76–89	>29	3
6–8	50–75	6–9	2
4–5	1–49	1–5	1
3	0	0	0

RTS = 0.9368 (GCSc) + 0.7326 (SBPc) + 0.2908 (RRc).

Table 2. Modified Early Warning Score.

	Modified Early Warning Score (MEWS)			
Score	0	1	2	3
Respiratory rate (min^{-1})	9–14	15–20	21–29 ≤ 8	≥ 30
Hear rate (min^{-1})	51–100	101–110 41–50	111–129 ≤ 40	≥ 130
Systolic BP (mmHg)	101–199	81–100	≥ 200 71–80	≤ 70
Temperature (°C)	35.1–38.4		≥ 38.5 ≤ 35	
Neurological	Alert	Responding to Voice	Responding to Pain	Unresponsive

The total score is the sum of each component.

2.3. Statistical Analysis

Continuous variables did not satisfy the normality test and are presented as median values with interquartile ranges (IQR). Categorical variables are presented as frequencies and percentages. Differences between survivors and non-survivors were tested using the Mann-Whitney *U*-test for continuous variables. Fisher's exact test or the chi-square test was used for the comparison of categorical variables, as appropriate. Receiver operating characteristic (ROC) curve analysis was performed to examine the prognostic performances of the ISS, RTS, SI, and MEWS for in-hospital mortality. The comparison of dependent ROC curves was performed using the DeLong method [17].

We conducted multivariate analysis using logistic regression of relevant covariates for in-hospital mortality. Variables with p values of <0.20 in univariate comparisons were included in the multivariate regression model. We used a backward stepwise approach, sequentially eliminating variables with a threshold p value of >0.10 to build the final adjusted regression model. We included one of the prognostic tools (MEWS, RTS, ISS, and SI) into the final model and performed the analysis separately in each group (all TBI, isolated TBI, and combined TBI groups). The results of logistic regression analysis are presented as odds ratios (ORs) and 95% confidence intervals (CIs). All analyses were performed using PASW/SPSS™ software, version 18 (IBM Inc., Chicago, IL, USA) and MedCalc version 19.0 (MedCalc Software, bvba, Ostend, Belgium). A two-sided significance level of 0.05 was used to indicate statistical significance.

3. Results

3.1. Patient Selection and Characteristics

In total, 1190 severe trauma patients were identified during the study period who met the inclusion criteria. Based on the exclusion criteria, 1108 patients were finally included in this study (Figure 1). There were 822 (74.2%) male patients, and the median age was 64.1 years (53.0–75.0 years). The in-hospital mortality rate was 16.5% ($n = 183$).

3.2. Comparison of Baseline and Clinical Characteristics between Survivors and Non-Survivors

Table 3 shows the comparison of baseline and clinical characteristics between survivors and non-survivors. Survivors had higher RTS, GCS score, and BT values and lower ISS, pulse rate, and SI values. SBP was not significantly different between survivors and non-survivors. The proportion of patients with hypothermia among non-survivors was higher than that among survivors. The MEWS (2 (1–3) vs. 5 (4–6); $p < 0.001$) was significantly lower in survivors than in non-survivors.

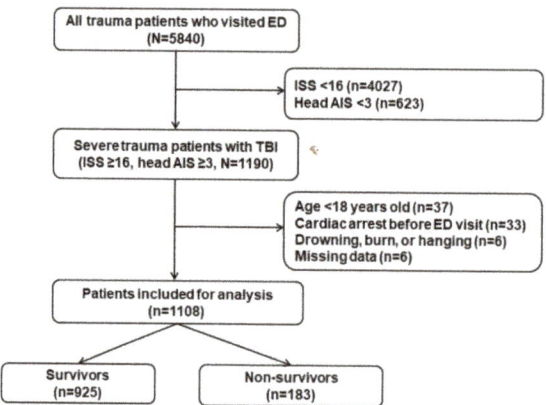

Figure 1. Schematic diagram showing the number of patients with TBI in the present study. TBI, traumatic brain injury; ISS, Injury Severity Score; AIS, Abbreviated Injury Scale.

Table 3. Comparison of baseline characteristics of TBI patients according to in-hospital mortality.

Variables	TBI Patients (N = 1108)	Survivors (N = 925)	Non-Survivors (N = 183)	p Value
Age, years, IQR	64.1 (53.0–75.0)	64.0 (53.0–75.0)	67.0 (53.0–76.1)	0.199
Male, n (%)	822 (74.2)	683 (73.8)	139 (76.0)	0.550
Mechanism of trauma				0.416
Blunt, n (%)	1,103 (99.5)	922 (99.7)	181 (98.9)	
Penetrating, n (%)	5 (0.5)	3 (0.3)	2 (1.1)	
Revised Trauma Score, IQR	5.97 (5.03–7.84)	5.97 (5.64–7.84)	4.09 (2.83–5.64)	<0.001
Injury Severity Score, IQR	22 (16–25)	21 (16–25)	25 (20–29)	<0.001
Glasgow Coma Scale, IQR	14 (7–15)	15 (10–15)	4 (3–9)	<0.001
Systolic BP, mmHg, IQR	130 (110–140)	130 (110–140)	120 (90–160)	0.050
Respiratory rate, /min, IQR	20 (20–20)	20 (20–20)	20 (20–22)	0.022
Pulse rate, /min, IQR	84 (74–96)	84 (74–94)	90 (72–104)	0.006
BT, °C, IQR	36.4 (36.1–36.7)	36.4 (36.2–36.8)	36.2 (36.0–36.5)	<0.001
BT ≤35 °C, n (%)	44 (4.0)	17 (1.8)	27 (14.8)	<0.001
PRC, unit	0 (0–2)	0 (0–1)	6 (5–12)	<0.001
FFP, unit	0 (0–2)	0 (0–0)	4 (2–8)	<0.001
PC, unit	0 (0–0)	0 (0–0)	6 (0–10)	<0.001
Shock Index	0.65 (0.54–0.82)	0.65 (0.54–0.80)	0.69 (0.54–1.13)	0.002
MEWS	2 (1–4)	2 (1–3)	5 (4–6)	<0.001

TBI, traumatic brain injury; IQR, interquartile range; BP, blood pressure; BT, body temperature; PRC, packed red blood cell; FFP, fresh frozen plasma; PC, platelet concentrates; MEWS, Modified Early Warning Score.

In the isolated TBI group, survivors had higher RTS, GCS score, and BT values and lower ISS and PR values than non-survivors. The MEWS (2 (1–3) vs. 4 (3–6); $p < 0.001$) was significantly lower in survivors than in non-survivors (Table 4).

In the combined TBI group, survivors had higher RTS, GCS score, SBP, and BT values and lower ISS and SI values than non-survivors. The MEWS (2 (1–4) vs. 6 (5–7); $p < 0.001$) was significantly lower in survivors than in non-survivors (Table 4).

Table 4. Comparison of baseline characteristics according to in-hospital mortality in isolated TBI and combined TBI groups.

Variables	Isolated TBI (N = 845)			Combined TBI (N = 263)		
	Survivors (N = 720)	Non-Survivors (N = 125)	p Value	Survivors (N = 205)	Non-Survivors (N = 58)	p Value
Age, years, IQR	65 (54–75)	67 (53–78)	0.366	60 (50–71)	65 (53–74)	0.104
Male, n (%)	533 (74.0)	93 (74.4)	1.000	150 (73.2)	46 (79.3)	0.437
Mechanism of trauma			0.927			0.920
Blunt, n (%)	718 (99.7)	124 (99.2)		204 (99.5)	57 (98.3)	
Penetrating, n (%)	2 (0.3)	1 (0.8)		1 (0.5)	1 (1.7)	
ISS, IQR	17 (16–25)	25 (16–25)	<0.001	25 (22–29)	31 (25–38)	<0.001
RTS, IQR	5.97 (5.64–7.84)	4.09 (2.83–5.97)	<0.001	6.38 (5.64–7.84)	4.09 (2.83–5.23)	<0.001
GCS, IQR	14 (9–15)	4 (3–10)	<0.001	15 (10–15)	4 (3–8)	<0.001
SBP, mmHg, IQR	130 (110–150)	140 (100–160)	0.224	110 (100–130)	90 (70–110)	<0.001
RR, /min, IQR	20 (20–20)	20 (20–22)	0.199	20 (20–22)	20 (20–24)	0.086
PR, /min, IQR	82 (72–92)	87 (71–103)	0.046	90 (79–104)	96 (76–110)	0.237
BT, °C, IQR	36.4 (36.2–36.8)	36.2 (36.0–36.5)	<0.001	36.4 (36.1–36.8)	36.2 (36.0–36.4)	<0.001
PRC, unit	0 (0–0)	1 (0–4)	<0.001	2 (0–4)	4 (2–10)	<0.001
FFP, unit	0 (0–0)	0 (0–2)	<0.001	0 (0–2)	3 (0–8)	<0.001
PC, unit	0 (0–0)	0 (0–0)	<0.001	0 (0–0)	0 (0–0)	<0.001
SI, IQR	0.62 (0.53–0.74)	0.63 (0.49–0.87)	0.726	0.81 (0.64–1.00)	1.09 (0.73–1.38)	<0.001
MEWS, IQR	2 (1–3)	4 (3–6)	<0.001	2 (1–4)	6 (5–7)	<0.001

TBI, traumatic brain injury; IQR, interquartile range; ISS, Injury Severity Score; RTS, Revised Trauma Score; GCS, Glasgow Coma Scale; SBP, systolic blood pressure; RR, respiratory rate; PR, pulse rate; BT, body temperature; PRC, packed red blood cell; FFP, fresh frozen plasma; PC, platelet concentrates; SI, Shock Index; MEWS, Modified Early Warning Score.

3.3. Prognostic Performance of the ISS, RTS, SI, and MEWS for in-Hospital Mortality

The areas under the curve (AUCs) of the ISS, RTS, SI, and MEWS for predicting in-hospital mortality were 0.638 (95% CI, 0.603–0.672), 0.742 (95% CI, 0.709–0.772), 0.524 (95% CI, 0.489–0.560), and 0.799 (95% CI, 0.769–0.827), respectively (Figure 2A).

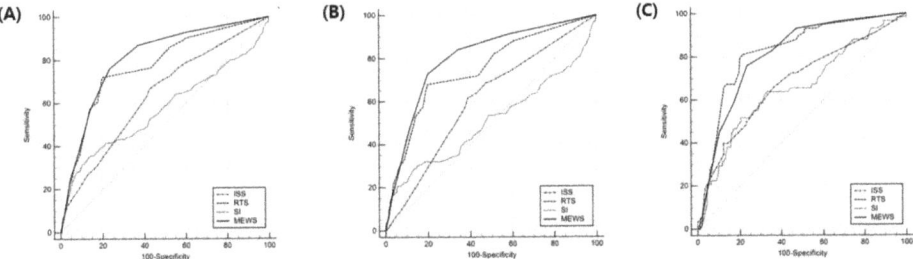

Figure 2. Receiver operating characteristic curve analyses of the ISS, RTS, SI, and MEWS for predicting in-hospital mortality. (**A**) Total TBI group: the AUCs of the ISS, RTS, SI, and MEWS were 0.638 (95% CI, 0.603–0.672), 0.742 (95% CI, 0.709–0.772), 0.524 (95% CI, 0.489–0.560), and 0.799 (95% CI, 0.769–0.827), respectively. (**B**) Isolated TBI group: the AUCs of the ISS, RTS, SI, and MEWS were 0.608 (95% CI, 0.574–0.641), 0.750 (95% CI, 0.719–0.778), 0.510 (95% CI, 0.476–0.544), and 0.803 (95% CI, 0.774–0.829), respectively. (**C**) Combined TBI group: the AUCs of the ISS, RTS, SI, and MEWS were 0.679 (95% CI, 0.619–0.735), 0.824 (95% CI, 0.773–0.868), 0.657 (95% CI, 0.597–0.715), and 0.809 (95% CI, 0.757–0.855), respectively. ISS, Injury Severity Score; RTS, Revised Trauma Score; SI, Shock Index; MEWS, Modified Early Warning Score; TBI, traumatic brain injury; AUC, area under curve; CI, confidence interval

The AUC of the MEWS was significantly different from the AUCs of the ISS, RTS, and SI (Table 5).

In the isolated TBI group, the AUCs of the ISS, RTS, SI, and MEWS for predicting in-hospital mortality were 0.608 (95% CI, 0.574–0.641), 0.750 (95% CI, 0.719–0.778), 0.510 (95%

CI, 0.476–0.544), and 0.803 (95% CI, 0.774–0.829), respectively (Figure 2B). The AUC of the MEWS in the isolated TBI group was significantly different from the AUCs of the ISS, RTS, and SI (Table 5).

In the combined TBI group, the AUCs of the ISS, RTS, SI, and MEWS for predicting in-hospital mortality were 0.679 (95% CI, 0.619–0.735), 0.824 (95% CI, 0.773–0.868), 0.657 (95% CI, 0.597–0.715), and 0.809 (95% CI, 0.757–0.855), respectively (Figure 2C). The AUC of the MEWS in the combined TBI group was significantly different from the AUCs of the ISS and SI but not from the AUC of the RTS (Table 5).

Table 5. Pairwise comparison test of the ROC curves including MEWS, RTS, ISS, and SI for in-hospital mortality in TBI patients.

	Difference between Areas	SE	95% CI	p Value
All TBI group				
MEWS vs. RTS	0.0575	0.0218	0.0147 to 0.100	0.0085
MEWS vs. ISS	0.161	0.0297	0.103 to 0.219	<0.0001
MEWS vs. SI	0.275	0.0311	0.214 to 0.336	<0.0001
RTS vs. ISS	0.104	0.0341	0.0368 to 0.170	0.0024
RTS vs. SI	0.217	0.0386	0.142 to 0.293	<0.0001
ISS vs. SI	0.114	0.0403	0.0347 to 0.193	0.0048
Isolated TBI group				
MEWS vs. RTS	0.0532	0.0217	0.0106 to 0.0958	0.0144
MEWS vs. ISS	0.195	0.0301	0.136 to 0.254	<0.0001
MEWS vs. SI	0.293	0.0324	0.229 to 0.356	<0.0001
RTS vs. ISS	0.142	0.0332	0.0770 to 0.207	<0.0001
RTS vs. SI	0.240	0.0390	0.163 to 0.316	<0.0001
ISS vs. SI	0.0976	0.0444	0.0107 to 0.185	0.0278
Combined TBI group				
MEWS vs. RTS	0.0147	0.0277	−0.0397 to 0.0691	0.5957
MEWS vs. ISS	0.130	0.0433	0.0453 to 0.215	0.0026
MEWS vs. SI	0.152	0.0350	0.0834 to 0.221	<0.0001
RTS vs. ISS	0.145	0.0445	0.0575 to 0.232	0.0011
RTS vs. SI	0.167	0.0479	0.0728 to 0.261	0.0005
ISS vs. SI	0.0220	0.0591	−0.0939 to 0.138	0.7104

MEWS, Modified Early Warning Score; RTS, Revised Trauma Score; ISS, Injury Severity Score; SI, Shock Index; ROC, receiver operator characteristic; SE, standard error; CI, confidence interval.

3.4. Multivariate Logistic Regression Analysis for in-Hospital Mortality

Table 6 shows the results of the multivariate analysis performed for in-hospital mortality. In all TBI group, age (OR, 1.013; 95% CI, 1.001–1.025), low GCS score (OR, 0.86; 95% CI, 0.54–0.820), low BT (OR, 0.537; 95% CI, 0.382–0.753), FFP (OR, 1.216; 95% CI, 1.129–1.310), and PC (OR, 1.018; 95% CI, 1.000–1.037) were independently associated with in-hospital mortality. In the isolated TBI group, low GCS score (OR, 0.792; 95% CI, 0.754–0.831), low BT (OR, 0.574; 95% CI, 0.398–0.830), FFP (OR, 1.226; 95% CI, 1.100–1.367), and PC (OR, 1.026; 95% CI, 1.002–1.049) were independently associated with in-hospital mortality (Table 6); while in the combined TBI group, age (OR, 1.033; 95% CI, 1.007–1.060), low GCS score (OR, 0.759; 95% CI, 0.698–0.824), low BT (OR, 0.424; 95% CI, 0.186–0.965), and PRC (OR, 1.153; 95% CI, 1.061–1.254) were independently associated with in-hospital mortality (Table 6).

Among the prognostic tools assessed, MEWS and RTS were associated with in-hospital mortality in all TBI, isolated TBI, and combined TBI groups, after adjusting for confounders (Table 7). ISS and SI were not associated with in-hospital mortality in all TBI, isolated TBI, and combined TBI groups.

Table 6. Multivariate logistic regression analysis for predicting in-hospital mortality in TBI patients.

	All TBI Group		Isolated TBI Group		Combined TBI Group	
	Adjusted OR (95% CI)	p Value	Adjusted OR (95% CI)	p Value	Adjusted OR (95% CI)	p Value
Age, years	1.013(1.001-1.025)	0.036			1.033 (1.007–1.060)	0.014
GCS score	0.786 (0.754–0.820)	<0.001	0.792 (0.754–0.831)	<0.001	0.759 (0.698–0.824)	<0.001
SBP, mmHg	1.002 (0.997–1.008)	0.428			1.003 (0.992–1.013)	0.616
RR, /min	1.038 (0.966–1.115)	0.315	1.020 (0.931–1.119)	0.670	1.086 (0.965–1.221)	0.173
PR, /min	1.006 (0.997–1.015)	0.203	1.006 (0.995–1.017)	0.324		
BT, °C	0.537 (0.382–0.753)	<0.001	0.574 (0.398–0.830)	0.003	0.424 (0.186–0.965)	0.041
PRC, unit	0.988 (0.897–1.087)	0.802	0.922 (0.814–1.043)	0.196	1.153 (1.061–1.254)	0.001
FFP, unit	1.216 (1.129–1.310)	<0.001	1.226 (1.100–1.367)	<0.001	1.047 (0.853–1.285)	0.661
PC, unit	1.018 (1.000–1.037)	0.048	1.026 (1.002–1.049)	0.030	1.002 (0.969–1.036)	0.914

TBI, traumatic brain injury; OR, odds ratio; CI, confidence interval; GCS, Glasgow Coma Scale; SBP, systolic blood pressure; RR, respiratory rate; PR, pulse rate; BT, body temperature; PRC packed red blood cell; FFP fresh frozen plasma; PC, platelet concentrates.

Table 7. Multivariate logistic regression analysis of MEWS, RTS, ISS, and SI for predicting in-hospital mortality in TBI [1] patients.

	All TBI Group		Isolated TBI Group		Combined TBI Group	
	Adjusted OR (95% CI)	p Value	Adjusted OR (95% CI)	p Value	Adjusted OR (95% CI)	p Value
MEWS	1.605 (1.470–1.753) [1]	<0.001	1.695 (1.519–1.891) [4]	<0.001	1.515 (1.302–1.762) [7]	<0.001
RTS	0.594 (0.534–0.659) [2]	<0.001	0.614 (0.544–0.693) [5]	<0.001	0.513 (0.408–0.644) [8]	<0.001
ISS	1.014 (0.984–1.045) [3]	0.357	1.015 (0.967–1.067) [6]	0.543	1.013 (0.964–1.065) [9]	0.605
SI	1.385 (0.840–2.282) [3]	0.202	1.479 (0.769–2.843) [6]	0.241	1.143 (0.469–2.787) [9]	0.769

Each prognostic tool was individually entered into the final model and analyzed separately. Each prognostic tool was not adjusted for other tools. TBI, traumatic brain injury; OR, odds ratio; CI, confidence interval; MEWS, Modified Early Warning Score; RTS, Revised Trauma Score; ISS, Injury Severity Score; SI, Shock Index; PRC packed red blood cell; FFP fresh frozen plasma; PC, platelet concentrates; GCS, Glasgow Coma Scale; BT, body temperature. [1] Adjusted for age, FFP, and PC. [2] Adjusted for age, BT, FFP, and PC. [3] Adjusted for age, GCS, BT, FFP, and PC. [4] Adjusted for FFP, and PC. [5] Adjusted for BT, FFP, and PC. [6] Adjusted for GCS, BT, FFP, and PC. [7] Adjusted for age and PRC. [8] Adjusted for age, BT, and PRC. [9] Adjusted for age, GCS, BT, and PRC.

4. Discussion

In the present study, the MEWS showed fair performance for predicting in-hospital mortality in patients with TBI. The GCS score and BT were associated with in-hospital mortality in all groups, including the total TBI, isolated TBI, and combined TBI groups.

The SI (the ratio of heart rate to SBP) showed poor performance for predicting in-hospital mortality in the present study. It was assumed that in all groups, SBP and heart rate had no relationship with the mortality of patients with TBI. McMahon et al. showed that the SI responded later to hemorrhage in the TBI group compared to the non-TBI group, and responded later in non-survivors compared to survivors [18]. Moreover, factors such as medication for hypertension and beta blockers can modulate SI at the compensation stage of the shock. The ISS was not associated with in-hospital mortality in all TBI, isolated TBI, and combined TBI groups. An important disadvantage of the ISS is that only one injury is considered in each body part. Since TBI patients with head AIS score of ≥ 3 were included in the present study, other injuries could have been overlooked. In contrast, previous studies have reported the association of ISS with mortality in TBI patients [19,20]. Thus, further research may be needed to clarify the relationship between ISS and prognosis of TBI. In this study, the RTS and MEWS were related to the mortality of patients with TBI. A previous study revealed that the RTS was related to the mortality of patients with TBI [20], and the MEWS was also likely to be related to the outcomes of patients with TBI in other studies [8,21]. As both the RTS and MEWS include the GCS score, which was associated with the prognosis of TBI, they were expected to show good performance for predicting mortality. However, the MEWS showed better performance than the RTS in the total TBI and isolated TBI groups in the present study. In our study, BT was associated with mortality in all groups. As the MEWS includes BT, which is not included in the RTS, the MEWS would be more accurate in predicting mortality than the RTS. In addition, since RTS includes GCS, there may be difficulties in measuring RTS when compared to measurements of MEWS, including AVPU. In particular, it is challenging to measure GCS-motor or GCS-verbal of intubated patients.

Several studies have demonstrated that the GCS score was related to the mortality of patients with TBI [3,22]. In a study by Han et al., a GCS score of ≤5 was associated with mortality in most groups, and the GCS score of non-survivors was 4 (3–9) in this study [22]. In another study on patients with TBI, the OR of the GCS score for mortality was 0.765, similar to that obtained in the present study [3], in which the GCS score of non-survivors corresponded to the unresponsiveness parameter in the AVPU scale [23]. Thus, it corresponded to 3 points in the MEWS and was believed to have played an important role in the performance of the MEWS [16].

Previous studies have revealed that a low BT was associated with mortality in patients with TBI [24–26]. In patients with severe trauma, including patients with TBI, bleeding caused hypovolemia, which can lead to lower BT; this accelerates coagulation disorders and eventually affects prognosis [27]. In contrast, low BT at the time of ED visit was related to mortality, even though the major injury was limited to a head injury, such as isolated TBI, in the present study. In other studies on isolated TBI, low BT at admission was associated with mortality [28,29]. This can be explained by the fact that a low BT at admission in patients with TBI reflects severe head injury. De Tanti et al. speculated that hypothalamic dysfunction due to brain injury may contribute to mortality in patients with severe TBI [30].

In the present study, the SBP of patients with isolated TBI was not associated with in-hospital mortality. A previous study also showed that SBP may be insufficient to predict the mortality of patients with TBI [31]. This could be attributed to the effect of cerebral autoregulation in patients with TBI with elevated intracranial pressure (ICP). Cerebral autoregulation is a homeostatic process that regulates and maintains cerebral blood flow across a range of blood pressures [32]. Thus, the elevation of ICP increases arterial blood pressure to maintain the perfusion pressure to the brain [33]. In contrast, SBP was associated with in-hospital mortality in the combined TBI group in the present study. The reason for this may be the difference in SBP between the combined TBI (110 (90–130) mmHg) and isolated TBI (130 (110–150) mmHg) groups. The combined TBI included bleeding from other body regions, such as the head, as well as head injury; thus, SBP would be lower in the combined TBI group than in the isolated TBI group. In a study of patients with TBI, including those with combined TBI, mortality increased when the SBP dropped from 110 to 100 mmHg [34].

This study had several limitations. First, it was a retrospective study that was performed at a single center. Therefore, its findings are not immediately generalizable to the overall population. Further multi-center studies with larger sample sizes and prospective designs are needed to substantiate our findings. Second, we did not analyze the effects of essential procedures (such as interventions, operations, and transfusions) on in-hospital mortality. Further research is needed to address these effects. Third, the measurements for vital signs and GCS scores may be inconsistent and vary from person-to-person. Although triage nurses have been constantly educated and trained, the results may be affected by individual medical experience. Fourth, we did not specifically record the site of temperature measurement as BT can vary depending on the region of the body. Thus, this may be considered as a confounder to our data analyses. Fifth, we did not consider the natural circadian rhythm of body temperature, although these effects would be limited during acute illnesses, such as TBI [35]. Sixth, the patient's clinical condition, such as the effects of comorbidities and drugs, was not investigated. Since such conditions can affect the patient's prognosis, these factors should be included in future research. Finally, we did not investigate the cause of death in patients with TBI. The most common causes of trauma-related death are central nervous injury and blood loss, and we did not compare and analyze the relationship between these causes and the various prediction tools, including the MEWS.

5. Conclusions

In the present study, the MEWS showed fair performance for predicting in-hospital mortality in patients with TBI. The GCS score and BT seemed to have a significant role in the discrimination ability of the MEWS. Therefore, the MEWS may be a useful tool for predicting in-hospital mortality in patients with TBI.

Author Contributions: Conceptualization, D.-K.K. and D.-H.L.; methodology, D.-K.K. and D.-H.L.; software, B.-K.L.; validation, Y.-S.C., S.-J.R., J.-H.L., and J.-H.H.; formal analysis, D.-K.K. and D.-H.L.; investigation, Y.-S.C., S.-J.R., and Y.-H.J.; data curation, D.-K.K., D.-H.L., and B.-K.L.; writing—original draft preparation, D.-K.K. and D.-H.L.; writing—review and editing, B.-K.L., Y.-S.C., S.-J.R., Y.-H.J., J.-H.L., and J.-H.H.; visualization, Y.-H.J.; supervision, B.-K.L.; project administration, D.-H.L. All authors have read and agreed to the published version of the manuscript.

Funding: This research received no external funding.

Institutional Review Board Statement: The study was conducted according to the guidelines of the Declaration of Helsinki, and approved by institutional review board of Chonnam National University Hospital (CNUH-2021-064).

Informed Consent Statement: Not applicable.

Data Availability Statement: The data presented in this study are available on request from the corresponding author. The data are not publicly available due to personal protection.

Conflicts of Interest: The authors have no conflicts of interest.

References

1. Rhee, P.; Joseph, B.; Pandit, V.; Aziz, H.; Vercruysse, G.; Kulvatunyou, N.; Friese, R.S. Increasing Trauma Deaths in the United States. *Ann. Surg.* **2014**, *260*, 13–21. [CrossRef]
2. van Breugel, J.M.M.; Menco, J.S.; Roderick, M.; Rolf, H.H.; Luke, P.H.; Karlijn, J.P. Global changes in mortality rates in polytrauma patients admitted to the ICU: A systematic review. *World J. Emerg. Surg.* **2020**, *15*, 55. [CrossRef]
3. Powers, A.Y.; Pinto, M.B.; Tang, O.Y.; Chen, J.-S.; Doberstein, C.; Asaad, W.F. Predicting mortality in traumatic intracranial hemorrhage. *J. Neurosurg.* **2020**, *132*, 552–559. [CrossRef]
4. Mahadewa, T.G.B.; Golden, N.; Saputra, A.; Ryalino, C. Modified Revised Trauma-Marshall score as a proposed tool in predicting the outcome of moderate and severe traumatic brain injury. *Open Access Emerg. Med.* **2018**, *10*, 135–139. [CrossRef]
5. Zhu, C.S.; Cobb, D.; Jonas, R.B.; Pokorny, D.; Rani, M.; Cotner-Pouncy, T.; Oliver, J.; Cap, A.; Cestero, R.; Nicholson, S.E.; et al. Shock index and pulse pressure as triggers for massive transfusion. *J. Trauma Acute Care Surg.* **2019**, *87*, S159–S164. [CrossRef]
6. Fröhlich, M.; Driessen, A.; Böhmer, A.; Nienaber, U.; Igressa, A.; Probst, C.; Bouillon, B.; Maegele, M.; Mutschler, M.; the TraumaRegister DGU. Is the shock index based classification of hypovolemic shock applicable in multiple injured patients with severe traumatic brain injury? An analysis of the TraumaRegister DGU®. *Scand. J. Trauma Resusc. Emerg. Med.* **2016**, *24*, 148. [CrossRef]
7. Wan-Ting, C.; Chin-Hsien, L.; Cheng-Yu, L.; Cheng-Yu, C.; Chi-Chun, L.; Keng-Wei, C.; Jiann-Hwa, C.; Wei-Lung, C.; Chien-Cheng, H.; Cherng-Jyr, L.; et al. Reverse shock index multiplied by Glasgow Coma Scale (rSIG) predicts mortality in severe trauma patients with head injury. *Sci. Rep.* **2020**, *10*, 1–7. [CrossRef]
8. Martín-Rodríguez, F.; López-Izquierdo, R.; Mohedano-Moriano, A.; Polonio-López, B.; Miquel, C.M.; Viñuela, A.; Fernández, C.D.; Correas, J.G.; Marques, G.; Martín-Conty, J.L. Identification of Serious Adverse Events in Patients with Traumatic Brain Injuries, from Prehospital Care to Intensive-Care Unit, Using Early Warning Scores. *Int. J. Environ. Res. Public Health* **2020**, *17*, 1504. [CrossRef]
9. Susman, M.; DiRusso, S.M.; Sullivan, T.; Risucci, D.; Nealon, P.; Cuff, S.; Haider, A.; Benzil, D. Traumatic Brain Injury in the Elderly: Increased Mortality and Worse Functional Outcome At Discharge Despite Lower Injury Severity. *J. Trauma Inj. Infect. Crit. Care* **2002**, *53*, 219–224. [CrossRef]
10. Zafonte, R.D.; Hammond, F.M.; Mann, N.R.; Wood, D.L.; Millis, S.R.; Black, K.L. Revised trauma score: An additive predictor of disability following traumatic brain injury? *Am. J. Phys. Med. Rehabil.* **1996**, *75*, 456–461. [CrossRef]
11. Kehoe, A.; Smith, J.E.; Bouamra, O.; Edwards, A.; Yates, D.; Lecky, F. Older patients with traumatic brain injury present with a higher GCS score than younger patients for a given severity of injury. *Emerg. Med. J.* **2016**, *33*, 381–385. [CrossRef]
12. Baker, S.P.; O'Neill, B.; Haddon, W.; Long, W.B. The injury severity score: A method for describing patients with multiple injuries and evaluating emergency care. *J. Trauma Inj. Infect. Crit. Care* **1974**, *14*, 187–196. [CrossRef]
13. Mellick, D.; Gerhart, K.A.; Whiteneck, G.G. Understanding outcomes based on the post-acute hospitalization pathways followed by persons with traumatic brain injury. *Brain Inj.* **2003**, *17*, 55–71. [CrossRef] [PubMed]
14. Dübendorfer, C.; Billeter, A.T.; Seifert, B.; Keel, M.; Turina, M. Serial lactate and admission SOFA scores in trauma: An analysis of predictive value in 724 patients with and without traumatic brain injury. *Eur. J. Trauma Emerg. Surg.* **2012**, *39*, 25–34. [CrossRef]

15. Kruisselbrink, R.; Kwizera, A.; Crowther, M.; Fox-Robichaud, A.; O'Shea, T.; Nakibuuka, J.; Ssinabulya, I.; Nalyazi, J.; Bonner, A.; Devji, T.; et al. Modified Early Warning Score (MEWS) Identifies Critical Illness among Ward Patients in a Resource Restricted Setting in Kampala, Uganda: A Prospective Observational Study. *PLoS ONE* **2016**, *11*, e0151408. [CrossRef]
16. Subbe, C.; Kruger, M.; Rutherford, P.; Gemmel, L. Validation of a modified Early Warning Score in medical admissions. *Qjm Int. J. Med.* **2001**, *94*, 521–526. [CrossRef]
17. Delong, E.R.; Delong, D.M.; Clarke-Pearson, D.L. Comparing the Areas under Two or More Correlated Receiver Operating Characteristic Curves: A Nonparametric Approach. *Biometrics* **1988**, *44*, 837. [CrossRef]
18. McMahon, C.G.; Kenny, R.; Bennett, K.; Little, R.; Kirkman, E. The Effect of Acute Traumatic Brain Injury on the Performance of Shock Index. *J. Trauma Inj. Infect. Crit. Care* **2010**, *69*, 1169–1175. [CrossRef]
19. Tucker, B.; Aston, J.; Dines, M.; Caraman, E.; Yacyshyn, M.; McCarthy, M.; Olson, J.E. Early Brain Edema is a Predictor of In-Hospital Mortality in Traumatic Brain Injury. *J. Emerg. Med.* **2017**, *53*, 18–29. [CrossRef]
20. Wagner, A.K.; Hammond, F.M.; Grigsby, J.H.; Norton, H.J. The value of trauma scores: Predicting discharge after traumatic brain injury. *Am. J. Phys. Med. Rehabil.* **2000**, *79*, 235–242. [CrossRef]
21. Najafi, Z.; Zakeri, H.; Mirhaghi, A. The accuracy of acuity scoring tools to predict 24-h mortality in traumatic brain injury patients: A guide to triage criteria. *Int. Emerg. Nurs.* **2018**, *36*, 27–33. [CrossRef] [PubMed]
22. Han, J.X.; See, A.A.Q.; Gandhi, M.; King, N.K.K. Models of Mortality and Morbidity in Severe Traumatic Brain Injury: An Analysis of a Singapore Neurotrauma Database. *World Neurosurg.* **2017**, *108*, 885–893. [CrossRef] [PubMed]
23. Kelly, C.A.; Upex, A.; Bateman, D. Comparison of consciousness level assessment in the poisoned patient using the alert/verbal/painful/unresponsive scale and the Glasgow coma scale. *Ann. Emerg. Med.* **2004**, *44*, 108–113. [CrossRef] [PubMed]
24. Rösli, D.; Schnüriger, B.; Candinas, D.; Haltmeier, T. The Impact of Accidental Hypothermia on Mortality in Trauma Patients Overall and Patients with Traumatic Brain Injury Specifically: A Systematic Review and Meta-Analysis. *World J. Surg.* **2020**, *44*, 4106–4117. [CrossRef]
25. Jeremitsky, E.; Omert, L.; Dunham, C.M.; Protetch, J.; Rodriguez, A. Harbingers of Poor Outcome the Day after Severe Brain Injury: Hypothermia, Hypoxia, and Hypoperfusion. *J. Trauma Inj. Infect. Crit. Care* **2003**, *54*, 312–319. [CrossRef]
26. Gaither, J.B.; Chikani, V.; Stolz, U.; Viscusi, C.; Denninghoff, K.R.; Barnhart, B.; Mullins, T.; Rice, A.D.; Mhayamaguru, M.; Smith, J.J.; et al. Body Temperature after EMS Transport: Association with Traumatic Brain Injury Outcomes. *Prehosp. Emerg. Care* **2017**, *21*, 575–582. [CrossRef]
27. Klauke, N.; Gräff, I.; Fleischer, A.; Boehm, O.; Guttenthaler, V.; Baumgarten, G.; Meybohm, P.; Wittmann, M. Effects of pre-hospital hypothermia on transfusion requirements and outcomes: A retrospective observatory trial. *BMJ Open.* **2016**, *6*, e009913. [CrossRef]
28. Bukur, M.; Kurtovic, S.; Berry, C.; Tanios, M.; Ley, E.J.; Salim, A. Pre-Hospital Hypothermia is Not Associated with Increased Survival After Traumatic Brain Injury. *J. Surg. Res.* **2012**, *175*, 24–29. [CrossRef]
29. Konstantinidis, A.; Inaba, K.; Dubose, J.; Barmparas, G.; Talving, P.; David, J.-S.; Lam, L.; Demetriades, D. The Impact of Nontherapeutic Hypothermia on Outcomes After Severe Traumatic Brain Injury. *J. Trauma Inj. Infect. Crit. Care* **2011**, *71*, 1627–1631. [CrossRef]
30. De Tanti, A.; Gasperini, G.; Rossini, M. Paroxysmal episodic hypothalamic instability with hypothermia after traumatic brain injury. *Brain Inj.* **2005**, *19*, 1277–1283. [CrossRef]
31. Asmar, S.; Chehab, M.; Bible, L.; Khurrum, M.; Castanon, L.; Ditillo, M.; Joseph, B. The Emergency Department Systolic Blood Pressure Relationship After Traumatic Brain Injury. *J. Surg. Res.* **2021**, *257*, 493–500. [CrossRef] [PubMed]
32. Petersen, L.G.; Ogoh, S. Gravity, intracranial pressure, and cerebral autoregulation. *Physiol. Rep.* **2019**, *7*, e14039. [CrossRef] [PubMed]
33. Guild, S.-J.; Saxena, U.A.; McBryde, F.D.; Malpas, S.C.; Ramchandra, R. Intracranial pressure influences the level of sympathetic tone. *Am. J. Physiol. Integr. Comp. Physiol.* **2018**, *315*, R1049–R1053. [CrossRef] [PubMed]
34. Spaite, D.W.; Hu, C.; Bobrow, B.J.; Chikani, V.; Sherrill, D.; Barnhart, B.; Gaither, J.B.; Denninghoff, K.R.; Viscusi, C.; Mullins, T.; et al. Mortality and Prehospital Blood Pressure in Patients With Major Traumatic Brain Injury: Implications for the Hypotension Threshold. *JAMA Surg.* **2017**, *152*, 360–368. [CrossRef] [PubMed]
35. Smith, C.M.; Adelson, P.D.; Chang, Y.-F.; Brown, S.D.; Kochanek, P.M.; Clark, R.S.B.; Bayir, H.; Hinchberger, J.; Bell, M.J. Brain-systemic temperature gradient is temperature-dependent in children with severe traumatic brain injury. *Pediatr. Crit. Care Med.* **2011**, *12*, 449–454. [CrossRef]

Article

Psychometric Characteristics of the Patient-Reported Outcome Measures Applied in the CENTER-TBI Study

Nicole von Steinbuechel [1,*], Katrin Rauen [2,3], Fabian Bockhop [1], Amra Covic [1], Ugne Krenz [1], Anne Marie Plass [1], Katrin Cunitz [1], Suzanne Polinder [4], Lindsay Wilson [5], Ewout W. Steyerberg [4,6], Andrew I. R. Maas [7], David Menon [8], Yi-Jhen Wu [1,†], Marina Zeldovich [1,†] and the CENTER-TBI Participants and Investigators [‡]

1. Institute of Medical Psychology and Medical Sociology, University Medical Center Göttingen, Waldweg 37A, 37073 Göttingen, Germany; fabian.bockhop@med.uni-goettingen.de (F.B.); amra.covic@med.uni-goettingen.de (A.C.); ugne.krenz@med.uni-goettingen.de (U.K.); annemarie.plass@med.uni-goettingen.de (A.M.P.); katrin.cunitz@med.uni-goettingen.de (K.C.); yi-jhen.wu@med.uni-goettingen.de (Y.-J.W.); marina.zeldovich@med.uni-goettingen.de (M.Z.)
2. Department of Geriatric Psychiatry, Psychiatric Hospital Zurich, University of Zurich, Minervastrasse 145, 8032 Zurich, Switzerland; katrin.rauen@uzh.ch or katrin.rauen@med.uni-muenchen.de
3. Institute for Stroke and Dementia Research (ISD), University Hospital, LMU Munich, Feodor-Lynen-Straße 17, 81377 Munich, Germany
4. Department of Public Health, Erasmus MC, University Medical Center Rotterdam, 3000 CA Rotterdam, The Netherlands; s.polinder@erasmusmc.nl (S.P.); e.steyerberg@erasmusmc.nl (E.W.S.)
5. Department of Psychology, University of Stirling, Stirling FK9 4LJ, UK; l.wilson@stir.ac.uk
6. Department of Biomedical Data Sciences, Leiden University Medical Center, 2333 RC Leiden, The Netherlands
7. Department of Neurosurgery, Antwerp University Hospital and University of Antwerp, 2650 Edegem, Belgium; andrew.maas@uza.be
8. Division of Anaesthesia, University of Cambridge/Addenbrooke's Hospital, Box 157, Cambridge CB2 0QQ, UK; dkm13@cam.ac.uk
* Correspondence: nvsteinbuechel@med.uni-goettingen.de; Tel.: +49-551-39-8192
† Shared last authorship.
‡ The full list of the CENTER-TBI participants and investigators is provided in the Online Supplement.

Abstract: Traumatic brain injury (TBI) may lead to impairments in various outcome domains. Since most instruments assessing these are only available in a limited number of languages, psychometrically validated translations are important for research and clinical practice. Thus, our aim was to investigate the psychometric properties of the patient-reported outcome measures (PROM) applied in the CENTER-TBI study. The study sample comprised individuals who filled in the six-months assessments (GAD-7, PHQ-9, PCL-5, RPQ, QOLIBRI/-OS, SF-36v2/-12v2). Classical psychometric characteristics were investigated and compared with those of the original English versions. The reliability was satisfactory to excellent; the instruments were comparable to each other and to the original versions. Validity analyses demonstrated medium to high correlations with well-established measures. The original factor structure was replicated by all the translations, except for the RPQ, SF-36v2/-12v2 and some language samples for the PCL-5, most probably due to the factor structure of the original instruments. The translation of one to two items of the PHQ-9, RPQ, PCL-5, and QOLIBRI in three languages could be improved in the future to enhance scoring and application at the individual level. Researchers and clinicians now have access to reliable and valid instruments to improve outcome assessment after TBI in national and international health care.

Keywords: psychometric properties; patient-reported outcome measures; traumatic brain injury; classical test theory

1. Introduction

Traumatic brain injury (TBI) causes alterations in brain function, as a result of an external force [1], for example, due to falls, road traffic accidents, sports, assaults, or violence. It is a considerable source of disability and death worldwide. The sequelae of TBI not only impact the lives of those affected and their relatives on many different levels [2], but they can also result in high direct and indirect costs [3,4].

Concerning the global prevalence of TBI, the vast majority of individuals experience mild TBI (70–90%), approximately 10% to 30% suffer from moderate or severe TBI [5,6]. Regardless of the severity, individuals after TBI may suffer from short- or long-term impairments in cognition [7,8], psychosocial functioning [9], health-related quality of life (HRQoL) [10,11], mental health [12,13], and/or functional disability [14]. These impairments can be assessed using domain-specific outcome measures.

The data analyzed in this study were collected in the international Collaborative European NeuroTrauma Effectiveness Research in TBI observational study (CENTER-TBI; clinicaltrials.gov NCT02210221), which has been conducted since 2014 in 18 European countries and Israel, with enrolment being completed at the six-month outcome assessment in 2018. This study aimed to capture a contemporary picture of TBI with respect to all severity groups, its care and outcome, to develop precision medicine approaches and apply comparative effectiveness research to identify best practices. It provides insights into the longitudinal detection of somatic, functional, behavioral, psychiatric, cognitive, psychological, and psychosocial sequelae after TBI and can serve as a basis for the development of a new multidimensional assessment approach [15,16].

An important criterion when selecting instruments for research and clinical practice is their psychometric quality. For most patient-reported outcome measures (PROMs) administered in the CENTER-TBI study this had not yet been examined in the field of TBI, nor had the newly translated versions of the instruments been psychometrically investigated. Hence, the present study aims to investigate the classical psychometric properties of the newly and previously translated PROMs in the field of TBI administered in the CENTER-TBI study.

In research and clinical contexts, instruments offer insights into outcome after TBI. The comparability of the translated instruments with their original version and the validation in the field of TBI enables the reliable and valid aggregation of data in multi-center national and international studies on outcomes after TBI.

The study aims are the investigation of:

1. The *reliability* (total score, scale, and item level) of the PROMs, comparing them with the values of the original instrument versions to ascertain the quality and comparability of the translations and applicability in the field of TBI;
2. The *convergent* and *discriminant validity* of the PROMs with established measures assessing functional recovery after TBI (GOSE), generic HRQoL (SF-36v2/SF-12v2), and TBI severity (GCS);
3. The *factorial validity* using confirmatory factor analyses (CFA) to replicate the original factorial structure of the translated instruments.

2. Materials and Methods

2.1. Participants

Participants were recruited at 63 centers across 18 countries, from 19 December 2014 to 17 December 2017. Ethical approval was secured for each site and informed consent was obtained from all patients or from their legal representatives. The inclusion criteria for the core study were a clinical diagnosis of TBI, presentation within 24 h after injury, and an indication for a computed tomography (CT) scan. Patients were differentiated into three strata: emergency room (ER; patients primarily evaluated at an ER), admission (ADM; patients admitted primarily to a hospital ward), and intensive care unit (ICU; patients who were primarily admitted to an ICU). Further details can be found elsewhere [16]. Data were retrieved from the core 2.1 of the CENTER-TBI database using the data access tool Neurobot.

The core study sample included 4509 individuals. In the present study, we focused on participants aged 16 years and above who had completed at least one outcome measure at the six months' assessment after the TBI. The data were collected either on-site at the hospital by personnel, by face-to-face or telephone interviews (clinical ratings), or via mail (PROMs) and centrally entered using a web-based electronic case report form.

2.2. Sample Charachteristics

Language, sex, age, education, employment, marital status, and living situation were selected as sociodemographic characteristics. Samples were then aggregated by language. More specifically, individuals from German-speaking communities in Austria, Belgium, and Germany were integrated into the German sample, individuals from French-speaking communities in Belgium and France into the French sample, and individuals from Dutch-speaking communities in Belgium or the Netherlands were merged into the Dutch sample. Only few participants ($N = 20$) received the outcome questionnaires in a language other than in the local language of the participating site. These individuals were classified according to their respective language group: Dutch (7), English (8), German (1), Romanian (3), and Swedish (1).

The following variables were used to characterize extracranial and brain injuries: the individuals' mental health status before the injury, clinical care pathways, cause of injury, loss of consciousness (LOC), post-traumatic amnesia (PTA), TBI severity (GCS), abnormalities on computed tomography (CT) scans, total injury severity score (ISS), and brain injury severity score from the Abbreviated Injury Scale (AIS) [17].

2.3. Pataient-Reported Outcome Measures (PROMs)

Since most instruments applied in the CENTER-TBI study only existed in English, they had to be translated into the languages of the participating countries following a formalized approach (i.e., linguistic validation) to ensure their linguistic, cultural and conceptual comparability in the respective languages [18,19]. For more details, see von Steinbuechel et al. [20].

The selection of the outcome measures was informed by the Common Data Elements (CDE) recommendations [21,22]. For six out of eight PROMs (see instrument description marked with an asterisk * below), at least one translation had to be performed. In this study, we report psychometrics for all eight PROMs newly and previously translated yet not validated instruments in the field of TBI.

The Generalized Anxiety Disorder 7 Item Scale (GAD-7)* [23] measures the level of generalized anxiety disorder using seven items and a four-point Likert scale (from 0 "not at all" to 3 "nearly every day"). The total score ranges from 0 to 21 with values of 10 and above indicating impairment and cut-offs of 5, 10, and 15 representing mild, moderate, and moderately severe to severe anxiety, respectively [23].

The Patient Health Questionnaire (PHQ-9)* [24] assesses self-reported symptoms of major depression using nine items and a four-point Likert scale (from 0 "not at all" to 3 "nearly every day"). The PHQ-9 total score ranges from 0 to 27 with a score of 10 and above indicating clinically relevant impairment and cut-offs of 5, 10, 15, and 20 indicating mild, moderate, moderately severe, and severe depression, respectively [24,25].

Both the GAD-7 and PHQ-9 were available in almost all languages except for Latvian (GAD-7 and PHQ-9) and Serbian (GAD-7 only). Nevertheless, we conducted analyses on both instruments to examine their psychometric properties in individuals after TBI.

The Posttraumatic Stress Disorder Checklist-5 (PCL-5)* [26] comprises 20 symptoms of post-traumatic stress disorder (PTSD) based on the Diagnostic and Statistical Manual of Mental Disorders, 5th edition (DSM-5) [27], using a five-point Likert scale (from 0 "not at all" to 4 "extremely"). The total score ranges from 0 to 80 with higher values indicating greater impairment. For clinical screening, either a cut-off score of 31 [28] or 33 is applied [29].

The Rivermead Post-Concussion Symptoms Questionnaire (RPQ)* [30] uses a five-point Likert scale (from 0 "not experienced at all" to 4 "a severe problem") to evaluate the following 16 post-concussion symptoms: headaches, dizziness, nausea and/or vomiting, noise sensitivity, sleep disturbance, fatigue, irritability, depression, frustration, forgetfulness and poor memory, poor concentration, slow thinking, blurred vision, light sensitivity, double vision, and restlessness. Participants rate how much they have been suffering from these symptoms during the past 24 h compared with their condition before the accident. The RPQ total score ranges from 0 to 64 with cut-offs of 13, 25, and 33 indicating mild, moderate, and severe symptoms, respectively [31].

The Quality of Life after Brain Injury Scale (QOLIBRI)* [32,33] measures TBI-specific HRQoL in individuals after TBI. It consists of six domains comprising 37 items using a five-point Likert scale (from 0 "not at all" to 4 "very"). The six domains comprise cognition, self, daily life and autonomy, social relationships, emotions, and physical conditions. The total score is transformed linearly to range from 0–100, whereby higher values indicate better TBI-specific HRQoL [34]. Patients after TBI with a score below 60 may be assumed to display impaired HRQoL [34]; country-specific reference values can be found elsewhere [35]. For the QOLIBRI, psychometric criteria of almost all target language versions involved in the present study (except for Swedish) had already been published [32,36]. The Spanish translation was published after CENTER-TBI had started [37]. To be congruent with the analyses of other PROMs, we replicated the psychometric analyses for the nine language versions of the QOLIBRI.

The Quality of Life after Brain Injury—Overall Scale (QOLIBRI-OS)* [38] is the short version of the QOLIBRI measuring the physical condition, cognition, emotions, daily life and autonomy, social relationships, and current and future prospects with using six items. The items are answered on a five-point Likert scale (from 0 "not at all" to 4 "very"). Patients after TBI with a score below 52 may be assumed to display impaired HRQoL [34]; country-specific reference values can be found elsewhere [39]. For the QOLIBRI-OS too, psychometric properties have already been examined in almost all languages, except for Spanish and Swedish [38]. Here, again, psychometric analyses were replicated in all languages to be congruent with the other PROMs.

The 36-item Short Form Health Survey—Version 2 (SF-36v2) [40,41]. The SF-36v2 measures subjective health status using 36 items with various response formats for each of the eight scales (from dichotomous "yes/no" to polytomous five-point Likert scale responses). The scales can be summed to produce the physical component score (PCS) and mental component score (MCS) measuring physical and mental functioning, respectively. Both scores range from 0 to 100 with higher values indicating better HRQoL. The values can be transformed into T-scores ($M = 50$, $SD = 10$) based on a normative U.S. sample. A value below 47 on a single health domain scale or component summary score is indicative of functional impairment in comparison to the U.S. population [40].

The 12-Item Short Form Survey—Version 2 (SF-12v2) [42] is a short, 12-item version of the SF-36v2. The scores range from 0 to 100 with higher values indicating better HRQoL. The raw values can be transformed into T-scores ($M = 50$, $SD = 10$) based on a normative U.S. sample. However, the authors recommend using country- and group-specific cut-off values as not every country/group has a mean health of 50 [42,43]. In the CENTER-TBI study, the SF-12v2 was found to have more missing data than the SF-36v2. Therefore, to increase the power for the calculation of the PCS and MCS of the SF-12v2, missing values were replaced by values derived from the respective items of the SF-36v2 and combined with reported data. For the analyses on the item level, only reported data were used.

The SF-36v2 and SF-12v2 translations were already available in the target languages and had to be purchased from Optum for one-time use [44]. However, since most translated versions of both the SF-36v2 and the SF-12v2 were not subjected to psychometric analyses in the field of TBI, they were included in the analyses of the present study. Both instruments were also used for validity analyses.

2.4. Clinician-Reported Outcome (ClinRo) and a Clinical Scale

The instruments listed below were used to analyze convergent and discriminant validity.

The Glasgow Outcome Scale Extended (GOSE) [45] is a clinician-reported outcome (ClinRo) of functional recovery after TBI using an eight-point scale (1 = dead, 2 = vegetative state, 3/4 = lower/upper severe disability, 5/6 = lower/upper moderate disability, 7/8 = lower/upper good recovery) and is based on structured interviews (GOSE) or self-ratings by individuals after TBI or their proxy (the questionnaire version; GOSE-Q [46]). Missing GOSE values were centrally replaced by values derived from the GOSE-Q. Since the GOSE-Q is not able to differentiate between vegetative state and lower severe disability, GOSE levels 2 and 3 were collapsed into one category. The missing values at six-months outcome assessments were imputed using a multi-state model; the imputation procedure is described elsewhere [47]. The GOSE was not subjected to reliability analyses, as it would require data from independent raters to provide interrater reliability, which was not available in the CENTER-TBI database.

The Glasgow Coma Scale (GCS) [48] allows healthcare professionals to consistently evaluate the level of consciousness of individuals after TBI, also classifying the severity of TBI. The GCS scores range from 3 (no response) to 15 (normal level) with higher values indicating less impaired consciousness and lower TBI severity. Scores of 13 to 15 indicate mild TBI, 9 to 12 moderate TBI, and 3 to 8 severe TBI.

2.5. Statistical Analyses

The present study focuses on the analyses of reliability, convergent and discriminant validity of eight PROMs in nine TBI language samples with enough participants (i.e., at least 50 participants in the Dutch, English, Finnish, French, German, Italian, Norwegian, Spanish, and Swedish samples) as well as factorial validity in six samples (i.e., at least 150 participants in the Dutch, English, Finnish, Italian, Norwegian, and Spanish samples). Figure 1 provides an overview of our psychometric analyses according to the classical test theoretical (CTT) criteria with the respective cut-off values [49].

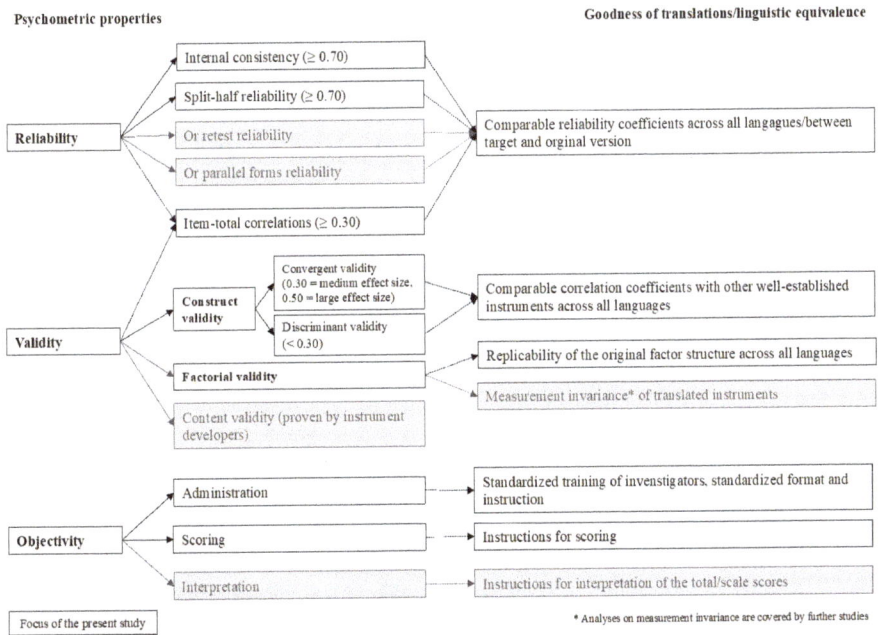

Figure 1. Criteria of classical test theoretical psychometric analyses and their application in this study. The white boxes indicate analyses performed in this study; the grey boxes describe psychometric properties investigated either during instrument development (i.e., content validity), or alternative methods of retest reliability or parallel form reliability, or analyses deferred to further studies (i.e., measurement invariance and interpretation).

2.6. Descriptive Statistics

Descriptive statistics include information on the sample sizes, percentage of missing data, mean (M), standard deviation (SD), skewness (SK), and kurtosis (KU) for each item per language version of an instrument and an average of the item characteristics across all languages. For skewness, values less than −1 or greater than 1 indicate a highly skewed distribution; values from ±1 to ±0.5 show that the distribution is moderately skewed; values from −0.5 to +0.5 denote a symmetrical distribution. For asymmetry and kurtosis, values between −2 and +2 are considered acceptable [50].

2.7. Reliability

For reliability analyses, researchers often accept data of 30 participants as being sufficient to detect a required minimal effect of 0.70 as a cut-off value for reliability coefficients [51]. However, some researchers argue that larger sample sizes are required to avoid bias [51,52]. In the present study, reliability coefficients were therefore only calculated if the sample size comprised at least 50 individuals per language, to provide more robust results.

To examine the reliability of each instrument, Cronbach's alpha, split-half reliability with the Spearman–Brown correction (odd vs. even items), and Cronbach's alpha if an item is omitted were reported. Both, the split-half reliability and the Cronbach's alpha if item omitted were calculated for scales with at least three items. Although different recommendations in terms of cut-off points for the Cronbach's alpha do exist, there is an agreement that in group comparisons Cronbach's alpha should reach at least a value of 0.70 implying acceptable internal consistency [53]; an alpha above 0.90 indicates excellent internal consistency [54]. The Cronbach's alpha value, if an item has been omitted, should not exceed the total Cronbach's alpha of a scale. A value higher than the total Cronbach's alpha indicates that the excluded item decreases the reliability of the instrument and requires further revision [55].

To evaluate the discriminating ability of the items, item–total correlations either at the scale or at the total score level, or both were calculated. A correlation coefficient of 0.30, corresponding to a medium effect size, was chosen as the cut-off criterion, based on the guidelines for effect size proposed by Cohen [56,57]. An item–total correlation below 0.30 implies that the item cannot discriminate well between high-performing and low-performing individuals. Furthermore, low item–total correlations, especially at the scale level, may identify irregularities of the factorial structure of an instrument.

2.8. Validity

2.8.1. Convergent and Discriminant Validity

All language samples analyzed in this study included at least 50 observations, which is recommended for validity analyses [58].

Spearman correlation coefficients were used to examine associations between the GOSE, physical (PCS) and the mental component score (MCS) of the SF-36v2 and SF-12v2, and the total scores/domain-specific scores of all other measures.

Discriminant validity was investigated by calculating Spearman correlation coefficients for the GCS and the total and scale scores of all instruments, to be in line with analyses already provided in the field of TBI [59]. To evaluate the strength of correlations, the Cohen criteria [56,57] were applied to identify small (0.10), medium (0.30), and large (0.50) effect sizes.

2.8.2. Factorial Validity

Factorial validity was examined by means of confirmatory factor analyses (CFA) and a robust weighted least squares estimator (WLSME) for ordinal data, whereby only the original factor structure of the instruments was analyzed. Therefore, one-factor solutions were estimated for the GAD-7 [23], the PHQ-9 [24], the RPQ [30], and the QOLIBRI-OS [38]. For the other instruments, respective multiple scale models were inspected: a four-factor model for the PCL-5 [26], a five-factor model for the QOLIBRI [32], an eight-factor model with two second-order factors for the SF-36v2 [40], and finally, a two-factor model for the SF-12v2 [42]. In CFA analyses, samples should comprise at least 150 observations to provide stable results [60]. Therefore, only language samples fulfilling this criterion were analyzed.

The model fit was evaluated based on the following fit indices using the respective cut-off values (in paratheses): χ^2 statistics with respective p-values ($p > 0.01$) [61], comparative fit index (CFI > 0.95) [62], Tucker–Lewis index (TLI > 0.95 [63]) root mean square error of approximation (RMSEA < 0.06) [64] with a 90-percent confidence interval (CI), and standardized root mean square residual (SRMR < 0.08) [63]. As some of the fit indices may be biased (e.g., χ^2 test can be influenced by large sample size [61]), all indices were considered simultaneously to evaluate the model fit. Furthermore, item loadings over 0.50 were considered acceptable and over 0.70 desirable [53].

Analyses were performed using the packages psych [65] for psychometric characteristics and lavaan [66] for the factorial validity analyses applying the R version 4.0.2 [67].

2.9. Comparability of the Translated Versions

To evaluate the quality of the translated versions of the eight PROMs, psychometric criteria obtained from the CENTER-TBI language samples were compared with those reported for the original English instrument versions. For this purpose, a systematic literature search was carried out. Psychometric characteristics were compared with those obtained from the original validation studies in the original populations, for which the respective instrument was developed. If available, they were also compared with the validation studies in the field of TBI. If the original articles did not provide information on all coefficients, these were retrieved from more recent studies.

These comparisons were confined to the reliability coefficients (i.e., Cronbach's alpha coefficients, split-half or test–retest reliability), as validity testing in the original studies was performed using instruments not applied in the CENTER-TBI study. Instruments showing reliability within the same ranges (i.e., <0.70—acceptable, 0.70–0.89—good, ≥0.90—excellent) or higher in both original and the PROMs applied in the CENTER-TBI study were considered comparable.

3. Results

3.1. Sample Characteristics

For the CENTER-TBI study, eight PROMs were translated or already available in 20 target languages (Figure 2). As some countries withdrew from the project early (Bulgarian and Czech centers) or no participants were recruited (Arabic and Russian), 16 countries participated in the study. Seven out of 16 language samples (i.e., Danish, Hungarian, Hebrew, Lithuanian, Latvian, Romanian, and Serbian) were not psychometrically analyzed due to a low number of observations ($N < 50$). Additionally, three language samples (French, Norwegian, Swedish) had to be excluded from the reliability analyses of the SF-12v2, also because of insufficient sample sizes. For the factorial validity, six language samples comprising at least $N = 150$ observations (i.e., Dutch, English, Finnish, Italian, Norwegian, and Spanish) were investigated for all instruments except for the SF-12v2, as only three SF-12v2 language samples (i.e., Dutch, Finnish, and Spanish) fulfilled the sample size criteria.

The number of participants varied between PROMs, since not every participant filled in each instrument at the six-months outcome assessment. Sample characteristics for each instrument and language are provided in the Online Supplement (OS 1: Sample characteristics, Tables S1–S8). A brief overview on the sample compositions used for the analyses is presented in Figure 2. Appendix A (Table A1) provides additional information on the number of participants for the validity analyses using the GOSE and the GCS.

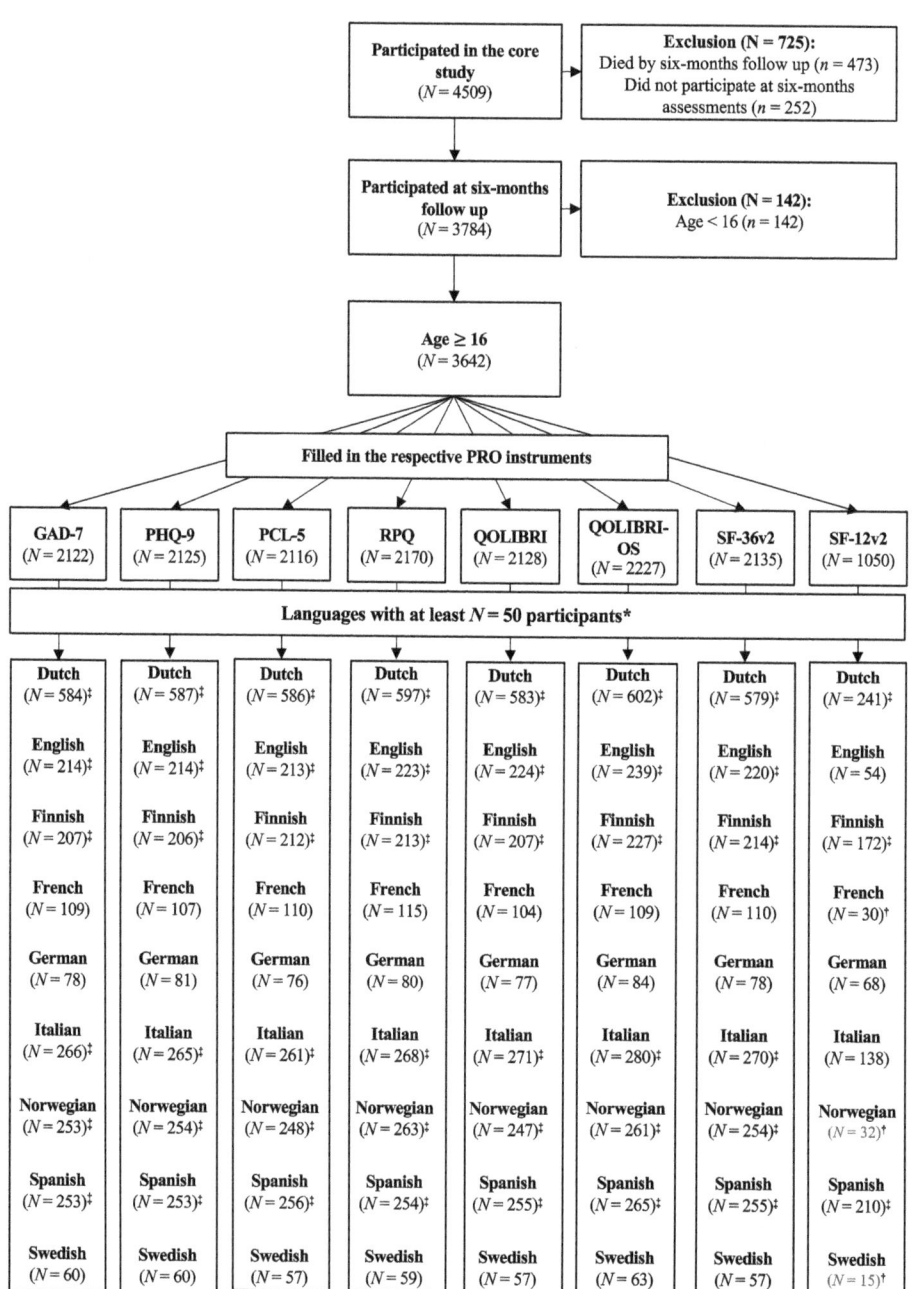

Figure 2. Number of participants for each PROM and language.

3.2. Reliability and Comparability of the PROMs

Reliability coefficients for the total and scale scores of the PROMs are shown below. Item characteristics as well as reliability coefficients on the item level are reported in the respective tables in the Online Supplement 2 (OS-2 Reliability, Tables S1–S8).

3.2.1. GAD-7

All translations analyzed were available prior to the CENTER-TBI study. Item scores for the GAD-7 were not normally distributed (SK: $M = 1.64$, $SD = 0.51$; KU: $M = 2.40$, $SD = 2.22$) across all languages. At the item level, most items were moderately to strongly correlated with the total score of the GAD-7 in most languages (0.36 to 0.89). When calculating Cronbach's alpha if item omitted, all values were smaller than the total Cronbach's alpha across all languages. The values of the split-half reliability ranged from 0.70 to 0.90 across all languages. On the total score level, all translations revealed Cronbach's alpha and split-half reliability values comparable to the results of the original English versions in a non-TBI population (i.e., patients from 15 primary care sites [23]) except for the Finnish, German, Spanish, and Swedish versions showing Cronbach's alpha values slightly lower than 0.90, but over 0.80. The reliability results were within the same or higher range (0.70 to 0.89 and ≥ 0.90) compared to the validation in an English TBI sample [68] (see Table 1).

Table 1. Reliability of the GAD-7: Comparison of the CENTER-TBI results with the values from the original English validation study and the first English validation study in the field of TBI.

GAD-7	CENTER-TBI [1]									Original English Version [2]	
	Dutch	English	Finnish	French	German	Italian	Norwegian	Spanish	Swedish	Non-TBI	TBI
N	584	214	207	109	78	266	253	253	60	2740	1838
Cronbach's alpha	0.92	0.90	0.86	0.94	0.84	0.92	0.90	0.89	0.86	0.92	0.88
N	584	214	207	109	78	266	253	253	60	591	-
Split-half or test–retest reliability [3]	0.93	0.91	0.89	0.95	0.85	0.95	0.93	0.93	0.83	0.83	-

Note. [1] Reliability coefficients obtained from the CENTER-TBI study sample. [2] Reliability coefficients from the original English validation of the GAD-7 in a non-TBI sample [23], and from the first English validation in a TBI sample [68]. [3] Split-half reliability (CENTER-TBI data), test–retest reliability provided by original studies; N = number of cases; values in **bold** represent at least satisfactory reliability (≥ 0.70).

3.2.2. PHQ-9

All analyzed PHQ-9 translations were available prior to the CENTER-TBI study. The items of the PHQ-9 were not normally distributed (SK: $M = 1.66$, $SD = 0.80$; KU: $M = 2.71$, $SD = 3.85$) across all languages. At the item level, all items were moderately to highly correlated with the total scores of the PHQ-9 across all languages, except for Swedish. Here, the item "Moving or speaking so slowly that other people could have noticed" had a low correlation ($r = 0.18$) with the total score. At the total score level, the Cronbach's alpha values were above 0.70 (0.78 to 0.89) in every language. When calculating Cronbach's alpha if item omitted, no value exceeded the total Cronbach's alpha. The values of the split-half reliability ranged from 0.85 to 0.90. Reliability coefficients were comparable (i.e., ranged from 0.70 to 0.89 and above) with those obtained from the original English publication in a non-TBI population (i.e., primary care patients from five general health clinics and three family practice clinics) [24]. The Cronbach's alpha coefficients calculated from CENTER-TBI data were slightly lower compared with the results from the first English validation study in a TBI sample [69], whereas the results of the split-half reliability were within a comparable range [70] (see Table 2).

Table 2. Reliability of the PHQ-9: Comparison of the CENTER-TBI results with the values from the original English validation study and the first English validation study in the field of TBI.

PHQ-9	CENTER-TBI [1]									Original English Version [2]	
	Dutch	English	Finnish	French	German	Italian	Norwegian	Spanish	Swedish	Non-TBI	TBI
N	587	214	206	107	81	265	254	253	60	3000	168 [†]
Cronbach's alpha	0.88	0.88	0.86	0.87	0.85	0.89	0.89	0.88	0.78	0.89	0.91 [†]
N	587	214	206	107	81	265	254	253	60	580	132 [‡]
Split-half or test–retest reliability [3]	0.90	0.90	0.92	0.91	0.90	0.91	0.91	0.91	0.85	0.84	0.76 [‡]

Note. [1] Reliability coefficients (CENTER-TBI study sample). [2] Reliability coefficients (original English validation of the PHQ-9 in a non-TBI sample [24] and from two English validations in TBI samples) [†] Cronbach's alpha [69] and [‡] test–retest reliability [70]. [3] Split-half reliability (CENTER-TBI data), test–retest reliability provided by original studies; N = number of cases; values in **bold** represent at least satisfactory reliability (≥ 0.70).

3.2.3. PCL-5

All but the Norwegian version of the PCL-5 were translated for the CENTER-TBI study. The items of the PCL-5 were not normally distributed (SK: M = 1.75, SD = 0.66; KU: M = 2.70, SD = 2.99) across all languages. At the scale (i.e., DSM-5 cluster) level, most items had medium to high correlations with the cluster total scores of the PCL-5 across all languages. Only the item "Trouble remembering important parts of the stressful experience" displayed borderline correlations with the total cluster scores in French ($r = 0.20$), Norwegian ($r = 0.28$), and Swedish ($r = 0.28$) language samples. The internal consistency was satisfactory to excellent (0.74 to 0.92) at the cluster level. All split-half reliability coefficients demonstrated at least satisfactory reliability (i.e., ≥ 0.70). At the total score level, the values of the Cronbach's alphas ranged from 0.91 to 0.94 in all languages. The Cronbach's alphas if item omitted did not exceed the values of the initial Cronbach's alpha except for the item "Trouble remembering important parts of the stressful experience" in all but English and German language samples. The split-half reliability was excellent (0.92 to 0.96) across all languages. Cronbach's alpha coefficients on the total score and the cluster level were comparable to the original English validation results in a non-TBI sample (i.e., undergraduate students having experienced a stressful life event [26] and military service members [71]) in all translations. No publications on psychometric properties of the PCL-5 in the field of TBI samples were found (see Table 3).

Table 3. Reliability of the PCL-5: Comparison of the CENTER-TBI results with the values from the original English validation study.

PCL-5	DSM-5 Cluster	CENTER-TBI [1]									Original English Version [2]	
		Dutch *	English	Finnish *	French *	German *	Italian *	Norwegian	Spanish *	Swedish *	Non-TBI	TBI
N	-	586	213	212	110	76	261	248	256	57	278 [†]	-
Cronbach's alpha	B	0.90	0.89	0.81	0.89	0.88	0.90	0.90	0.88	0.88	0.80	
	C	0.79	0.83	0.78	0.92	0.77	0.90	0.82	0.82	0.82	0.83	
	D	0.85	0.84	0.79	0.83	0.78	0.83	0.79	0.87	0.80	0.82	
	E	0.79	0.81	0.83	0.83	0.74	0.83	0.82	0.84	0.76	0.75	
	Total	0.93	0.94	0.92	0.93	0.92	0.95	0.93	0.94	0.91	0.94 [†]/0.92	
N	-	586	213	212	110	76	261	248	256	57	53/912	-
Split-half or test–retest reliability [3]	B	0.92	0.91	0.86	0.91	0.91	0.92	0.92	0.88	0.84	0.80	
	C	-	-	-	-	-	-	-	-	-	0.83	
	D	0.87	0.87	0.83	0.84	0.86	0.85	0.83	0.89	0.85	0.82	
	E	0.84	0.85	0.84	0.85	0.78	0.85	0.86	0.90	0.88	0.75	
	Total	0.96	0.95	0.94	0.94	0.92	0.95	0.95	0.96	0.92	0.82 [†]/0.91	

Note. * Instruments translated and linguistically validated for the CENTER-TBI study. [1] Reliability coefficients (CENTER-TBI study sample). [2] Reliability coefficients (original English validation of the PCL-5 in a non-TBI sample on the [†] total score level [26]) and on the total score and cluster level [71]. [3] Split-half reliability (CENTER-TBI data), test–retest reliability provided by original studies; DSM-5 clusters: B = Intrusion; C = Avoidance; D = Negative alterations in cognition and mood; E = Hyperarousal; Cronbach's alpha and split-half reliability not reported due to the scale length (two items); N = number of cases; values in **bold** represent at least satisfactory reliability (≥ 0.70).

3.2.4. RPQ

All but the German and Norwegian versions of the RPQ were translated for the CENTER-TBI study. The item score distributions of the RPQ were skewed (SK: M = 1.31, SD = 0.83; KU: M = 1.37, SD = 4.07) across all languages. At the item level, most items displayed medium to high correlations with the total scores of the RPQ. In the German translation, the item "*Double Vision*" had a borderline correlation with the total score of the RPQ (r = 0.25). The item "*Nausea*" of the German and Swedish translations displayed rather low correlations (r = 0.25 and r = 0.24, respectively) with the total score.

At the scale level, however, the values of the Cronbach's alpha and the split-half reliability were above 0.70 across all languages. No comparisons between the original and the translated language versions can be provided for the internal consistency, as no information was available concerning Cronbach's alpha in the English RPQ version investigated in a TBI sample. Moreover, further studies on the RPQ [31,72,73] provided no information on the internal consistency, as they focused on the factorial structure of the questionnaire. The test–retest reliability scores in the original study were comparable to the split-half reliability results of the English and Finnish language samples from the CENTER-TBI study. The split-half reliability of all other translations was slightly above 0.90 except for the Swedish version ($\alpha_{Cronbach}$ = 0.82). For details, see Table 4.

Table 4. Reliability of the RPQ: Comparison of the CENTER-TBI results with the values from the original English validation study in the field of TBI.

RPQ	CENTER-TBI [1]									Original English Version [2]
	Dutch *	English	Finnish *	French *	German	Italian *	Norwegian	Spanish *	Swedish *	TBI
N	597	223	213	115	80	268	263	254	59	41
Cronbach's alpha	**0.93**	**0.92**	**0.92**	**0.92**	**0.89**	**0.91**	**0.92**	**0.92**	**0.89**	-
N	597	223	213	115	80	268	263	254	59	-
Split-half or test–retest reliability [3]	**0.94**	**0.95**	**0.95**	**0.94**	**0.93**	**0.94**	**0.93**	**0.92**	**0.82**	**0.90**

Note. * Instruments translated and linguistically validated for the CENTER-TBI study. [1] Reliability coefficients (CENTER-TBI study sample). [2] Reliability coefficients from the original English validation of the RPQ in a TBI sample [30]. [3] Split-half reliability (CENTER-TBI data), test–retest reliability (original validation study); N = number of cases; values in **bold** represent at least satisfactory reliability (≥ 0.70).

3.2.5. QOLIBRI

At the total score level, Cronbach's alpha and the split-half reliability coefficients of all translated QOLIBRI versions were above 0.90. Item–total correlations displayed medium to high correlations with the total score except for the German version. Here, the item "*How bothered are you by feeling angry or aggressive*" revealed a low correlation with the total score (r = 0.25). Below, item distributions and reliabilities are reported for each subscale.

Cognition. The items were almost normally distributed (SK: M = −0.91, SD = 0.34; KU: M = 0.46, SD = 0.78) across all languages and highly correlated with the total score of the Cognition scale across all languages (0.62 to 0.84). At the scale level, all reliability coefficients were excellent (Cronbach's alpha: 0.91 to 0.93; split-half-reliability: 0.90 to 0.94).

Self. The items were approximately normally distributed (SK: M = −0.68, SD = 0.27; KU: M = −0.11, SD = 0.65) in all languages and correlated highly with the scale score (0.64 to 0.88). Reliability coefficients were excellent (Cronbach's alpha: 0.92 to 0.94; split-half reliability: 0.92 to 0.96).

Daily Life and Autonomy. Across all languages, items were nearly normally distributed (SK: M = −0.97, SD = 0.36; KU: M = 0.18, SD = 0.91). Items correlated highly with the scale scores (0.61 to 0.86). Reliability coefficients were excellent (Cronbach's alpha: 0.90 to 0.94; split-half reliability: 0.92 to 0.96).

Social Relationships. In general, item scores were normally distributed (SK: M = −1.02, SD = 0.40; KU: M = 0.61, SD = 1.25) across all languages. Correlations for item and scale scores ranged from 0.39 to 0.80. Reliability results were satisfactory to excellent for all translated versions (Cronbach's alpha: 0.76 to 0.89; split-half reliability: 0.86 to 0.95).

Emotions. On average, the items were nearly normally distributed (SK: $M = -1.01$, $SD = 0.48$; KU: $M = 0.25$, $SD = 1.20$) for all languages. All items were moderately to highly correlated with the total scores of the scale across all languages (0.52 to 0.82). At the scale level, reliability results were good to excellent (Cronbach's alpha: 0.82 to 0.89; split-half reliability: 0.86 to 0.90).

Physical. The item distributions were close to a normal distribution (SK: $M = -0.89$, $SD = 0.38$; KU: $M = -0.23$, $SD = 0.88$) across all languages. All coefficients were satisfactory to good across all languages on the item (item–total correlation: 0.35 to 0.74) as well as on the scale level (Cronbach's alpha: 0.76 to 0.88; split-half reliability: 0.76 to 0.88).

All reliability coefficients were comparable (i.e., within the same or higher range) to those reported in the original publication on a TBI population. As the QOLIBRI was developed for use in the TBI field, no validation studies in non-TBI populations are reported (see Table 5).

Table 5. Reliability of the QOLIBRI: Comparison of the CENTER-TBI results with the values from the original English validation study in the field of TBI.

QOLIBRI	Scale	CENTER-TBI [1]									Original English Version [2]
		Dutch	English	Finnish	French	German	Italian	Norwegian	Spanish	Swedish	TBI
N	-	583	224	207	104	77	271	247	255	57	97
Cronbach's alpha	Cognition	0.92	0.92	0.92	0.93	0.91	0.93	0.93	0.92	0.92	0.92
	Self	0.92	0.92	0.94	0.94	0.92	0.94	0.93	0.93	0.92	0.90
	Daily life	0.93	0.93	0.92	0.93	0.93	0.94	0.90	0.94	0.92	0.93
	Social	0.86	0.88	0.85	0.89	0.87	0.88	0.84	0.84	0.76	0.88
	Emotions	0.87	0.85	0.82	0.89	0.86	0.86	0.85	0.86	0.86	0.88
	Physical	0.79	0.79	0.79	0.81	0.76	0.85	0.82	0.84	0.75	0.80
	Total	0.96	0.96	0.96	0.97	0.96	0.97	0.96	0.96	0.95	0.97
N	-	583	224	207	104	77	271	247	255	57	56
Split-half or test–retest reliability [3]	Cognition	0.90	0.91	0.93	0.94	0.92	0.94	0.92	0.91	0.92	0.80
	Self	0.93	0.94	0.96	0.95	0.92	0.95	0.94	0.94	0.93	0.83
	Daily life	0.95	0.95	0.94	0.94	0.95	0.94	0.92	0.95	0.96	0.77
	Social	0.88	0.91	0.86	0.95	0.90	0.89	0.86	0.89	0.86	0.79
	Emotions	0.89	0.86	0.87	0.90	0.89	0.88	0.88	0.89	0.88	0.76
	Physical	0.78	0.76	0.78	0.80	0.83	0.88	0.83	0.86	0.77	0.83
	Total	0.97	0.98	0.98	0.98	0.98	0.98	0.98	0.97	0.98	0.88

Note. [1] Reliability coefficients (CENTER-TBI study sample). [2] Reliability coefficients (original English validation of the QOLIBRI in a TBI sample [32]). [3] Split-half reliability (CENTER-TBI data), test–retest reliability (original study); N = number of cases; values in **bold** represent at least satisfactory reliability (≥ 0.70).

3.2.6. QOLIBRI-OS

The items of the QOLIBRI-OS were close to being normally distributed (SK: $M = -0.71$, $SD = 0.23$; KU: $M = -0.05$, $SD = 0.53$) and were moderately to highly correlated with the total scores of the QOLIBRI-OS (0.59 to 0.83) across all languages. At the total score level, the Cronbach' alpha values were close to or above 0.90 (0.88 to 0.92), and the split-half reliability ranged from 0.90 to 0.94. Moreover, the values of the Cronbach's alpha if item omitted were smaller than the Cronbach's alpha in each language. The reliabilities of the translated versions were in general within the same range as those of the original ones. The split-half coefficients were greater than the test–retest reliability of the original QOLIBRI-OS. For details, see Table 6.

Table 6. Comparison of the CENTER-TBI results with the values from the original English validation study in the field of TBI.

QOLIBRI-OS	CENTER-TBI [1]									Original English Version [2]
	Dutch	English	Finnish	French	German	Italian	Norwegian	Spanish	Swedish	TBI
N	602	239	227	109	84	280	261	265	63	97
Cronbach's alpha	0.91	0.90	0.92	0.90	0.88	0.91	0.92	0.90	0.91	0.91
N	602	239	227	109	84	280	261	265	63	54
Split-half or test–retest reliability [3]	0.92	0.92	0.94	0.94	0.90	0.92	0.92	0.93	0.93	0.69

Note. [1] Reliability coefficients (CENTER-TBI study sample). [2] Reliability coefficients (original English validation of the QOLIBRI-OS in a TBI sample [38]). [3] Split-half reliability (CENTER-TBI data), test–retest reliability (original study); N = number of cases; values in **bold** represent at least satisfactory reliability (≥ 0.70).

3.2.7. SF-36v2

All SF-36v2 translations were available prior to the CENTER-TBI study. The instrument was investigated on the scale and item level and with respect to the mental (MCS) and physical (PCS) component score.

Physical Functioning (PF). The items were not normally distributed (SK: $M = -1.46$, $SD = 0.88$; KU: $M = 1.65$, $SD = 3.27$) across all languages. Items were moderately to highly correlated with the scale score across all languages (0.56 to 0.91). At the scale level, all reliability coefficients showed excellent results (Cronbach's alpha: 0.92 to 0.95; split-half-reliability: 0.95 to 0.98).

Role-Physical (RP). The items were almost normally distributed (SK: $M = -0.50$, $SD = 0.35$; KU: $M = -0.90$, $SD = 0.45$) across all languages and highly correlated with the scale score across all languages (0.83 to 0.93). At the scale level, all reliability coefficients were excellent (Cronbach's alpha: 0.94 to 0.96; split-half-reliability: 0.94 to 0.97).

Bodily Pain (BP). The items were almost normally distributed (SK: $M = -0.65$, $SD = 0.33$; KU: $M = -0.60$, $SD = 0.59$) across all languages and highly correlated with the scale score across all languages (0.78 to 0.83). At the scale level, all reliability coefficients showed were good to excellent (Cronbach's alpha: 0.86 to 0.89). The split-half reliability was not calculated because of the scale length (two items).

General Health (GH). The items were normally distributed (SK: $M = -0.60$, $SD = 0.53$; KU: $M = -0.31$, $SD = 0.88$) across all languages. Items were moderately to highly correlated with the scale score across all languages (0.37 to 0.78). At the scale level, Cronbach's alpha was satisfactory to good (0.73 to 0.84). The split-half reliability of the English, German, Norwegian, Spanish, and Swedish samples was low to borderline (0.59 to 0.69) and satisfactory for the other languages (0.70 to 0.78).

Vitality (VT). The items were normally distributed (SK: $M = -0.28$, $SD = 0.25$; KU: $M = -0.50$, $SD = 0.37$) across all languages and moderately to highly correlated with the scale score across all languages (0.48 to 0.78). At the scale level, all reliability coefficients were good to excellent (Cronbach's alpha: 0.83 to 0.88; split-half reliability: 0.85 to 0.95).

Social Functioning (SF). The items were normally distributed (SK: $M = -0.89$, $SD = 0.34$; KU: $M = -0.12$, $SD = 0.83$) across all languages. The items were highly correlated with the scale score across all languages (0.69 to 0.81). Cronbach's alpha was good to excellent (0.81 to 0.90); split-half reliability was not calculated because of the scale length (two items).

Role Emotional (RE). Across all languages, items were nearly normally distributed (SK: $M = -1.00$, $SD = 0.40$; KU: $M = 0.09$, $SD = 0.91$) in all language samples. They were highly correlated with the scale score across all languages (0.72 to 0.92). At the scale level, all reliability coefficients were excellent (Cronbach's alpha: 0.90 to 0.95; split-half reliability: 0.91 to 0.96).

Mental Health (MH). The items were close to being normally distributed (SK: $M = -0.80$, $SD = 0.45$; KU: $M = 0.22$, $SD = 1.11$) across all languages. They were moderately to highly correlated with the scale score across all languages (0.48 to 0.83). At the scale level, all reliability coefficients were good to excellent (Cronbach's alpha: 0.83 to 0.89; split-half reliability: 0.81 to 0.92).

The internal consistency of the translated versions of the SF-36v2 was comparable to the original English version, which was validated in a U.S. general population [40,41]. The Cronbach's alpha coefficients on the scale levels were within the same ranges or above. The split-half reliability coefficients were within the same or higher ranges compared to the original version. Despite the wide application of the SF-36v2, no studies on psychometric properties of the English version in the field of TBI for the English version were found.

Physical Component Score (PCS). Items were moderately to highly correlated with the PCS (0.35 to 0.87) except for the item "*I expect my health to get worse*" in the English version ($r = 0.23$). Cronbach's alpha ranged from 0.32 to 0.95 and the split-half reliability coefficients from 0.93 to 0.95. When omitting an item, the newly calculated Cronbach's alpha did not exceed the initial value in any language sample. The reliability coefficients were within the same or higher range compared with the psychometric properties of the original SF-36v2.

Mental Component Score (MCS). The items were moderately to highly correlated with the MCS (0.43 to 0.88). Cronbach's alpha (0.92 to 0.95) and split-half coefficients (0.95 to 0.98) indicted a high reliability. When omitting an item, the newly calculated Cronbach's alpha values did not exceed the initial one. Here, again, the reliability of the instrument translations was comparable (i.e., was within the same or higher range) with the results obtained from the original validation study (see Table 7).

Table 7. Reliability of the SF-36v2: Comparison of the CENTER-TBI results with the values from the original English validation study.

SF-36v2	Scale	CENTER-TBI [1]									Original English Version [2]	
		Dutch	English	Finnish	French	German	Italian	Norwegian	Spanish	Swedish	Non-TBI	TBI
N	-	579	220	214	110	78	270	254	255	57	4024–4036	-
Cronbach's alpha	PF	0.94	0.94	0.93	0.94	0.92	0.95	0.93	0.94	0.95	0.94	
	RP	0.95	0.95	0.94	0.95	0.95	0.96	0.96	0.96	0.95	0.96	
	BP	0.89	0.87	0.88	0.88	0.89	0.88	0.87	0.87	0.86	0.87	
	GH	0.81	0.81	0.84	0.84	0.77	0.81	0.79	0.79	0.73	0.82	
	VT	0.83	0.87	0.88	0.85	0.85	0.86	0.86	0.83	0.88	0.87	
	SF	0.82	0.87	0.87	0.90	0.81	0.82	0.87	0.87	0.88	0.84	
	RE	0.94	0.90	0.91	0.94	0.92	0.94	0.95	0.94	0.93	0.93	
	MH	0.87	0.83	0.87	0.89	0.85	0.87	0.85	0.86	0.89	0.87	
	HT	-	-	-	-	-	-	-	-	-	-	
	PCS	0.94	0.94	0.94	0.94	0.93	0.95	0.93	0.95	0.94	0.96	
	MCS	0.94	0.93	0.94	0.95	0.94	0.94	0.94	0.94	0.94	0.93	
N	-	579	220	214	110	78	270	254	255	57	147	-
Split-half or test–retest reliability [3]	PF	0.97	0.97	0.97	0.97	0.95	0.98	0.96	0.97	0.97	0.85	
	RP	0.96	0.94	0.95	0.95	0.97	0.97	0.97	0.97	0.97	0.78	
	BP	-	-	-	-	-	-	-	-	-	0.71	
	GH	0.72	0.69	0.78	0.75	0.65	0.74	0.68	0.67	0.59	0.87	
	VT	0.85	0.90	0.94	0.95	0.89	0.89	0.89	0.91	0.92	0.75	
	SF	-	-	-	-	-	-	-	-	-	0.70	
	RE	0.95	0.93	0.91	0.96	0.95	0.95	0.95	0.93	0.93	0.61	
	MH	0.86	0.82	0.86	0.84	0.86	0.85	0.81	0.83	0.92	0.76	
	HT	-	-	-	-	-	-	-	-	-	-	
	PCS	0.96	0.96	0.97	0.97	0.94	0.97	0.95	0.97	0.96	0.88	
	MCS	0.96	0.95	0.96	0.97	0.97	0.97	0.96	0.97	0.98	0.79	

Note. [1] Reliability coefficients (CENTER-TBI study sample). [2] Reliability coefficients (original English validation of the QOLIBRI in a non-TBI sample [41]). [3] Split-half reliability (CENTER-TBI data), test–retest reliability (original validation study); Cronbach's alpha and split-half reliability are not reported due to the scale length (two items); PF = Physical functioning; BP = Bodily Pain; GH = General Health; VT = Vitality; SF = Social Functioning; RE = Role-Emotional; MH = Mental Health; HT = Reported Health Transition; PCS = Physical Component Score; MCS = Mental Component Score; split-half reliability not reported for the BP and SF scales due to the scale length (two items); no psychometric properties reported for the HT scale due to the scale length (one item); N = number of cases; values in **bold** represent at least satisfactory reliability (≥ 0.70).

3.2.8. SF-12v2

All SF-12v2 translations were available prior to the CENTER-TBI study. Many of the scales of the SF-12v2 consist of two items (PF, RP, RE, MH), and some include one item (BP, VT, SF, GH); therefore, the reliability coefficients are provided on the physical (PCS) and mental (MCS) component score level.

Physical Component Score (PCS). The items were close to being normally distributed (SK: $M = -0.54$, $SD = 0.47$; KU: $M = -0.64$, $SD = 0.55$) across all languages. On the item level, all items correlated moderately to highly with the PCS (0.55 to 0.89). At the scale level, all reliability coefficients were good to excellent (Cronbach's alpha: 0.86 to 0.94; split-half-reliability: 0.88 to 0.92).

Mental Component Score (MCS). The items were close to being normally distributed (SK: $M = -0.67$, $SD = 0.35$; KU: $M = -0.32$, $SD = 0.49$) across all languages and correlated moderately to highly with the MCS (0.55 to 0.89). At the scale level, all reliability coefficients were good to excellent (Cronbach's alpha: 0.86 to 0.94; split-half-reliability: 0.88 to 0.92).

The reliability of the translated versions of the SF-12v2 was comparable to the original English version, which was validated in a general U.S. population [42]. The split-half reliability coefficients (using the CENTER-TBI data) were within the higher range for both component scores compared with the original version. Despite the wide application of the SF-12v2, no studies on psychometric properties of the English version in the field of TBI were found (see Table 8).

Table 8. Reliability of the SF-12v2: Comparison of the CENTER-TBI results with the values from the original English validation study.

SF-12v2	Component Score	CENTER-TBI [1]						Original English Version [2]	
		Dutch	English	Finnish	German	Italian	Spanish	Non-TBI	TBI
N	-	241	54	172	68	138	210	4002	-
Cronbach's alpha	PCS	0.86	0.91	0.90	0.89	0.89	0.91	0.92	-
	MCS	0.89	0.90	0.86	0.94	0.89	0.89	0.88	-
N	-	241	54	172	68	138	210	215	-
Split-half or test–retest reliability [3]	PCS	0.91	0.95	0.92	0.92	0.94	0.95	0.85	-
	MCS	0.89	0.90	0.88	0.92	0.89	0.92	0.67	-

Note. French, Norwegian, and Swedish language samples were excluded from the reliability analyses due to the low number of participants ($N < 50$). [1] Reliability coefficients (CENTER-TBI study sample). [2] Reliability coefficients (original English validation of the SF-12v2 in a non-TBI sample [42]). [3] Split-half reliability (CENTER-TBI study), test–retest reliability (original validation study); N = number of cases; PCS = Physical Component Score; MCS = Mental Component Score; values in **bold** represent at least satisfactory reliability (≥ 0.70).

3.3. Validity

3.3.1. Convergent and Discriminant Validity

Validity coefficients for all PROMs and the PCS and MCS of the SF-36v2 and the SF-12v2 are provided on the total score level (see Table 9). For details concerning the validity of the PCL-5, the QOLIBRI, and the SF-36v2 on the scale level, see Appendix B Tables A2–A4.

Most instruments indicating a degree of impairment (i.e., GAD-7, PHQ-9, PCL-5, and RPQ) displayed medium to high negative correlations with the PCS of the SF-36v2 (-0.30 to -0.82). Some exceptions were observed in the English ($r_S = -0.15$) and the Swedish ($r_S = -0.12$) versions of the GAD-7, as well as in the French version ($r_S = -0.25$) of the PCL-5 which demonstrated low negative correlations. For the instruments measuring disease-specific HRQoL after TBI (i.e., the QOLIBRI and the QOLIBRI-OS) medium to high positive correlations with the SF-36v2 PCS domain (0.49 to 0.65) were found across all languages.

Table 9. Convergent and discriminant validity of the GAD-7, PHQ-9, PCL-5, RPQ, QOLIBRI, and QOLIBRI-OS with the SF-36v2, the SF-12v2, the GOSE, and the GCS.

Instrument	Language/Value	Convergent Validity				Discriminant Validity	
		SF-36v2 PCS	SF-36v2 MCS	SF-12v2 PCS	SF-12v2 MCS	GOSE	GCS
GAD-7	Dutch	−0.31	−0.71	−0.27	−0.70	−0.41	−0.11
	English	−0.15	−0.76	−0.15	−0.71	−0.36	−0.04
	Finnish	−0.35	−0.73	−0.34	−0.69	−0.52	−0.20
	French	−0.33	−0.78	−0.26	−0.74	−0.35	−0.09
	German	−0.45	−0.74	−0.31	−0.72	−0.24	0.01
	Italian	−0.31	−0.77	−0.27	−0.74	−0.30	0.06
	Norwegian	−0.33	−0.74	−0.29	−0.72	−0.32	0.07
	Spanish	−0.38	−0.72	−0.40	−0.68	−0.39	−0.04
	Swedish	−0.12	−0.65	−0.22	−0.63	−0.54	−0.30
	M	−0.30	−0.73	−0.28	−0.70	−0.38	−0.07
	Max	−0.12	−0.65	−0.15	−0.63	−0.24	0.07
	Min	−0.45	−0.78	−0.40	−0.74	−0.54	−0.30
	SD	0.10	0.04	0.07	0.04	0.10	0.12
PHQ-9	Dutch	−0.46	−0.74	−0.43	−0.71	−0.49	−0.14
	English	−0.33	−0.77	−0.32	−0.74	−0.47	−0.13
	Finnish	−0.47	−0.77	−0.50	−0.71	−0.56	−0.07
	French	−0.39	−0.83	−0.36	−0.79	−0.41	−0.19
	German	−0.60	−0.61	−0.56	−0.68	−0.45	0.06
	Italian	−0.45	−0.73	−0.43	−0.70	−0.41	−0.01
	Norwegian	−0.44	−0.76	−0.38	−0.76	−0.37	0.02
	Spanish	−0.49	−0.76	−0.49	−0.74	−0.44	−0.04
	Swedish	−0.43	−0.68	−0.52	−0.67	−0.63	−0.33
	M	−0.45	−0.74	−0.44	−0.72	−0.47	−0.09
	Max	−0.33	−0.61	−0.32	−0.67	−0.37	0.06
	Min	−0.60	−0.83	−0.56	−0.79	−0.63	−0.33
	SD	0.07	0.06	0.08	0.04	0.08	0.12
PCL-5	Dutch *	−0.39	−0.63	−0.36	−0.62	−0.45	−0.20
	English	−0.29	−0.71	−0.28	−0.66	−0.44	−0.14
	Finnish *	−0.38	−0.66	−0.40	−0.61	−0.49	−0.20
	French *	−0.25	−0.69	−0.20	−0.65	−0.31	−0.07
	German *	−0.44	−0.68	−0.37	−0.62	−0.16	0.17
	Italian *	−0.35	−0.71	−0.32	−0.67	−0.33	0.07
	Norwegian	−0.42	−0.66	−0.37	−0.65	−0.42	−0.06
	Spanish *	−0.32	−0.61	−0.33	−0.55	−0.44	−0.10
	Swedish *	−0.30	−0.54	−0.37	−0.48	−0.52	−0.24
	M	−0.35	−0.65	−0.33	−0.61	−0.40	−0.09
	Max	−0.25	−0.54	−0.20	−0.48	−0.16	0.17
	Min	−0.44	−0.71	−0.40	−0.67	−0.52	−0.24
	SD	0.06	0.05	0.06	0.06	0.11	0.13
RPQ	Dutch *	−0.48	−0.64	−0.45	−0.62	−0.54	−0.19
	English	−0.43	−0.63	−0.47	−0.62	−0.60	−0.26
	Finnish *	−0.54	−0.60	−0.55	−0.54	−0.63	−0.19
	French *	−0.44	−0.71	−0.40	−0.67	−0.39	−0.07
	German	−0.50	−0.44	−0.47	−0.46	−0.52	−0.07
	Italian *	−0.43	−0.62	−0.44	−0.56	−0.47	−0.07
	Norwegian	−0.51	−0.59	−0.47	−0.57	−0.58	−0.11
	Spanish *	−0.52	−0.61	−0.52	−0.56	−0.63	−0.21
	Swedish *	−0.38	−0.45	−0.44	−0.42	−0.59	−0.34
	M	−0.47	−0.59	−0.47	−0.56	−0.55	−0.17
	Max	−0.38	−0.44	−0.40	−0.42	−0.39	−0.07
	Min	−0.54	−0.71	−0.55	−0.67	−0.63	−0.34
	SD	0.05	0.09	0.04	0.08	0.08	0.09

Table 9. Cont.

Instrument	Language/Value	Convergent Validity				Discriminant Validity	
		SF-36v2 PCS	SF-36v2 MCS	SF-12v2 PCS	SF-12v2 MCS	GOSE	GCS
QOLIBRI	Dutch	0.58	0.71	0.56	0.69	0.54	0.23
	English	0.51	0.74	0.53	0.71	0.60	0.21
	Finnish	0.59	0.80	0.59	0.72	0.59	0.12
	French	0.53	0.76	0.49	0.74	0.53	0.11
	German	0.62	0.68	0.56	0.68	0.37	−0.09
	Italian	0.55	0.74	0.56	0.71	0.52	0.00
	Norwegian	0.53	0.73	0.51	0.71	0.44	−0.01
	Spanish	0.65	0.63	0.65	0.61	0.56	0.16
	Swedish	0.59	0.66	0.60	0.61	0.64	0.34
	M	0.57	0.72	0.56	0.69	0.53	0.12
	Max	0.65	0.80	0.65	0.74	0.64	0.34
	Min	0.51	0.63	0.49	0.61	0.37	−0.09
	SD	0.05	0.05	0.05	0.05	0.08	0.14
QOLIBRI-OS	Dutch	0.58	0.65	0.57	0.66	0.50	0.19
	English	0.49	0.72	0.52	0.72	0.53	0.17
	Finnish	0.51	0.74	0.55	0.66	0.48	−0.01
	French	0.63	0.66	0.60	0.62	0.56	0.25
	German	0.63	0.57	0.55	0.67	0.40	−0.08
	Italian	0.57	0.65	0.59	0.61	0.44	−0.04
	Norwegian	0.49	0.69	0.48	0.66	0.47	0.01
	Spanish	0.59	0.58	0.61	0.58	0.55	0.19
	Swedish	0.57	0.61	0.59	0.61	0.62	0.40
	M	0.56	0.65	0.56	0.64	0.51	0.12
	Max	0.63	0.74	0.61	0.72	0.62	0.40
	Min	0.49	0.57	0.48	0.58	0.40	−0.08
	SD	0.05	0.06	0.04	0.04	0.07	0.16

Note. * Instrument translated and linguistically validated for the CENTER-TBI study; M = mean, Max = maximum, Min = minimum; SD = standard deviation; SF-36v2-PCS = physical component score; SF-36v2—MCS = mental component score; SF-12v2—PCS = physical component score SF-12v2—MCS = mental component score.; GCS = Glasgow Coma Scale; GOSE = Glasgow Outcome Scale—Extended. Values in **bold** represent an at least medium effect size ($\geq |0.30|$), significant at $\alpha = 0.05$.

All PROMs indicating a degree of impairment correlated negatively and moderately to highly with the MCS of the SF-36v2 (−0.44 to −0.83). The ones capturing disease specific HRQoL displayed medium to high positive correlations (0.57 to 0.80) with the MCS across all languages.

The PCS of the SF-12v2 was negatively correlated at a low to medium level with the PHQ-9 (−0.32 to −0.56) and RPQ (−0.40 to −0.55) and positively with the QOLIBRI (0.49 to 0.65) and the QOLIBRI-OS (0.48 to 0.61) across all languages. The GAD-7 revealed significant medium correlations with the PCS of the SF-12v2 in Finnish ($r_S = -0.34$), in German ($r_S = -0.31$), and in Spanish ($r_S = -0.40$); all other values ranged from −0.29 to −0.15.

All PROMs indicating a degree of impairment were negatively and moderately to highly correlated with the MCS of the SF-12v2 (−0.42 to −0.79) and positively with the QOLIBRI and the QOLIBRI-OS (0.58 to 0.74).

Significant medium to high correlations were found between the PROMs and the GOSE total score, whereby greater impairment was associated with lower functional recovery status in almost all languages across all instruments (from −0.30 to −0.63). Only the German version of the GAD-7 ($r_S = -0.24$) and the German version of the PCL-5 ($r_S = -0.16$) demonstrated low associations with the GOSE. Higher TBI-specific HRQoL was associated with a better functional recovery status across all languages (0.37 to 0.64).

The associations of the PROMs and the GCS were weak and not significant in most languages. Only the Swedish translations of the GAD-7 ($r_S = -0.30$), the PHQ-9 ($r_S = -0.33$), the RPQ ($r_S = -0.34$), the QOLIBRI ($r_S = 0.34$), and the QOLIBRI-OS ($r_S = 0.40$) displayed medium correlations with the GCS.

3.3.2. Factorial Validity

Table 10 gives an overview on the goodness of fit statistics for the estimated models. Factor loadings are provided in the Online Supplement (OS-3 Factorial validity, Tables S1–S8).

Table 10. Factorial validity: results of the CFA.

Instrument	Language	χ^2	df	p	CFI	TLI	RMSEA	90% CI	SRMR
GAD-7	Dutch	27.90	14	0.015	**1.00**	**1.00**	**0.04**	[0.02,0.06]	**0.03**
	English	38.69	14	<0.001	**1.00**	**0.99**	0.09	[0.06,0.13]	**0.06**
	Finnish	15.82	14	0.325	**1.00**	**1.00**	**0.03**	[0.00,0.07]	**0.05**
	Italian	49.29	14	<0.001	**1.00**	**1.00**	0.10	[0.07,0.13]	**0.05**
	Norwegian	9.28	14	0.813	**1.00**	**1.00**	**0.00**	[0.00,0.04]	**0.03**
	Spanish	57.87	14	<0.001	**0.99**	**0.99**	0.11	[0.08,0.14]	**0.06**
PHQ-9	Dutch	54.56	27	0.001	**1.00**	**1.00**	**0.04**	[0.03,0.06]	**0.05**
	English	46.62	27	0.011	**1.00**	**0.99**	**0.06**	[0.03,0.09]	**0.07**
	Finnish	54.38	27	0.001	**0.99**	**0.99**	0.07	[0.04,0.10]	0.08
	Italian	17.65	27	0.914	**1.00**	**1.00**	**0.00**	[0.00,0.02]	**0.04**
	Norwegian	18.63	27	0.883	**1.00**	**1.00**	**0.00**	[0.00,0.02]	**0.04**
	Spanish	42.95	27	0.026	**1.00**	**1.00**	**0.05**	[0.02,0.08]	**0.06**
PCL-5	Dutch *	264.37	164	<0.001	**1.00**	**1.00**	**0.03**	[0.03,0.04]	**0.05**
	English	241.20	164	<0.001	**1.00**	**1.00**	**0.05**	[0.03,0.06]	**0.07**
	Finnish *	NA	NA	NA	NA	NA	NA	NA	NA
	Italian *	305.80	164	<0.001	**1.00**	**1.00**	**0.06**	[0.05,0.07]	**0.07**
	Norwegian	201.45	164	0.025	**1.00**	**1.00**	**0.03**	[0.01,0.04]	**0.06**
	Spanish *	373.92	164	<0.001	**0.99**	**0.99**	0.07	[0.06,0.08]	**0.07**
RPQ	Dutch *	786.30	104	<0.001	**0.99**	**0.99**	0.11	[0.10,0.11]	0.08
	English	345.83	104	<0.001	**0.99**	**0.98**	0.10	[0.09,0.12]	0.09
	Finnish *	280.16	104	<0.001	**0.99**	**0.99**	0.09	[0.08,0.10]	0.09
	Italian *	429.59	104	<0.001	**0.98**	**0.98**	0.11	[0.10,0.12]	0.09
	Norwegian	230.42	104	<0.001	**0.99**	**0.99**	0.07	[0.06,0.08]	0.08
	Spanish *	285.93	104	<0.001	**0.98**	**0.98**	0.08	[0.07,0.10]	0.09
QOLIBRI	Dutch	1299.37	614	<0.001	**1.00**	**1.00**	**0.05**	[0.04,0.05]	**0.05**
	English	NA	NA	NA	NA	NA	NA	NA	NA
	Finnish	NA	NA	NA	NA	NA	NA	NA	NA
	Italian	932.84	614	<0.001	**1.00**	**1.00**	**0.05**	[0.04,0.05]	**0.05**
	Norwegian	793.74	614	<0.001	**1.00**	**1.00**	**0.04**	[0.03,0.04]	**0.06**
	Spanish	889.15	614	<0.001	**1.00**	**1.00**	**0.04**	[0.04,0.05]	**0.06**
QOLIBRI-OS	Dutch	37.15	9	<0.001	**1.00**	**1.00**	0.07	[0.05,0.10]	**0.03**
	English	15.22	9	0.085	**1.00**	**1.00**	**0.05**	[0.00,0.10]	**0.04**
	Finnish	11.17	9	0.264	**1.00**	**1.00**	**0.03**	[0.00,0.09]	**0.03**
	Italian	32.07	9	<0.001	**1.00**	**1.00**	0.10	[0.06,0.13]	**0.04**
	Norwegian	10.39	9	0.320	**1.00**	**1.00**	**0.03**	[0.00,0.08]	**0.02**
	Spanish	32.14	9	<0.001	**1.00**	**0.99**	0.10	[0.06,0.14]	**0.04**
SF-36v2	Dutch	2552.88	551	<0.001	**0.99**	**0.99**	0.08	[0.08,0.08]	**0.07**
	English	1239.59	551	<0.001	**0.99**	**0.99**	0.08	[0.07,0.08]	0.09
	Finnish	NA	NA	NA	NA	NA	NA	NA	NA
	Italian	NA	NA	NA	NA	NA	NA	NA	NA
	Norwegian	1300.94	551	<0.001	**1.00**	**0.99**	0.07	[0.07,0.08]	0.09
	Spanish	NA	NA	NA	NA	NA	NA	NA	NA
SF-12v2	Dutch	295.82	53	<0.001	**0.99**	**0.98**	0.14	[0.13,0.16]	0.09
	Finnish	162.88	53	<0.001	**0.99**	**0.99**	0.11	[0.09,0.13]	0.08
	Spanish	113.38	53	<0.001	**1.00**	**1.00**	0.07	[0.06,0.09]	**0.06**

Note. * Instrument translated and linguistically validated for the CENTER-TBI study; χ^2 = Chi-square statistic, df = degrees of freedom, p = p-value, CFI = comparative fit index, TLI = Tucker–Lewis index, RMSEA = root mean square error of approximation; 95% CI = 95% confidence interval (lower and upper bound); SRMR = standardized root mean square residual; values in bold indicate satisfactory results according to the respective cut-off values. NA means that the respective model did not converge; no models were estimated for the English, French, German, Italian, Norwegian, and the Swedish SF12-v2 due to the sample size being too small (N < 150).

GAD-7. Except for the χ^2 statistic and the RMSEA in the Dutch (χ^2 only), English, Italian, and Spanish samples, the fit indices demonstrated that the data fitted the one-factor model well across the languages. The item loadings were above 0.50 (0.68 to 0.96) indicating that all items measured a unidimensional construct across the languages.

PHQ-9. Almost all indices exhibited a satisfactory model fit across the languages except for the χ^2 statistic in the Dutch and Finnish translations and RMSEA and SRMR in the Finnish translation. The item loadings were above 0.50 (0.58 to 0.94) across all languages. Overall, the one-factor solution was acceptable.

PCL-5. Almost all fit measures exhibited a satisfactory model fit. The χ^2 test of all translations was significant and the RMSEA of the Spanish translation was above the cut-off value. The model for the Finnish sample did not converge. Average item loadings on the scale (DSM-cluster) level were above 0.70 (B—*Intrusion*: 0.84 to 0.91; C—*Avoidance*: 0.88 to 0.91; D—*Negative alterations*: 0.75 to 0.81; E—*Hyperarousal*: 0.73 to 0.79) denoting an appropriate fit of the four-factor structure of the PCL-5 across all countries. However, the loadings of the item "Trouble remembering important parts" in the English (0.49) and Norwegian (0.38) translations were below the cut-off of 0.50.

RPQ. All RPQ translations revealed significant χ^2 statistics and the RMSEA and SRMR values (except for the Dutch and Norwegian versions) were above the respective cut-offs. The factor loadings varied from 0.41 to 0.92. The item "Headaches" of the Finnish RPQ and the item "Double Vision" of the Norwegian RPQ reached values below the cut-off. Overall, the one-factor solution demonstrated a rather poor fit.

QOLIBRI. All but two (the English and Finnish) QOLIBRI translations had satisfactory fit indices, except for the χ^2 statistic, which was significant across all translations. The English and Finnish models did not converge. The item loadings of the scales were above 0.70 (*Cognition*: 0.74 to 0.92; *Self*: 0.75 to 0.93; *Daily Life and Autonomy*: 0.76 to 0.96; *Social*: 0.65 to 0.92; *Emotions*: 0.63 to 0.97; *Physical*: 0.59 to 0.92). Overall, the original five-factor structure fitted the data well.

QOLIBRI-OS. For the most part, the CFA results of the QOLIBRI-OS translations displayed acceptable fit indices, with the RMSEA values of the Dutch, Italian, and Spanish translations slightly above the cut-off value and significant χ^2 statistics. All other indices were within acceptable ranges. The factor loadings ranged from 0.73 to 0.92 indicating the unidimensionality of the TBI-specific HRQoL construct across the QOLIBRI-OS translations.

SF-36v2. Two out of six models did not converge (Finnish and Italian). The CFI and the TLI of the other translations were satisfactory; nevertheless, χ^2 statistics were significant, and the RMSEA and the SRMR (except for the Dutch translation) were above the respective cut-off values. All factor loadings on the scale level were above 0.50; one item of the Dutch version of the SF-36v2 ("Walking several hundred yards") was exceedingly highly correlated with the *Physical Functioning* scale and therefore also with the PCS (r = 1.0). Overall, the factorial structure of the SF-36v2 with eight scales and two second-order factors did not show evidence of a good fit.

SF-12v2. The models displayed satisfactory CFI and TLI values across all languages as well as the SRMR of the Spanish translation. The χ^2 statistics were significant and the RMSEA and SRMR were above permissible cut-off values. The item loadings of the PCS ranged from 0.69 to 0.97 and of the MCS from 0.67 to 0.95.

4. Discussion

The present study examined psychometric properties of the eight PROMs administered in the CENTER-TBI study in individuals after TBI. Many of them were translated and linguistically validated for this study; others had not yet been psychometrically investigated in the field of TBI. Therefore, a classical test theoretical framework was applied.

The results of the reliability and validity analyses performed on the PROMs indicate that most newly translated and already existing questionnaires generally displayed satisfactory to excellent psychometric characteristics in the field of TBI and were comparable to each other as well as to the original English versions investigated predominantly in non-TBI samples, in individuals after TBI, or both. On the scale level, high internal consistency and scale reliability of the newly translated and already existing instruments across all languages were observed. On the item level, only very few items from a few questionnaires demonstrated irregularities, mostly in no more than one language. However, the factorial validity analyses of the original instruments revealed some difficulties in the replicating the original factorial structures, indicating a need for further investigations.

Some translations displayed problems at the item level, displaying lower correlations with the respective total scale scores: the item *"Moving or speaking so slowly that other people could have noticed"* from the Swedish PHQ-9, the items *"Nausea"* in the Swedish and the German RPQ and *"Double Vision"* in the German RPQ, and the item *"How bothered are you by feeling angry or aggressive"* from the German QOLIBRI. Item–total correlations are directly related to the factorial structure of a questionnaire; therefore, low correlations may indicate that the questionnaire does not measure unidimensionally. The QOLIBRI consists of five scales; thus, the low correlation of the item *"How bothered are you by feeling angry or aggressive"* in the German translation is not problematic, as the scale level and total score level characteristics were satisfactory. Moreover, the low item–total correlations of the RPQ translations are not unexpected, as the questionnaire underwent several revisions regarding the scoring by different authors [30,72,73], whereby the items *"Nausea"* and *"Double Vision"* were assigned to different domains. Nevertheless, the low correlation of the item *"Moving or speaking so slowly that other people could have noticed"* in the Swedish PHQ-9 is more difficult to explain, as the PHQ-9 is a unidimensional measure. Problems with the wording might be a possible explanation, or more likely the composition of the respective language sample. The Swedish sample contained the most severely impaired patients (GCS), with the lowest functional level of recovery (GOSE) and the highest injury severity score (AIS). Thus, individuals in the Swedish sample seem to be more severely injured compared to other language samples. Therefore, the low correlation of this PHQ-9 item may be attributable to the particularities of the Swedish sample. Future research could review the wording of this item and examine the Swedish PHQ-9 in a broader spectrum of TBI severities.

Additionally, one item from the PCL-5 (*"Trouble remembering important parts of the stressful experience"*) did not distinguish well between low and high levels of PTSD across all languages and displayed low correlations with the scale score (i.e., DSM-5 cluster) in French, Norwegian, and Swedish translations. The factorial structure of the original PCL-5 has been examined on several occasions [74,75], whereby this item was re-assigned to different dimensions. The results of the present study indicate that PCL-5 translations have adopted the methodological problem of the original questionnaire version. Thus, further investigation of the factorial structure of the PCL-5 could lead to an amelioration of the questionnaire's psychometric characteristics.

As expected, the validity inspection of the PROMs (newly translated and available prior to the CENTER-TBI study) indicated medium to strong correlations with the SF-36v2, the SF-12v2, and the GOSE in most languages. The PCS and MCS of the SF-36v2 and SF-12v2 generally demonstrated negatively medium to strong negative correlations with the GAD-7, PHQ-9, PCL-5, and RPQ. One exception was the GAD-7, which revealed a low correlation with the PCS of the SF-36v2 in English and Swedish and the PCS of the SF-12v2 in six out of nine languages (Dutch, English, French, Italian, Norwegian, and Swedish). This might be attributable to the items of the SF-12v2 constituting the PCS in the original version. While the items of the SF-36v2 cover a wider range of physical activities and activity-related problems, the items of the SF-12v2 focus on a limited number of physical problems that are most probably associated less with anxiety. Nevertheless, the results are generally in line with previous findings suggesting that negative emotions (i.e., anxiety, depression, or stress) are highly correlated with generic HRQoL, especially with the MCS [76,77]. Moreover, the assumption that the mental and physical components of the SF-36v2 and the SF-12v2 would have strong positive correlations with the QOLIBRI and the QOLIBRI-OS was affirmed across all languages, supporting results from previous studies [34,78].

Generally, the GAD-7 (except for the German language sample), the PHQ-9, the PCL-5 (except for the German language sample), and the RPQ exhibited medium to strong negative correlations with the GOSE. The German individuals after TBI had a relatively high recovery rate with 50% of full recovery after six months (i.e., GOSE = 8); they suffered a less severe TBI (50% had GCS of 15) and were, consequently, less impaired, as reflected by the low correlation. These results are in line with previous research showing that the functional recovery status after TBI is frequently associated with the absence of mental health problems [79] and post-concussion symptoms [80], and vice versa. The GOSE also revealed medium to strong positive correlations with the QOLIBRI and QOLIBRI-OS across all languages, indicating that higher disease-specific HRQoL is associated with better functional outcomes, which is in line with previous research findings [34,38,81].

Further, the TBI severity as assessed by the GCS rating the degree of consciousness displayed a low association with both the psychological and health-related PROMs in almost all languages except for the Swedish translations of the PHQ-9, the RPQ, the QOLIBRI, and the QOLIBRI-OS. Previously published validity results in the field of TBI [59] found no association between GCS and psychological outcomes and post-concussion symptoms. These populations contained a lower number of more severely injured individuals, as measured by the ISS, and therefore, smaller or no correlations were found. In the Swedish translations, the higher association of the GCS and the outcomes in the Swedish sample might be explained by the higher injury severity and stronger polytrauma of the participants.

Overall, the original factorial structures suggested by the instrument developers were replicated for the GAD-7, the PHQ-9, and the QOLIBRI-OS. The translations of the PCL-5 displayed an acceptable model fit, indicating that the initial factorial structure describes the data well. Nevertheless, we recommend a further investigation of the item *"Trouble remembering important parts of the stressful experience"* which displayed irregularities in both reliability analyses across all languages and the factor loadings of the CFA in some translations. The five-factor structure of the original QOLIBRI was replicated in all but two language samples; the English and Finnish models did not converge. This could be due to several reasons: extreme response categories rarely chosen by the participants, relatively large number of parameters that must be estimated in relation to the sample size, or (unconsidered) correlations between latent factors [61].

The original factor solutions could not be replicated for the RPQ translations; this is in line with previous research findings, as several factor solutions have been proposed for the RPQ [30,31,72,73]. Since the RPQ has primarily been developed for TBI populations, further investigation of the factorial structure and thus implementation of an appropriate scoring are strongly recommended.

The SF-36v2 (except for the Dutch version showing an acceptable model fit) and the SF-12v2 presented a poor model fit. Neither of these instruments were specifically developed for populations after TBI, and they use a wide range of different response scales formats, which might be confusing and tiring, especially for respondents with cognitive deficits, and affect their response behavior [82] resulting in less good fit of the estimated models [83,84]. For the assessment of generic HRQoL in TBI populations, further investigation of the factorial structure of both PROMs seems appropriate.

Objectivity. The layout and instructions for administering the newly translated PROMs were internationally harmonized and are therefore similar across all language versions. Moreover, instructions for the assessment, scoring, and interpretation were provided (see the SOPs of the CENTER-TBI study). For the interpretation of results, general population-based norms or reference values are helpful. For example, for the QOLIBRI, population-based reference values for the UK and the Netherlands have recently been made available [35].

Strengths and limitations of the study. The main strength of the present study is the broad overview of the psychometric properties of the various previous and newly translated and linguistically validated PROMs in the TBI field [20], which had not yet been carried out.

The psychometric results allow researchers and clinicians to rate the quality of the translated questionnaires before selecting them for national and international studies and clinical practice to evaluate outcomes after TBI.

Because of the small sample sizes in some languages, further modern test theoretical analyses cannot be reported here. Additional research concerning the assumption of measurement invariance (MI) across languages could increase the quality of the instruments even further with respect to the international administration and pooling of international data. MI analysis evaluates whether the same construct is understood and measured across different languages. Some of our recent studies have already shown that the PHQ-9 and GAD-7 [85], QOLIBRI [35], and QOLIBRI-OS [39] applied in the field of TBI measure one and the same construct across languages. Furthermore, follow-up studies will focus on assessing measurement invariance comparisons of the different constructs in the individual PROMs in the different languages and the sensitivity and responsiveness of the PROMs for different patient groups and risk factors.

The present study also has some limitations. Despite the large number of participants in the CENTER-TBI core study, the psychometric properties of some translations could not be examined because of the limited number of participants. Consequently, the Danish, Hebrew, Hungarian, Latvian, Lithuanian, Romanian, and Serbian translations of the PROMs need further investigation with a larger number of patients. Furthermore, given the range of TBI severity (mild to severe) covered, we observed that even six months after TBI, participants with higher TBI severity with and without extracranial injuries and polytrauma were not always able to complete the PROMs. To provide robust psychometric analyses in more severe patient groups, future assessments should be also conducted at later time points.

5. Conclusions

This study provides psychometric characteristics of the PROMs administered in the CENTER-TBI study for individuals after TBI. The psychometric properties of these PROMs are satisfactory to excellent on the scale level in nine European languages. These results highlight the value of a rigid process of translation and linguistic and cultural adaptation of questionnaires that goes far beyond a literal translation and that ensures the cultural comparability of the translated versions. Therefore, researchers and clinicians can now select reliable and valid instruments for clinical use, data collection, and aggregation, when evaluating outcomes after TBI in international studies, thus improving outcome assessment in national and international healthcare.

Supplementary Materials: The following materials are available online at https://www.mdpi.com/article/10.3390/jcm10112396/s1. List of the CENTER-TBI participants and investigators; Online Supplement 1 (OS-1: Sociodemographic characteristics); Online Supplement 2 (OS-2: Reliability); Online Supplement 3 (OS-3: Factorial validity), Online Supplement 4 (OS-4: Participants and Investigators).

Author Contributions: Conceptualization: N.v.S., Y.-J.W. and M.Z.; formal analysis: F.B., Y.-J.W. and M.Z.; funding acquisition: N.v.S., S.P., A.I.R.M. and D.M.; methodology: N.v.S., Y.-J.W. and M.Z.; project administration: N.v.S.; software: F.B., Y.-J.W. and M.Z.; supervision: N.v.S., A.I.R.M. and D.M.; visualization: M.Z., writing—original draft: N.v.S., K.R., U.K., Y.-J.W. and M.Z.; writing—review and editing: N.v.S., K.R., F.B., A.C., U.K., A.M.P., K.C., S.P., L.W., E.W.S., A.I.R.M., D.M., Y.-J.W. and M.Z. All authors have read and agreed to the published version of the manuscript.

Funding: CENTER-TBI was supported by the European Union 7th Framework programme (EC grant 602150). Additional funding was obtained from the Hannelore Kohl Stiftung (Germany), from OneMind (USA), and from Integra LifeSciences Corporation (USA). The funders of the study had no role in study design, data collection, data analysis, data interpretation, or writing of the report.

Institutional Review Board Statement: The CENTER-TBI study (EC grant 602150) has been conducted in accordance with all relevant laws of the European Union (EU) if directly applicable or of direct effect and all relevant laws of the country where the recruiting sites were located. Informed consent by the patients and/or the legal representative/next of kin was obtained, accordingly to the local legislations, for all patients recruited in the Core Dataset of CENTER-TBI and documented in the electronic case report form (e-CRF). For the full list of sites, ethical committees, and ethical approval details, see the official CENTER-TBI website (https://www.center-tbi.eu/project/ethical-approval).

Informed Consent Statement: Informed consent was obtained from all subjects involved in the study.

Data Availability Statement: All relevant data are available upon request from CENTER-TBI, and the authors are not legally allowed to share it publicly. The authors confirm that they received no special access privileges to the data. CENTER-TBI is committed to data sharing and in particular to responsible further use of the data. Hereto, we have a data sharing statement in place: https://www.center-tbi.eu/data/sharing. The CENTER-TBI Management Committee, in collaboration with the General Assembly, established the Data Sharing policy, and Publication and Authorship Guidelines to assure correct and appropriate use of the data as the dataset is hugely complex and requires help of experts from the Data Curation Team or Bio- Statistical Team for correct use. This means that we encourage researchers to contact the CENTER-TBI team for any research plans and the Data Curation Team for any help in appropriate use of the data, including sharing of scripts. Requests for data access can be submitted online: https://www.center-tbi.eu/data. The complete manual for data access is also available online: https://www.center-tbi.eu/files/SOP-Manual-DAPR-20181101.pdf.

Acknowledgments: We gratefully thank all CENTER-TBI participants and investigators. We are immensely grateful to our patients with TBI for helping us in our efforts to improve care and outcomes for TBI.

Conflicts of Interest: The authors declare no conflict of interest.

Abbreviations

GAD-7	Generalized Anxiety Disorder 7 Item Scale
HRQoL	Health-related quality of life
PHQ-9	Patient Health Questionnaire
PCL-5	Posttraumatic Stress Disorder Checklist-5
RPQ	Rivermead Post-Concussion Symptoms Questionnaire
QOLIBRI	Quality of Life after Traumatic Brain Injury
QOLIBRI-OS	Quality of Life after Traumatic Brain Injury—Overall Scale
SF-36v2	36-item Short Form Health Survey—Version 2
SF-12v2	12-Item Short Form Survey—Version 2
PCS	Physical component score
MCS	Mental component score
MI	Measurement invariance
PF	Physical functioning
RP	Role—Physical
GH	General Health
VT	Vitality
SF	Social functioning
RE	Role—Emotional
MH	Mental health
GOSE	Glasgow Outcome Scale—Extended
GCS	Glasgow Coma Scale

Appendix A. Number of Participants (GOSE and GCS)

Table A1. Number of participants for convergent (assessed with the GOSE) and discriminant (assessed with the GCS) validity per language and outcome instrument.

Instrument	Language	GOSE	GCS
GAD-7	Dutch	584	569
	English	213	213
	Finnish	207	199
	French	109	100
	German	78	77
	Italian	266	266
	Norwegian	253	251
	Spanish	253	251
	Swedish	60	57
PHQ-9	Dutch	587	572
	English	213	213
	Finnish	206	198
	French	107	99
	German	81	80
	Italian	265	265
	Norwegian	254	252
	Spanish	253	251
	Swedish	60	57
PCL-5	Dutch	586	570
	English	212	212
	Finnish	212	204
	French	110	103
	German	76	75
	Italian	261	261
	Norwegian	248	246
	Spanish	256	254
	Swedish	57	54
RPQ	Dutch	597	582
	English	222	222
	Finnish	213	205
	French	115	107
	German	80	79
	Italian	268	268
	Norwegian	263	261
	Spanish	254	252
	Swedish	59	56
QOLIBRI	Dutch	583	568
	English	223	222
	Finnish	207	199
	French	104	96
	German	77	76
	Italian	270	271
	Norwegian	247	245
	Spanish	255	253
	Swedish	57	54
QOLIBRI-OS	Dutch	602	585
	English	238	238
	Finnish	227	219
	French	109	99
	German	84	83
	Italian	279	280
	Norwegian	261	259
	Spanish	265	263
	Swedish	63	60

Table A1. Cont.

Instrument	Language	GOSE	GCS
SF-36v2	Dutch	579	564
	English	219	218
	Finnish	214	206
	French	110	100
	German	78	77
	Italian	269	270
	Norwegian	254	252
	Spanish	255	253
	Swedish	57	54
SF-12v2 *	Dutch	241	229
	English	54	54
	Finnish	172	168
	French	30	27
	German	68	67
	Italian	138	138
	Norwegian	32	32
	Spanish	210	209
	Swedish	15	12
SF-12v2 combined **	Dutch	605	588
	English	242	241
	Finnish	231	223
	French	110	100
	German	82	81
	Italian	275	276
	Norwegian	259	257
	Spanish	257	255
	Swedish	58	55

Note. * Reported SF-12v2 values used for the reliability analyses. ** Combined SF-12v2 values (i.e., reported values and derived from the respective items of the SF-36v2) were used for the convergent and divergent validity analyses; **bold** values represent samples with $N \geq 50$.

Appendix B. Validity on Scale Level

Table A2. Convergent and discriminant validity of the PCL-5 scales.

Cluster	Language/Value	Convergent Validity				Discriminant Validity	
		SF-36v2 PCS	SF-36v2 MCS	SF-12v2 PCS	SF-12v2 MCS	GOSE	GCS
B	Dutch	−0.33	−0.46	−0.32	−0.45	−0.29	−0.15
	English	−0.24	−0.47	−0.24	−0.43	−0.18	−0.03
	Finnish	−0.38	−0.43	−0.33	−0.39	−0.27	−0.09
	French	−0.24	−0.43	−0.18	−0.44	−0.21	0.02
	German	−0.28	−0.61	−0.20	−0.47	0.02	0.26
	Italian	−0.30	−0.57	−0.27	−0.53	−0.24	0.13
	Norwegian	−0.33	−0.49	−0.29	−0.49	−0.27	−0.04
	Spanish	−0.25	−0.40	−0.24	−0.33	−0.28	0.03
	Swedish	−0.20	−0.27	−0.26	−0.19	−0.35	−0.13
Total	M	−0.28	−0.46	−0.26	−0.41	−0.23	0.00
	Max	−0.20	−0.27	−0.18	−0.19	0.02	0.26
	Min	−0.38	−0.61	−0.33	−0.53	−0.35	−0.15
	SD	0.06	0.10	0.05	0.10	0.11	0.13

Table A2. Cont.

Cluster	Language/Value	Convergent Validity				Discriminant Validity	
		SF-36v2 PCS	SF-36v2 MCS	SF-12v2 PCS	SF-12v2 MCS	GOSE	GCS
C	Dutch	−0.26	**−0.36**	−0.23	**−0.37**	−0.23	−0.09
	English	−0.18	**−0.38**	−0.19	**−0.34**	−0.12	0.00
	Finnish	−0.27	**−0.42**	−0.26	**−0.39**	−0.28	−0.14
	French	−0.13	**−0.45**	−0.11	**−0.39**	−0.10	0.10
	German	−0.27	**−0.48**	−0.21	**−0.42**	−0.03	0.26
	Italian	−0.19	**−0.48**	−0.17	**−0.46**	−0.15	0.09
	Norwegian	−0.23	**−0.38**	−0.20	**−0.38**	−0.21	−0.03
	Spanish	−0.21	−0.29	−0.17	−0.28	−0.20	0.01
	Swedish	−0.26	−0.24	−0.26	−0.15	−0.26	−0.03
Total	M	−0.22	−0.39	−0.20	−0.35	−0.18	0.02
	Max	−0.13	−0.24	−0.11	−0.15	−0.03	0.26
	Min	−0.27	−0.48	−0.26	−0.46	−0.28	−0.14
	SD	0.05	0.08	0.05	0.09	0.08	0.12
D	Dutch	**−0.33**	**−0.57**	**−0.31**	**−0.57**	**−0.41**	−0.22
	English	−0.22	**−0.67**	−0.21	**−0.62**	**−0.45**	−0.19
	Finnish	−0.24	**−0.59**	−0.26	**−0.57**	**−0.46**	−0.18
	French	−0.20	**−0.61**	−0.15	**−0.57**	−0.29	−0.12
	German	**−0.39**	**−0.60**	**−0.33**	**−0.56**	−0.17	0.14
	Italian	**−0.32**	**−0.68**	−0.28	**−0.65**	**−0.34**	−0.01
	Norwegian	**−0.39**	**−0.57**	**−0.34**	**−0.56**	**−0.41**	−0.06
	Spanish	−0.29	**−0.58**	**−0.30**	**−0.54**	**−0.49**	−0.20
	Swedish	−0.25	**−0.51**	−0.29	**−0.44**	**−0.45**	−0.28
Total	M	−0.29	−0.60	−0.27	−0.56	−0.39	−0.12
	Max	−0.20	−0.51	−0.15	−0.44	−0.17	0.14
	Min	−0.39	−0.68	−0.34	−0.65	−0.49	−0.28
	SD	0.07	0.05	0.06	0.06	0.10	0.13
E	Dutch	**−0.37**	**−0.61**	**−0.34**	**−0.60**	**−0.43**	−0.17
	English	−0.28	**−0.67**	−0.29	**−0.64**	**−0.36**	−0.09
	Finnish	**−0.42**	**−0.61**	**−0.43**	**−0.55**	**−0.44**	−0.20
	French	−0.25	**−0.70**	−0.21	**−0.66**	**−0.35**	−0.07
	German	**−0.47**	**−0.60**	**−0.42**	**−0.60**	−0.22	0.11
	Italian	**−0.33**	**−0.69**	−0.29	**−0.65**	−0.29	0.12
	Norwegian	**−0.36**	**−0.64**	**−0.31**	**−0.63**	**−0.37**	0.00
	Spanish	**−0.32**	**−0.63**	**−0.33**	**−0.59**	**−0.36**	−0.03
	Swedish	−0.20	**−0.51**	**−0.30**	**−0.48**	**−0.42**	−0.20
Total	M	−0.33	−0.63	−0.32	−0.60	−0.36	−0.06
	Max	−0.20	−0.51	−0.21	−0.48	−0.22	0.12
	Min	−0.47	−0.70	−0.43	−0.66	−0.44	−0.20
	SD	0.08	0.06	0.07	0.06	0.07	0.12

Note. Cluster B = Intrusion; Cluster C = Avoidance; Cluster D = Negative alterations in cognition and mood; Cluster E = Hyperarousal; M = mean, Max = maximum, Min = minimum; SD = standard deviation; SF-36v2/SF-12v2—PCS = Physical Component Score; SF-36v2/SF-12v2—MCS = Mental Component Score; GCS = Glasgow Coma Scale; GOSE = Glasgow Outcome Scale—Extended. Values in **bold** represent an at least medium effect size ($\geq |0.30|$), significant at $\alpha = 0.05$.

Table A3. Convergent and divergent validity of the QOLIBRI scales.

Scale	Language/Values	Convergent Validity				Discriminant Validity	
		SF-36v2 PCS	SF-36v2 MCS	SF-12v2 PCS	SF-12v2 MCS	GOSE	GCS
Cognition	Dutch	0.40	0.58	0.38	0.57	0.43	0.21
	English	0.34	0.61	0.37	0.58	0.43	0.20
	Finnish	0.49	0.69	0.49	0.62	0.50	0.07
	French	0.33	0.58	0.34	0.59	0.48	0.10
	German	0.46	0.53	0.39	0.52	0.26	−0.05
	Italian	0.44	0.61	0.46	0.58	0.40	0.02
	Norwegian	0.42	0.54	0.41	0.52	0.34	−0.06
	Spanish	0.41	0.52	0.43	0.49	0.33	0.07
	Swedish	0.33	0.42	0.41	0.40	0.44	0.21
	M	0.40	0.56	0.41	0.54	0.40	0.09
	Max	0.49	0.69	0.49	0.62	0.50	0.21
	Min	0.33	0.42	0.34	0.40	0.26	−0.06
	SD	0.06	0.07	0.05	0.07	0.08	0.11
Self	Dutch	0.51	0.66	0.50	0.66	0.43	0.19
	English	0.38	0.72	0.40	0.70	0.45	0.09
	Finnish	0.50	0.78	0.52	0.69	0.50	0.04
	French	0.49	0.73	0.42	0.71	0.46	0.07
	German	0.49	0.70	0.41	0.71	0.29	−0.15
	Italian	0.51	0.70	0.51	0.68	0.43	−0.07
	Norwegian	0.45	0.68	0.43	0.65	0.35	−0.07
	Spanish	0.57	0.61	0.61	0.59	0.46	0.13
	Swedish	0.43	0.74	0.40	0.72	0.43	0.06
	M	0.48	0.70	0.47	0.68	0.42	0.03
	Max	0.57	0.78	0.61	0.72	0.50	0.19
	Min	0.38	0.61	0.40	0.59	0.29	−0.15
	SD	0.05	0.05	0.07	0.04	0.06	0.11
Daily Life and Autonomy	Dutch	0.61	0.59	0.61	0.58	0.56	0.31
	English	0.58	0.56	0.59	0.54	0.63	0.30
	Finnish	0.63	0.65	0.61	0.58	0.55	0.14
	French	0.62	0.69	0.58	0.66	0.59	0.18
	German	0.63	0.58	0.55	0.58	0.41	0.06
	Italian	0.64	0.65	0.64	0.61	0.62	0.15
	Norwegian	0.50	0.64	0.49	0.62	0.48	0.05
	Spanish	0.70	0.48	0.69	0.46	0.54	0.21
	Swedish	0.62	0.58	0.64	0.54	0.66	0.39
	M	0.61	0.60	0.60	0.57	0.56	0.20
	Max	0.70	0.69	0.69	0.66	0.66	0.39
	Min	0.50	0.48	0.49	0.46	0.41	0.05
	SD	0.05	0.06	0.06	0.06	0.08	0.12
Social Relationships	Dutch	0.29	0.57	0.30	0.55	0.29	0.12
	English	0.29	0.63	0.33	0.57	0.34	0.06
	Finnish	0.34	0.71	0.37	0.59	0.33	0.10
	French	0.35	0.61	0.32	0.58	0.33	0.01
	German	0.36	0.56	0.31	0.51	0.11	−0.12
	Italian	0.30	0.57	0.30	0.55	0.28	−0.15
	Norwegian	0.23	0.50	0.21	0.48	0.15	−0.11
	Spanish	0.34	0.52	0.35	0.51	0.31	0.11
	Swedish	0.22	0.47	0.21	0.44	0.22	0.24
	M	0.30	0.57	0.30	0.53	0.26	0.03
	Max	0.36	0.71	0.37	0.59	0.34	0.24
	Min	0.22	0.47	0.21	0.44	0.11	−0.15
	SD	0.05	0.07	0.06	0.05	0.08	0.13

Table A3. Cont.

Scale	Language/Values	SF-36v2 PCS	SF-36v2 MCS	SF-12v2 PCS	SF-12v2 MCS	GOSE	GCS
			Convergent Validity			Discriminant Validity	
Emotions	Dutch	0.33	**0.71**	0.29	**0.71**	**0.36**	0.12
	English	0.20	**0.69**	0.20	**0.66**	**0.46**	0.09
	Finnish	**0.31**	**0.70**	**0.30**	**0.65**	**0.39**	0.11
	French	0.26	**0.71**	0.19	**0.68**	0.29	0.00
	German	0.28	**0.64**	0.23	**0.63**	0.09	−0.20
	Italian	0.23	**0.58**	0.22	**0.56**	0.21	−0.10
	Norwegian	**0.34**	**0.73**	0.27	**0.72**	**0.30**	−0.02
	Spanish	0.26	**0.44**	0.24	**0.43**	0.28	0.04
	Swedish	0.17	**0.67**	0.23	**0.61**	**0.45**	0.24
	M	0.26	0.65	0.24	0.63	0.31	0.03
	Max	0.34	0.73	0.30	0.72	0.46	0.24
	Min	0.17	0.44	0.19	0.43	0.09	−0.20
	SD	0.06	0.09	0.04	0.09	0.12	0.13
Physical	Dutch	**0.70**	**0.48**	**0.66**	**0.47**	**0.53**	0.14
	English	**0.64**	**0.44**	**0.65**	**0.45**	**0.57**	0.28
	Finnish	**0.66**	**0.44**	**0.62**	**0.43**	**0.58**	0.19
	French	**0.72**	**0.48**	**0.65**	**0.48**	**0.43**	0.07
	German	**0.73**	**0.35**	**0.69**	**0.42**	**0.56**	−0.04
	Italian	**0.56**	**0.55**	**0.55**	**0.54**	**0.47**	0.04
	Norwegian	**0.70**	**0.54**	**0.67**	**0.52**	**0.57**	0.14
	Spanish	**0.68**	**0.45**	**0.64**	**0.42**	**0.58**	0.12
	Swedish	**0.67**	0.26	**0.67**	0.19	**0.61**	**0.36**
	M	0.67	0.44	0.64	0.44	0.54	0.15
	Max	0.73	0.55	0.69	0.54	0.61	0.36
	Min	0.56	0.26	0.55	0.19	0.43	−0.04
	SD	0.05	0.09	0.04	0.10	0.06	0.12

Note. M = mean, Max = maximum, Min = minimum; SD = standard deviation; SF-36v2/SF-12v2—PCS = Physical Component Score; SF-36v2/SF-12v2—MCS = Mental Component Score; GCS = Glasgow Coma Scale; GOSE = Glasgow Outcome Scale—Extended. Values in **bold** represent an at least medium effect size ($\geq |0.30|$), significant at $\alpha = 0.05$.

Table A4. Convergent and divergent validity of the SF-36v2 scales.

Scale	Language/Value	Convergent Validity	Discriminant Validity
		GOSE	GCS
PF	Dutch	**0.45**	0.12
	English	**0.54**	0.22
	Finnish	**0.49**	0.08
	French	**0.36**	0.07
	German	**0.37**	−0.07
	Italian	**0.61**	0.13
	Norwegian	**0.52**	0.24
	Spanish	**0.52**	0.20
	Swedish	**0.43**	0.20
Total	M	0.48	0.13
	Max	0.61	0.24
	Min	0.36	−0.07
	SD	0.08	0.10

Table A4. Cont.

Scale	Language/Value	Convergent Validity GOSE	Discriminant Validity GCS
RP	Dutch	0.63	0.26
	English	0.67	0.34
	Finnish	0.58	0.19
	French	0.48	0.24
	German	0.24	0.06
	Italian	0.67	0.22
	Norwegian	0.61	0.24
	Spanish	0.60	0.22
	Swedish	0.64	0.41
Total	M	0.57	0.24
	Max	0.67	0.41
	Min	0.24	0.06
	SD	0.14	0.10
BP	Dutch	0.39	0.00
	English	0.32	0.04
	Finnish	0.36	−0.04
	French	0.26	0.06
	German	0.43	−0.08
	Italian	0.37	0.04
	Norwegian	0.27	−0.06
	Spanish	0.44	0.08
	Swedish	0.24	0.12
Total	M	0.34	0.02
	Max	0.44	0.12
	Min	0.24	−0.08
	SD	0.07	0.07
GH	Dutch	0.33	0.06
	English	0.36	0.11
	Finnish	0.50	0.03
	French	0.39	0.10
	German	0.26	0.00
	Italian	0.42	−0.02
	Norwegian	0.39	−0.03
	Spanish	0.42	0.10
	Swedish	0.38	0.20
Total	M	0.38	0.06
	Max	0.50	0.20
	Min	0.26	−0.03
	SD	0.07	0.08
VT	Dutch	0.45	0.16
	English	0.43	0.06
	Finnish	0.52	0.02
	French	0.37	0.08
	German	0.23	−0.08
	Italian	0.43	0.03
	Norwegian	0.35	−0.03
	Spanish	0.38	0.06
	Swedish	0.47	0.15
Total	M	0.40	0.05
	Max	0.52	0.16
	Min	0.23	−0.08
	SD	0.08	0.08

Table A4. Cont.

Scale	Language/Value	Convergent Validity GOSE	Discriminant Validity GCS
SF	Dutch	0.55	0.21
	English	0.61	0.25
	Finnish	0.53	0.14
	French	0.49	0.21
	German	0.24	−0.03
	Italian	0.57	0.13
	Norwegian	0.57	0.14
	Spanish	0.54	0.24
	Swedish	0.50	0.13
Total	M	0.51	0.16
	Max	0.61	0.25
	Min	0.24	−0.03
	SD	0.11	0.09
RE	Dutch	0.43	0.20
	English	0.46	0.11
	Finnish	0.47	0.11
	French	0.37	0.24
	German	0.13	−0.05
	Italian	0.52	0.13
	Norwegian	0.37	0.07
	Spanish	0.48	0.12
	Swedish	0.46	0.19
Total	M	0.41	0.12
	Max	0.52	0.24
	Min	0.13	−0.05
	SD	0.12	0.08
MH	Dutch	0.38	0.12
	English	0.33	0.04
	Finnish	0.44	0.12
	French	0.34	−0.04
	German	0.14	−0.07
	Italian	0.30	−0.12
	Norwegian	0.31	−0.09
	Spanish	0.37	0.10
	Swedish	0.50	0.10
Total	M	0.35	0.02
	Max	0.50	0.12
	Min	0.14	−0.12
	SD	0.10	0.10
PCS	Dutch	0.49	0.11
	English	0.52	0.22
	Finnish	0.51	0.06
	French	0.37	0.14
	German	0.38	−0.03
	Italian	0.60	0.17
	Norwegian	0.53	0.18
	Spanish	0.53	0.17
	Swedish	0.46	0.30
Total	M	0.49	0.15
	Max	0.60	0.30
	Min	0.37	−0.03
	SD	0.07	0.09

Table A4. Cont.

		Convergent Validity	Discriminant Validity
Scale	Language/Value	GOSE	GCS
MCS	Dutch	**0.40**	0.19
	English	**0.42**	0.10
	Finnish	**0.46**	0.11
	French	**0.39**	0.15
	German	0.07	−0.10
	Italian	**0.37**	0.00
	Norwegian	**0.35**	−0.04
	Spanish	**0.37**	0.10
	Swedish	**0.50**	0.14
Total	M	0.37	0.07
	Max	0.50	0.19
	Min	0.07	−0.10
	SD	0.12	0.10

Note. M = mean, Max = maximum, Min = minimum; SD = standard deviation; PF = Physical functioning; BP = Bodily Pain; GH = General Health; VT = Vitality; SF = Social Functioning; RE = Role-Emotional; MH = Mental Health; PCS = Physical Component Score; MCS = Mental Component Score; GCS = Glasgow Coma Scale; GOSE = Glasgow Outcome Scale—Extended. No correlations with the Reported Health Transition (HT) scale reported because of the scale length (one item); values in bold represent an at least medium effect size ($\geq |0.30|$), significant at $\alpha = 0.05$.

References

1. Menon, D.K.; Schwab, K.; Wright, D.W.; Maas, A.I. Position Statement: Definition of Traumatic Brain Injury. *Arch. Phys. Med. Rehabil.* **2010**, *91*, 1637–1640. [CrossRef]
2. Verhaeghe, S.; Defloor, T.; Grypdonck, M. Stress and Coping among Families of Patients with Traumatic Brain Injury: A Review of the Literature. *J. Clin. Nurs.* **2005**, *14*, 1004–1012. [CrossRef] [PubMed]
3. Humphreys, I.; Wood, R.L.; Phillips, C. Macey. The Costs of Traumatic Brain Injury: A Literature Review. *Clin. Outcomes Res.* **2013**, *5*, 281. [CrossRef]
4. Leibson, C.L.; Brown, A.W.; Long, K.H.; Ransom, J.E.; Mandrekar, J.; Osler, T.M.; Malec, J.F. Medical Care Costs Associated with Traumatic Brain Injury over the Full Spectrum of Disease: A Controlled Population-Based Study. *J. Neurotrauma* **2012**, *29*, 2038–2049. [CrossRef]
5. Cassidy, J.D.; Carroll, L.; Peloso, P.; Borg, J.; von Holst, H.; Holm, L.; Kraus, J.; Coronado, V. Incidence, risk factors and prevention of mild traumatic brain injury: Results of the WHO collaborating centre task force on mild traumatic brain injury. *J. Rehabil. Med.* **2004**, *36*, 28–60. [CrossRef]
6. Dewan, M.C.; Rattani, A.; Gupta, S.; Baticulon, R.E.; Hung, Y.-C.; Punchak, M.; Agrawal, A.; Adeleye, A.O.; Shrime, M.G.; Rubiano, A.M.; et al. Estimating the global incidence of traumatic brain injury. *J. Neurosurg.* **2019**, *130*, 1080–1097. [CrossRef]
7. Rabinowitz, A.R.; Levin, H.S. Cognitive Sequelae of Traumatic Brain Injury. *Psychiatr. Clin. N. Am.* **2014**, *37*, 1–11. [CrossRef]
8. Bamdad, M.J.; Ryan, L.M.; Warden, D.L. Functional Assessment of Executive Abilities Following Traumatic Brain Injury. *Brain Inj.* **2003**, *17*, 1011–1020. [CrossRef]
9. Hoofien, D.; Gilboa, A.; Vakil, E.; Donovick, P.J. Traumatic Brain Injury (TBI) 10-20 Years Later: A Comprehensive Outcome Study of Psychiatric Symptomatology, Cognitive Abilities and Psychosocial Functioning. *Brain Inj.* **2001**, *15*, 189–209. [CrossRef]
10. Sasse, N.; Gibbons, H.; Wilson, L.; Martinez-Olivera, R.; Schmidt, H.; Hasselhorn, M.; von Wild, K.; von Steinbüchel, N. Self-Awareness and Health-Related Quality of Life after Traumatic Brain Injury. *J. Head Trauma Rehabil.* **2013**, *28*, 464–472. [CrossRef]
11. Rauen, K.; Reichelt, L.; Probst, P.; Schäpers, B.; Müller, F.; Jahn, K.; Plesnila, N. Quality of Life up to 10 Years after Traumatic Brain Injury: A Cross-Sectional Analysis. *Health Qual. Life Outcomes* **2020**, *18*, 166. [CrossRef]
12. Bombardier, C.H.; Fann, J.R.; Temkin, N.R.; Esselman, P.C.; Barber, J.; Dikmen, S.S. Rates of major depressive disorder and clinical outcomes following traumatic brain injury. *JAMA* **2010**, *303*, 1938–1945. [CrossRef] [PubMed]
13. Bryant, R.A.; O'Donnell, M.L.; Creamer, M.; McFarlane, A.C.; Clark, C.R.; Silove, D. The Psychiatric Sequelae of Traumatic Injury. *AJP* **2010**, *167*, 312–320. [CrossRef] [PubMed]
14. Ponsford, J.; Draper, K.; Schönberger, M. Functional Outcome 10 Years after Traumatic Brain Injury: Its Relationship with Demographic, Injury Severity, and Cognitive and Emotional Status. *J. Inter. Neuropsych. Soc.* **2008**, *14*, 233–242. [CrossRef]
15. Maas, A.I.R.; Menon, D.K.; Steyerberg, E.W.; Citerio, G.; Lecky, F.; Manley, G.T.; Hill, S.; Legrand, V.; Sorgner, A. Collaborative European NeuroTrauma Effectiveness Research in Traumatic Brain Injury (CENTER-TBI): A Prospective Longitudinal Observational Study. *Neurosurgery* **2015**, *76*, 67–80. [CrossRef]

16. Steyerberg, E.W.; Wiegers, E.; Sewalt, C.; Buki, A.; Citerio, G.; De Keyser, V.; Ercole, A.; Kunzmann, K.; Lanyon, L.; Lecky, F.; et al. Case-Mix, Care Pathways, and Outcomes in Patients with Traumatic Brain Injury in CENTER-TBI: A European Prospective, Multicentre, Longitudinal, Cohort Study. *Lancet Neurol.* **2019**, *18*, 923–934. [CrossRef]
17. Gennarelli, T.A.; Wodzin, E. AIS 2005: A Contemporary Injury Scale. *Injury* **2006**, *37*, 1083–1091. [CrossRef]
18. Acquadro, C.; Conway, K.; Hareendran, A.; Aaronson, N. Literature Review of Methods to Translate Health-Related Quality of Life Questionnaires for Use in Multinational Clinical Trials. *Value Health* **2008**, *11*, 509–521. [CrossRef]
19. Acquadro, C. *Linguistic Validation Manual for Health Outcome Assessments*; MAPI Research Institute: Lyon, France, 2012.
20. Steinbuechel, N.; Rauen, K.; Krenz, U.; Wu, Y.-J.; Covic, A.; Plass, A.M.; Cunitz, K.; Bockhop, F.; Polinder, S.; Wilson, L.; et al. Translation and linguistic validation of outcome instruments for traumatic brain injury research and clinical practice: A step-by-step approach within the observational CENTER-TBI study. *J. Clin. Med.*. Not published.
21. NINDS Common Data Elements. Available online: http://www.commondataelements.ninds.nih.gov/ (accessed on 1 February 2021).
22. Wilde, E.A.; Whiteneck, G.G.; Bogner, J.; Bushnik, T.; Cifu, D.X.; Dikmen, S.; French, L.; Giacino, J.T.; Hart, T.; Malec, J.F.; et al. Recommendations for the Use of Common Outcome Measures in Traumatic Brain Injury Research. *Arch. Phys. Med. Rehabil.* **2010**, *91*, 1650–1660.e17. [CrossRef]
23. Spitzer, R.L.; Kroenke, K.; Williams, J.B.W.; Löwe, B. A Brief Measure for Assessing Generalized Anxiety Disorder: The GAD-7. *Arch. Intern. Med.* **2006**, *166*, 1092–1097. [CrossRef]
24. Kroenke, K.; Spitzer, R.L.; Williams, J.B.W. The PHQ-9: Validity of a Brief Depression Severity Measure. *J. Gen. Intern. Med.* **2001**, *16*, 606–613. [CrossRef]
25. Kroenke, K.; Spitzer, R.L. The PHQ-9: A New Depression Diagnostic and Severity Measure. *Psychiatr. Ann.* **2002**, *32*, 509–515. [CrossRef]
26. Blevins, C.A.; Weathers, F.W.; Davis, M.T.; Witte, T.K.; Domino, J.L. The Posttraumatic Stress Disorder Checklist for DSM-5 (PCL-5): Development and Initial Psychometric Evaluation. *J. Trauma. Stress* **2015**, *28*, 489–498. [CrossRef]
27. American Psychiatric Association. *Diagnostic and Statistical Manual of Mental Disorders: DSM-5*, 5th ed.; American Psychiatric Publishing: Washington, DC, USA, 2013; ISBN 978-0-89042-555-8.
28. Ashbaugh, A.R.; Houle-Johnson, S.; Herbert, C.; El-Hage, W.; Brunet, A. Psychometric Validation of the English and French Versions of the Posttraumatic Stress Disorder Checklist for DSM-5 (PCL-5). *PLoS ONE* **2016**, *11*, e0161645. [CrossRef] [PubMed]
29. Stein, M.B.; Jain, S.; Giacino, J.T.; Levin, H.; Dikmen, S.; Nelson, L.D.; Vassar, M.J.; Okonkwo, D.O.; Diaz-Arrastia, R.; Robertson, C.S.; et al. Risk of Posttraumatic Stress Disorder and Major Depression in Civilian Patients After Mild Traumatic Brain Injury: A TRACK-TBI Study. *Jama Psychiatry* **2019**, *76*, 249. [CrossRef]
30. King, N.S.; Crawford, S.; Wenden, F.J.; Moss, N.E.; Wade, D.T. The Rivermead Post Concussion Symptoms Questionnaire: A Measure of Symptoms Commonly Experienced after Head Injury and Its Reliability. *J. Neurol.* **1995**, *242*, 587–592. [CrossRef]
31. Potter, S.; Leigh, E.; Wade, D.; Fleminger, S. The Rivermead Post Concussion Symptoms Questionnaire: A Confirmatory Factor Analysis. *J. Neurol.* **2006**, *253*, 1603–1614. [CrossRef]
32. von Steinbuechel, N.; Wilson, L.; Gibbons, H.; Hawthorne, G.; Höfer, S.; Schmidt, S.; Bullinger, M.; Maas, A.; Neugebauer, E.; Powell, J.; et al. Quality of Life after Brain Injury (QOLIBRI): Scale Development and Metric Properties. *J. Neurotrauma* **2010**, *27*, 1167–1185. [CrossRef]
33. von Steinbuechel, N.; Wilson, L.; Gibbons, H.; Hawthorne, G.; Höfer, S.; Schmidt, S.; Bullinger, M.; Maas, A.; Neugebauer, E.; Powell, J.; et al. Quality of Life after Brain Injury (QOLIBRI): Scale Validity and Correlates of Quality of Life. *J. Neurotrauma* **2010**, *27*, 1157–1165. [CrossRef] [PubMed]
34. Wilson, L.; Marsden-Loftus, I.; Koskinen, S.; Bakx, W.; Bullinger, M.; Formisano, R.; Maas, A.; Neugebauer, E.; Powell, J.; Sarajuuri, J.; et al. Interpreting Quality of Life after Brain Injury Scores: Cross-Walk with the Short Form-36. *J. Neurotrauma* **2017**, *34*, 59–65. [CrossRef]
35. Gorbunova, A.; Zeldovich, M.; Voormolen, D.C.; Krenz, U.; Polinder, S.; Haagsma, J.A.; Hagmayer, Y.; Covic, A.; Real, R.G.L.; Asendorf, T.; et al. Reference Values of the QOLIBRI from General Population Samples in the UK and The Netherlands. *JCM* **2020**, *9*, 2100. [CrossRef]
36. Siponkoski, S.; Wilson, L.; Steinbüchel, N.; Sarajuuri, J.; Koskinen, S. Quality of Life after Traumatic Brain Injury: Finnish Experience of the QOLIBRI in Residential Rehabilitation. *J. Rehabil. Med.* **2013**, *45*, 835–842. [CrossRef]
37. Castaño-León, A.M.; Navarro-Main, B.; Gomez, P.A.; Gil, A.; Soler, M.D.; Lagares, A.; Bernabeu, M.; Steinbüchel, N.; Real, R.G.L. Quality of Life After Brain Injury: Psychometric Properties of the Spanish Translation of the QoLIBRI. *Eval. Health Prof.* **2018**, *41*, 456–473. [CrossRef]
38. von Steinbuechel, N.; Wilson, L.; Gibbons, H.; Muehlan, H.; Schmidt, H.; Schmidt, S.; Sasse, N.; Koskinen, S.; Sarajuuri, J.; Höfer, S.; et al. QOLIBRI Overall Scale: A Brief Index of Health-Related Quality of Life after Traumatic Brain Injury. *J. Neurol. Neurosurg. Psychiatry* **2012**, *83*, 1041–1047. [CrossRef]
39. Wu, Y.-J.; Rauen, K.; Zeldovich, M.; Voormolen, D.C.; Gorbunova, A.; Covic, A.; Cunitz, K.; Plass, A.M.; Polinder, S.; Haagsma, J.A.; et al. Reference Values and Psychometric Properties of the Quality of Life after Traumatic Brain Injury Overall Scale in Italy, the Netherlands, and the United Kingdom. *Value Health* **2021**, in press.
40. Ware, J.E.; Kosinski, M.; Bjorner, J.B.; Turner-Bowker, D.M.; Gandek, B.; Maruish, M.E. *User's Manual for the 36v2 Health Survey*, 2nd ed.; Quality Metric Incorporated: Lincoln, RI, USA, 2007.

41. Maruish, M.E.; Maruish, M.; Kosinski, M.; Bjorner, J.B.; Gandek, B.; Turner-Bowker, D.M.; Ware, J.E. *User's Manual for the SF-36v2 Health Survey*, 3rd ed.; Quality Metric Incorporated: Lincoln, RI, USA, 2011.
42. Ware, J.E.; Kosinski, M.; Turner-Bowker, D.M.; Gandek, B. *User's Manual for the SF12v2 Health Survey*; Quality Metric Incorporated: Lincoln, RI, USA, 2009.
43. Fukuhara, S.; Ware, J.E.; Kosinski, M.; Wada, S.; Gandek, B. Psychometric and Clinical Tests of Validity of the Japanese SF-36 Health Survey. *J. Clin. Epidemiol.* **1998**, *51*, 1045–1053. [CrossRef]
44. Optum The Optum®SF-36v2®Health Survey. Available online: https://www.optum.com/solutions/life-sciences/answer-research/patient-insights/sf-health-surveys/sf-36v2-health-survey.html (accessed on 1 February 2021).
45. Wilson, J.T.L.; Pettigrew, L.E.L.; Teasdale, G.M. Structured Interviews for the Glasgow Outcome Scale and the Extended Glasgow Outcome Scale: Guidelines for Their Use. *J. Neurotrauma* **1998**, *15*, 573–585. [CrossRef]
46. Wilson, L.; Edwards, P.; Fiddes, H.; Stewart, E.; Teasdale, G.M. Reliability of Postal Questionnaires for the Glasgow Outcome Scale. *J. Neurotrauma* **2002**, *19*, 999–1005. [CrossRef]
47. Kunzmann, K.; Wernisch, L.; Richardson, S.; Steyerberg, E.W.; Lingsma, H.; Ercole, A.; Maas, A.I.R.; Menon, D.; Wilson, L. Imputation of Ordinal Outcomes: A Comparison of Approaches in Traumatic Brain Injury. *J. Neurotrauma* **2021**, *38*, 455–463. [CrossRef]
48. Teasdale, G.; Jennett, B. Assessment of Coma and Impaired Consciousness. A Practical Scale. *Lancet* **1974**, *304*, 81–84. [CrossRef]
49. McDonald, R.P. *Test Theory: A Unified Treatment*; L. Erlbaum Associates: Mahwah, NJ, USA, 1999; ISBN 978-0-8058-3075-0.
50. Bulmer, M.G. *Principles of Statistics*; Dover Publications, Inc.: New York, NY, USA, 1979; ISBN 0-486-63760-3.
51. Bujang, M.A.; Omar, E.D.; Baharum, N.A. A Review on Sample Size Determination for Cronbach's Alpha Test: A Simple Guide for Researchers. *MJMS* **2018**, *25*, 85–99. [CrossRef]
52. Yurdugül, H. Minimum Sample Size for Cronbach's Coefficient Alpha. *Hacettepe Üniversitesi Eğitim Fakültesi Dergisi* **2008**, *35*, 397–405.
53. Hair, J.F.; Black, W.C.; Babin, B.J.; Anderson, R.E. *Multivariate Data Analysis*; Pearson College Division: London, UK, 2010.
54. Fayers, P.; Machin, D. *Quality of Life the Assessment, Analysis and Interpretation of Patient-Reported Outcomes*; John Wiley & Sons: New York, NY, USA, 2013; ISBN 978-1-118-69945-4.
55. Cho, E.; Kim, S. Cronbach's Coefficient Alpha: Well Known but Poorly Understood. *Organ. Res. Methods* **2015**, *18*, 207–230. [CrossRef]
56. Cohen, J. A Power Primer. *Psychol. Bull.* **1992**, *112*, 155–159. [CrossRef]
57. Cohen, J. *Statistical Power Analysis for the Behavioral Sciences*, 2nd ed.; L. Erlbaum Associates: Hillsdale, NJ, USA, 1988; ISBN 978-0-8058-0283-2.
58. Terwee, C.B.; Bot, S.D.M.; de Boer, M.R.; van der Windt, D.A.W.M.; Knol, D.L.; Dekker, J.; Bouter, L.M.; de Vet, H.C.W. Quality Criteria Were Proposed for Measurement Properties of Health Status Questionnaires. *J. Clin. Epidemiol.* **2007**, *60*, 34–42. [CrossRef]
59. Nelson, L.D.; Ranson, J.; Ferguson, A.R.; Giacino, J.; Okonkwo, D.O.; Valadka, A.B.; Manley, G.T.; McCrea, M.A.; the TRACK-TBI Investigators. Validating Multi-Dimensional Outcome Assessment Using the Traumatic Brain Injury Common Data Elements: An Analysis of the TRACK-TBI Pilot Study Sample. *J. Neurotrauma* **2017**, *34*, 3158–3172. [CrossRef]
60. Wolf, E.J.; Harrington, K.M.; Clark, S.L.; Miller, M.W. Sample Size Requirements for Structural Equation Models: An Evaluation of Power, Bias, and Solution Propriety. *Educ. Psychol. Meas.* **2013**, *73*, 913–934. [CrossRef]
61. Brown, T.A. Confirmatory Factor Analysis for Applied Research. In *Methodology in the Social Sciences*, 2nd ed.; The Guilford Press:: New York, NY, USA; London, UK, 2015; ISBN 978-1-4625-1779-4.
62. Bentler, P.M. Comparative Fit Indexes in Structural Models. *Psychol. Bull.* **1990**, *107*, 238–246. [CrossRef]
63. Hu, L.; Bentler, P.M. Cutoff Criteria for Fit Indexes in Covariance Structure Analysis: Conventional Criteria versus New Alternatives. *Struct. Equ. Modeling A Multidiscip. J.* **1999**, *6*, 1–55. [CrossRef]
64. Browne, M.; Cudeck, R. Alternative ways of assessing model fit. In *Testing Structural Equation*; Bollen, K.A., Long, S.J., Eds.; Sage Focus Editions; Sage Publications: Newbury Park, CA, USA, 1993; Volume 154, pp. 136–162. ISBN 978-0-8039-4507-4.
65. Revelle, W. Psych: Procedures for Psychological, Psychometric, and Personality Research. Northwestern University: Evanston, IL, USA, R Package Version 2.0.12; 2020.
66. Rosseel, Y. Lavaan: An R Package for Structural Equation Modeling. *J. Stat. Soft.* **2012**, *48*. [CrossRef]
67. R Core Team. *R: A Language and Environment for Statistical Computing*; R Foundation for Statistical Computing: Vienna, Austria, 2020.
68. Hart, T.; Fann, J.R.; Chervoneva, I.; Juengst, S.B.; Rosenthal, J.A.; Krellman, J.W.; Dreer, L.E.; Kroenke, K. Prevalence, Risk Factors, and Correlates of Anxiety at 1 Year After Moderate to Severe Traumatic Brain Injury. *Arch. Phys. Med. Rehabil.* **2016**, *97*, 701–707. [CrossRef]
69. Donders, J.; Darland, K. Psychometric Properties and Correlates of the PHQ-2 and PHQ-9 after Traumatic Brain Injury. *Brain Inj.* **2017**, *31*, 1871–1875. [CrossRef]
70. Fann, J.R.; Bombardier, C.H.; Dikmen, S.; Esselman, P.; Warms, C.A.; Pelzer, E.; Rau, H.; Temkin, N. Validity of the Patient Health Questionnaire-9 in Assessing Depression Following Traumatic Brain Injury. *J. Head Trauma Rehabil.* **2005**, *20*, 501–511. [CrossRef]
71. Wortmann, J.H.; Jordan, A.H.; Weathers, F.W.; Resick, P.A.; Dondanville, K.A.; Hall-Clark, B.; Foa, E.B.; Young-McCaughan, S.; Yarvis, J.S.; Hembree, E.A.; et al. Psychometric Analysis of the PTSD Checklist-5 (PCL-5) among Treatment-Seeking Military Service Members. *Psychol. Assess.* **2016**, *28*, 1392–1403. [CrossRef]

72. Eyres, S.; Carey, A.; Gilworth, G.; Neumann, V.; Tennant, A. Construct Validity and Reliability of the Rivermead Post-Concussion Symptoms Questionnaire. *Clin. Rehabil.* **2005**, *19*, 878–887. [CrossRef]
73. Smith-Seemiller, L.; Fow, N.R.; Kant, R.; Franzen, M.D. Presence of Post-Concussion Syndrome Symptoms in Patients with Chronic Pain vs Mild Traumatic Brain Injury. *Brain Inj.* **2003**, *17*, 199–206. [CrossRef]
74. Miller, M.W.; Wolf, E.J.; Kilpatrick, D.; Resnick, H.; Marx, B.P.; Holowka, D.W.; Keane, T.M.; Rosen, R.C.; Friedman, M.J. The Prevalence and Latent Structure of Proposed DSM-5 Posttraumatic Stress Disorder Symptoms in U.S. National and Veteran Samples. *Psychol. Trauma Theory Res. Pract. Policy* **2013**, *5*, 501–512. [CrossRef]
75. Biehn, T.L.; Elhai, J.D.; Seligman, L.D.; Tamburrino, M.; Armour, C.; Forbes, D. Underlying Dimensions of DSM-5 Posttraumatic Stress Disorder and Major Depressive Disorder Symptoms. *Psychol. Inj. Law* **2013**, *6*, 290–298. [CrossRef]
76. Teymoori, A.; Gorbunova, A.; Haghish, F.E.; Real, R.; Zeldovich, M.; Wu, Y.-J.; Polinder, S.; Asendorf, T.; Menon, D.; CENTER-TBI Investigators and Participants CENTER-TBI Investigators and Participants. Factorial Structure and Validity of Depression (PHQ-9) and Anxiety (GAD-7) Scales after Traumatic Brain Injury. *JCM* **2020**, *9*, 873. [CrossRef]
77. Geier, T.J.; Hunt, J.C.; Hanson, J.L.; Heyrman, K.; Larsen, S.E.; Brasel, K.J.; deRoon-Cassini, T.A. Validation of Abbreviated Four- and Eight-Item Versions of the PTSD Checklist for *DSM-5* in a Traumatically Injured Sample: Abbreviated PCL-5 Validation in Traumatic Injury. *J. Trauma. Stress* **2020**, *33*, 218–226. [CrossRef] [PubMed]
78. von Steinbuechel, N.; Covic, A.; Polinder, S.; Kohlmann, T.; Cepulyte, U.; Poinstingl, H.; Backhaus, J.; Bakx, W.; Bullinger, M.; Christensen, A.-L.; et al. Assessment of Health-Related Quality of Life after TBI: Comparison of a Disease-Specific (QOLIBRI) with a Generic (SF-36) Instrument. *Behav. Neurol.* **2016**, *2016*, 1–14. [CrossRef]
79. Zahniser, E.; Nelson, L.D.; Dikmen, S.S.; Machamer, J.E.; Stein, M.B.; Yuh, E.; Manley, G.T.; Temkin, N.R. TRACK-TBI Investigators the Temporal Relationship of Mental Health Problems and Functional Limitations Following MTBI: A TRACK-TBI and TED Study. *J. Neurotrauma* **2019**, *36*, 1786–1793. [CrossRef]
80. Polinder, S.; Cnossen, M.C.; Real, R.G.L.; Covic, A.; Gorbunova, A.; Voormolen, D.C.; Master, C.L.; Haagsma, J.A.; Diaz-Arrastia, R.; von Steinbuechel, N. A Multidimensional Approach to Post-Concussion Symptoms in Mild Traumatic Brain Injury. *Front. Neurol.* **2018**, *9*, 1113. [CrossRef]
81. Von Steinbüchel, N.; Meeuwsen, M.; Zeldovich, M.; Vester, J.C.; Maas, A.; Koskinen, S.; Covic, A. Differences in Health-Related Quality of Life after Traumatic Brain Injury between Varying Patient Groups: Sensitivity of a Disease-Specific (QOLIBRI) and a Generic (SF-36) Instrument. *J. Neurotrauma* **2020**, *37*, 1242–1254. [CrossRef]
82. Rockwood, T.H.; Sangster, R.L.; Dillman, D.A. The Effect of Response Categories on Questionnaire Answers: Context and Mode Effects. *Sociol. Methods Res.* **1997**, *26*, 118–140. [CrossRef]
83. Maydeu-Olivares, A.; Kramp, U.; García-Forero, C.; Gallardo-Pujol, D.; Coffman, D. The Effect of Varying the Number of Response Alternatives in Rating Scales: Experimental Evidence from Intra-Individual Effects. *Behav. Res. Methods* **2009**, *41*, 295–308. [CrossRef]
84. Maydeu-Olivares, A.; Fairchild, A.J.; Hall, A.G. Goodness of Fit in Item Factor Analysis: Effect of the Number of Response Alternatives. *Struct. Equ. Modeling Multidiscip. J.* **2017**, *24*, 495–505. [CrossRef]
85. Teymoori, A.; Real, R.; Gorbunova, A.; Haghish, E.F.; Andelic, N.; Wilson, L.; Asendorf, T.; Menon, D.; von Steinbüchel, N. Measurement Invariance of Assessments of Depression (PHQ-9) and Anxiety (GAD-7) across Sex, Strata and Linguistic Backgrounds in a European-Wide Sample of Patients after Traumatic Brain Injury. *J. Affect. Disord.* **2020**, *262*, 278–285. [CrossRef]

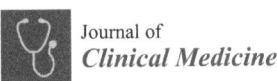

Article

Translation and Linguistic Validation of Outcome Instruments for Traumatic Brain Injury Research and Clinical Practice: A Step-by-Step Approach within the Observational CENTER-TBI Study

Nicole von Steinbuechel [1,*], Katrin Rauen [2,3], Ugne Krenz [1], Yi-Jhen Wu [1], Amra Covic [1], Anne Marie Plass [1], Katrin Cunitz [1], Isabelle Mueller [1], Fabian Bockhop [1], Suzanne Polinder [4], Lindsay Wilson [5], Ewout W. Steyerberg [4,6], Andrew I. R. Maas [7], David Menon [8], Marina Zeldovich [1] and The Linguistic Validation Group of CENTER-TBI [†]

1. Institute of Medical Psychology and Medical Sociology, University Medical Center Göttingen, Waldweg 37A, 37073 Göttingen, Germany; ugne.krenz@med.uni-goettingen.de (U.K.); yi-jhen.wu@med.uni-goettingen.de (Y.-J.W.); amra.covic@med.uni-goettingen.de (A.C.); annemarie.plass@med.uni-goettingen.de (A.M.P.); katrin.cunitz@med.uni-goettingen.de (K.C.); isabelle.mueller@med.uni-goettingen.de (I.M.); fabian.bockhop@med.uni-goettingen.de (F.B.); marina.zeldovich@med.uni-goettingen.de (M.Z.)
2. Department of Geriatric Psychiatry, Psychiatric Hospital Zurich, University of Zurich, Minervastrasse 145, 8032 Zurich, Switzerland; katrin.rauen@uzh.ch or katrin.rauen@med.uni-muenchen.de
3. Institute for Stroke and Dementia Research (ISD), University Hospital, LMU Munich, Feodor-Lynen-Straße 17, 81377 Munich, Germany
4. Department of Public Health, Erasmus MC, University Medical Center Rotterdam, 3000 CA Rotterdam, The Netherlands; s.polinder@erasmusmc.nl (S.P.); e.steyerberg@erasmusmc.nl (E.W.S.)
5. Department of Psychology, University of Stirling, Stirling FK9 4LJ, UK; l.wilson@stir.ac.uk
6. Department of Biomedical Data Sciences, Leiden University Medical Center, 2333 RC Leiden, The Netherlands
7. Department of Neurosurgery, Antwerp University Hospital and University of Antwerp, 2650 Edegem, Belgium; andrew.maas@uza.be
8. Division of Anaesthesia, University of Cambridge, Addenbrooke's Hospital, Box 157, Cambridge CB2 0QQ, UK; dkm13@cam.ac.uk

* Correspondence: nvsteinbuechel@med.uni-goettingen.de; Tel.: +49-551-39-8192

† The full list of the Linguistic Validation Group is provided in the Appendix A.

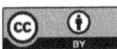

Abstract: Assessing outcomes in multinational studies on traumatic brain injury (TBI) poses major challenges and requires relevant instruments in languages other than English. Of the 19 outcome instruments selected for use in the observational Collaborative European NeuroTrauma Effectiveness Research in TBI (CENTER-TBI) study, 17 measures lacked translations in at least one target language. To fill this gap, we aimed to develop well-translated linguistically and psychometrically validated instruments. We performed translations and linguistic validations of patient-reported measures (PROMs), clinician-reported (ClinRO), and performance-based (PerfO) outcome instruments, using forward and backward translations, reconciliations, cognitive debriefings with up to 10 participants, iterative revisions, and international harmonization with input from over 150 international collaborators. In total, 237 translations and 211 linguistic validations were carried out in up to 20 languages. Translations were evaluated at the linguistic and cultural level by coding changes when the original versions are compared with subsequent translation steps, using the output of cognitive debriefings, and using comprehension rates. The average comprehension rate per instrument varied from 88% to 98%, indicating a good quality of the translations. These outcome instruments provide a solid basis for future TBI research and clinical practice and allow the aggregation and analysis of data across different countries and languages.

Keywords: translation; linguistic validation; outcome instruments; traumatic brain injury

1. Introduction

Traumatic brain injury (TBI) is a major cause of lifelong disability worldwide [1]. It is defined as "an alteration in brain function, or other evidence of brain pathology, caused by an external force" [2] (p. 1637). A TBI may result in a variety of consequences, such as temporary or persisting functional disability [3]; neurological problems [4,5], including sensory-motor disorders [6,7], as well as neuropsychological [8,9], psychosocial, and psychiatric sequelae [10–12]; and reduced health-related quality of life (HRQOL) [13].

Given the broad range of areas affected, the complexity and heterogeneity of TBI and its consequences cannot be adequately captured by unidimensional outcome assessments [14]. The paradigm shift in classifying and treating TBI not only as an acute but rather as a chronic brain disease emphasizes the need for a multi-level outcome assessment [1,15,16], which should cover the various outcome domains and reflect the perspectives of both patients and healthcare professionals.

Over the past 35 years, outcome instruments have been developed for different clinical fields [17,18] and, during the last decade, TBI research has started to apply combinations of them [13,14,19]. Outcomes after TBI can be assessed using instruments based on clinician-reported outcomes (ClinROs), patient-reported outcomes measures (PROMs), and performance-based physical and cognitive outcomes (PerfOs). PROMs use patients' self-ratings regarding their subjective perspective of their health condition and/or medical treatment [20,21]. In ClinRO instruments and clinical tests, the patients' status is assessed by trained healthcare professionals, while PerfO instruments capture the "objective" functional performance through standardized tests, mostly carried out by psychologists or other clinical personnel [21].

Multicenter multinational studies that investigate outcomes multidimensionally by using these types of instruments are required to comprehensively characterize outcome and recovery trajectories after TBI. A prerequisite for reliable and valid national and international multidimensional investigations of outcomes after TBI is the availability of well-translated, linguistically validated, and internationally harmonized ClinRO, PerfO instruments, and PROMs to assess cognitive, psychological, and psychosocial outcomes, HRQOL, recovery, and amnesia in multiple languages. Many of these are, however, only available in a limited number of languages [22].

To overcome this limitation, the instruments need to be translated and linguistically validated in the target languages for international studies on TBI outcome. The linguistic validation of instruments is challenging as it needs to address the cultural and conceptual differences between the respective language while maintaining the contents of each instrument on a conceptual level across the different languages [23]. A systematic review found that no standardized international guidelines exist for the linguistic validation of health-related outcome instruments [24]. Nevertheless, several guidelines and recommendations for iterative translation procedures are in use, published by the MAPI Research Trust [25], the International Society for Pharmacoeconomics and Outcomes Research (ISPOR) [26,27], and others [23,28,29]. Moreover, further research is addressing the issue of the cross-linguistic adaptation of PROMs [26], ClinRO and PerfO instruments [30], and clinical ratings (e.g., Reference [31]). To date, general principles include the following steps:

First, the team coordinating the translation of an instrument should identify and clarify the concepts behind the instructions, items, and response formats (together with the developer) [25]. The translation of the original instrument into the target language should be performed by two independent native speakers, living in the country, fluent in English, briefed concerning the translation of health-related outcome instruments, and ideally having already performed this kind of translation before [25,26]. Second, the two translations should be combined to form a single forward version [25,28]. This reconciled version is back-translated by one independent linguist—a native speaker in the language of the original instrument and fluent in the target language—living in the respective country [24]. The reconciled target version is then revised considering the backward translation. Third, the target version should be cognitively debriefed in five to ten patients [25]. The amendments suggested by the target language translators are reviewed by the language translation coordinating team, discussed with the team and the target language translators (and the developer); then the translated instrument is finalized [25]. Finally, if an instrument is simultaneously translated into several languages, these translations should be internationally harmonized to ensure they are comparable, a process that is performed in the translation coordinating center together with the instrument's authors [24]. These steps are meant to ensure that an instrument translation is "conceptually and linguistically equivalent to the source measure and allows data pooling and analysis/comparison across countries" [25] (p. 21).

While designing the Collaborative European NeuroTrauma Effectiveness Research study (CENTER-TBI; EC grant 602150; clinicaltrials.gov NCT02210221), a large international observational European study on TBI, we found that 17 of the 19 selected instruments or subtests were not available in at least one target language. To deal with this challenge, we decided to conduct translations and linguistic validations of these outcome instruments into up to 20 target languages, following most of the recommendations mentioned above. These translated instruments have been made available to the international scientific and clinical community. The present study describes the first part of the linguistic validation process of the outcome instruments administered in the CENTER-TBI study. The second part, concerning the psychometric properties of the PROMs is also published in the same issue of this journal [32].

2. Methods

2.1. Languages

The CENTER-TBI study was conducted from 2015 to 2017, across 18 countries in Europe and in Israel. The study protocol has been published and descriptive results have been presented [33,34]. The target languages for the linguistic validation were determined by the language(s) spoken in those countries that had expressed an interest in participating (Table 1).

Table 1. Target languages for the linguistic validation of the countries that participated in the CENTER-TBI study.

No.	Target Languages	Country
1	Arabic	Israel
2	Bosnian/Croatian/Serbian	Bosnia/Croatia/Serbia
3	Bulgarian	Bulgaria
4	Czech	Czech Republic
5	Danish	Denmark
6	Dutch	Belgium, the Netherlands
7	Finnish	Finland
8	French	Belgium, France
9	German	Austria, Belgium, Germany
10	Hebrew	Israel
11	Hungarian	Hungary
12	Italian	Italy
13	Latvian	Latvia
14	Lithuanian	Lithuania
15	Norwegian	Norway
16	Romanian	Romania
17	Russian	Israel
18	Slovakian	Slovakia
19	Spanish	Spain
20	Swedish	Sweden

Note. As the Bulgarian and Czech centers dropped out of the CENTER-TBI study early on, not all linguistic validation steps could be performed (see results and discussion). Moreover, cognitive debriefings were not carried out for the Arabic and Russian language. Thus, these languages are not available on the CENTER-TBI website, but from nvsteinbuechel@med.uni-goettingen.de for further linguistic validation.

2.2. Instruments

The selection of the outcome instruments was informed by the Common Data Elements (CDE) recommendations [35,36] taking into consideration TBI specificity and the free availability of instruments. As a result, the following outcome instruments were administered in the CENTER-TBI study (see Table 2). For a detailed description, see Appendix B.

Table 2. Outcome instruments administered in the CENTER-TBI study.

Abbreviation	Instrument	Outcome Domain	No. of Items	Response Format	Response Categories
clinician-reported outcome instrument (ClinRO), its questionnaire version, and a clinical amnesia test					
GOSE *	Glasgow Outcome Scale Extended [37]	Functional outcome and level of disability	19	Dichotomous and polytomous	"yes"/"no" (**16 items**) and item-specific rating scales and response categories (**three items**)
GOSE-Q	Glasgow Outcome Scale Extended—Questionnaire version [38]	Functional outcome and level of disability	14	Dichotomous and polytomous	"yes"/"no" (**five items**) and item-specific rating scales and response categories (**nine items**)
GOAT	Galveston Orientation Amnesia Test [39]	Post-traumatic amnesia	10 and 3 sub-items	Dichotomous	Error evaluation by clinician
Patient-reported outcome measures (PROMs)					
GAD-7	Generalized Anxiety Disorder 7 item scale [40]	Psychological outcome (generalized anxiety disorder)	7	Polytomous	"not at all" "several days" "more than half the days" "nearly every day"
PHQ-9	Patient Health Questionnaire 9 [41]	Psychological outcome (depression)	9 items and 1 additional question	Polytomous	"not at all" "several days" "more than half the days" "nearly every day" (**nine items**) and "not difficult at all" "somewhat difficult" "very difficult" "extremely difficult" (**one item**)
PCL-5	Posttraumatic Stress Disorder Checklist [42]	Psychological outcome (post-traumatic stress disorder)	20 items and 1 additional question	Polytomous and one dichotomous item	"not at all" "a little bit" "moderately" "quite a bit" "extremely" **and** "yes"/"no" (**one item**)
RPQ	Rivermead Post-concussion Symptoms Questionnaire [43]	Psychological, cognitive, and behavioral outcome	16 and 1 additional question	Polytomous and two semi-open questions	"no more of a problem" "a mild problem" "a moderate problem" "a severe problem" **and** the possibility of listing two further difficulties and rating them on the same scale
QOLIBRI	Quality of Life after Brain Injury Scale [44,45]	TBI-specific HRQOL	37 items	Polytomous	"not at all" "slightly" "moderately" "quite" "very"

Table 2. Cont.

Abbreviation	Instrument	Outcome Domain	No. of Items	Response Format	Response Categories
QOLIBRI-OS *	Quality of Life after Brain Injury—Overall Scale [46]	TBI-specific HRQOL	6 items	Polytomous	"not at all" "slightly" "moderately" "quite" "very"
SF-36v2	Short Form Health Survey—Version 2 [47]	Generic HRQOL	36 items	Polytomous	Different kinds of Likert scales and item-related rating scales and response categories
SF-12v2 *	12-Item Short Form Survey—Version 2 [48]	Generic HRQOL	12 items	Polytomous	Different kinds of Likert scales and item-related rating scales and response categories
Performance-based outcomes (PerfO)					
CANTAB	Cambridge Neuropsychological Test Automated Battery ** [49]	Neuropsychological outcome	6 subtests (RTI, SWM, PAL, RVP, AST, SOC)	-	-
RAVLT	Rey Auditory Verbal Learning Test [50]	Neuropsychological outcome	-	-	Three versions of two respective word lists, 15 words each (A and B, four versions of the instrument for repeated testing)
TMT-A, B	Trail-Making Test A, B [51]	Neuropsychological outcome	-	-	TMT-A: numbers from 1 to 25 TMT-B: letters (A–L) and numbers (1–13)

* Instruments marked with an asterisk were selected as core instruments of the CENTER-TBI study [33]. ** For the computer-based CANTAB tests, the instructions and procedure descriptions were subjected to translation. The responses are language free as the test battery consists of visual and auditory stimuli to which subjects react on the behavioral level: RTI = reaction time, SWM = spatial working memory, PAL = paired associate learning, RVP = rapid visual processing, AST = attention switching task, SOC = stockings of Cambridge. HRQOL = health-related quality of life. Bold was used to highlight the number of items in the questionnaire.

2.3. Translation and Linguistic Validation Procedure

Outcome instruments were identified for which published translations and linguistic validations were not available in the languages required for the countries participating in the CENTER-TBI study. For these instruments, translations and linguistic validations were performed between October 2013 and October 2015. Table 3 gives an overview of the pre-existing translations and the translated and linguistically validated versions in the target languages of the participating countries.

Table 3. Pre-existing translations and translated and linguistically validated versions in the target languages of the participating countries.

No.	Language	ClinRO, Its Questionnaire Version, and a Clinical Amnesia Test								PROMs																	PerfO	
		GOSE*		GOSE-Q*		GOAT		GAD-7		PHQ-9		PCL-5*		RPQ		QOLIBRI*		QOLIBRI-OS*		SF-36v2		SF-12v2*		RAVLT		TMT A/B		CANTAB (Subtests)	
		T	LV	T	LV	T	LV	T	LV	T	LV	T	LV	T	LV	T	LV	T	LV	T	LV	T	LV	T	LV	T	LV	T	LV
1	Arabic (for Israel)	✓	✓	✓	✓	✓	✓	-	-	-	-	✓	✓	✓	✓	✓	✓	✓	✓	-	-	-	-	✓	✓	✓	✓	1,3,4,5,6	1,3,4,5,6
2	Bosnian/Croatian/Serbian	✓	✓	✓	✓	✓	✓	✓	✓	-	-	✓	✓	✓	✓	✓	✓	✓	✓	-	-	-	-	✓	✓	✓	✓	1,3,4,5,6	1,3,4,5,6
3	Bulgarian	✓	-	✓	-	✓	-	-	-	-	-	✓	-	✓	-	✓	-	✓	-	-	-	-	-	✓	-	✓	-	1,2,3,4,5,6	-
4	Czech	✓	-	✓	-	✓	-	-	-	-	-	✓	-	✓	-	✓	-	✓	-	-	-	-	-	✓	-	-	-	1,4,5	-
5	Danish	-	-	✓	✓	✓	✓	-	-	-	-	✓	✓	-	-	-	-	-	-	-	-	-	-	✓	✓	-	-	1,2,3,4,5,6	1,2,3,4,5,6
6	Dutch	-	-	✓	✓	✓	✓	-	-	-	-	✓	✓	✓	✓	✓	✓	✓	✓	-	-	-	-	✓	✓	✓	✓	1,3	1,3
7	Finnish	-	-	✓	✓	✓	✓	-	-	-	-	✓	✓	✓	✓	-	-	-	-	-	-	-	-	✓	✓	✓	✓	1,2,3,4,5,6	1,2,3,4,5,6
8	French	-	-	✓	✓	✓	✓	-	-	-	-	✓	✓	✓	✓	-	-	-	-	-	-	-	-	✓	✓	✓	✓	1,3	1,3
9	German	-	-	✓	✓	✓	✓	-	-	-	-	✓	✓	-	-	-	-	-	-	-	-	-	-	✓	✓	✓	✓	1	1
10	Hebrew	✓	✓	✓	✓	✓	✓	-	-	-	-	✓	✓	✓	✓	✓	✓	✓	✓	-	-	-	-	✓	✓	✓	✓	1,3,4,5,6	1,3,4,5,6
11	Hungarian	✓	✓	✓	✓	✓	✓	-	-	-	-	✓	✓	✓	✓	✓	✓	✓	✓	-	-	-	-	✓	✓	✓	✓	1,3,4,5,6	1,3,4,5,6
12	Italian	✓	-	✓	✓	✓	-	-	-	-	-	✓	✓	✓	-	-	-	-	-	-	-	-	-	✓	✓	✓	✓	1,3	1,3
13	Latvian	✓	✓	✓	✓	✓	✓	✓	✓	✓	✓	✓	✓	✓	✓	✓	✓	✓	✓	-	-	-	-	✓	✓	✓	✓	1,2,3,4,5,6	1,2,3,4,5,6
14	Lithuanian	✓	-	✓	✓	✓	✓	-	-	-	-	-	-	✓	✓	✓	✓	✓	✓	-	-	-	-	✓	✓	✓	✓	1,2,3,4,5,6	1,2,3,4,5,6
15	Norwegian	-	-	✓	✓	✓	✓	-	-	-	-	-	-	✓	✓	✓	✓	✓	✓	-	-	-	-	✓	✓	✓	✓	1,2,3,4,5,6	1,2,3,4,5,6
16	Romanian	✓	✓	✓	✓	✓	✓	-	-	-	-	✓	-	✓	✓	✓	✓	✓	✓	-	-	-	-	✓	✓	✓	✓	1,2,4,5	1,2,4,5

Table 3. *Cont.*

No.	Language	GOSE* T	GOSE* LV	GOSE-Q* T	GOSE-Q* LV	GOAT T	GOAT LV	GAD-7 T	GAD-7 LV	PHQ-9 T	PHQ-9 LV	PCL-5* T	PCL-5* LV	RPQ T	RPQ LV	QOLIBRI* T	QOLIBRI* LV	QOLIBRI-OS* T	QOLIBRI-OS* LV	SF-36v2 T	SF-36v2 LV	SF-12v2* T	SF-12v2* LV	RAVLT T	RAVLT LV	TMT A/B T	TMT A/B LV	CANTAB (Subtests) T	CANTAB (Subtests) LV
17	Russian (for Israel)	✓	✓	✓	✓	✓	✓	-	-	-	-	-	-	✓	✓	✓	✓	✓	✓	-	-	-	-	✓	✓	✓	✓	1,4,5	1,4,5
18	Slovakian	✓	✓	✓	✓	✓	✓	-	-	-	-	✓	✓	✓	✓	✓	✓	✓	✓	-	-	-	-	✓	✓	✓	✓	1,4,5	1,4,5
19	Spanish	✓	✓	✓	✓	✓	✓	-	-	-	-	✓	✓	✓	✓	✓	✓	✓	✓	-	-	-	-	✓	✓	✓	✓	1	1
20	Swedish	✓	✓	✓	✓	✓	✓	✓	✓	✓	✓	✓	✓	✓	✓	✓	✓	✓	✓	-	-	✓	✓	✓	✓	✓	-	1,2,3,4,5,6	1,2,3,4,5,6

Note: ✓ = instruments translated and linguistically validated for the CENTER-TBI study; – = already existing translated and linguistically validated instruments; empty cells or missing instruments marked with an asterisk were selected as core instruments (GOSE, QOLIBRI-OS, SF-12v2) [30], complemented by the GOSE-Q, the PCL-5, and the QOLIBRI, and were translated by two translators and cognitively debriefed. ClinROs = clinician-reported outcome instrument; PROMs = patient-reported outcome measures; PerfOs = performance-based outcome instruments; T = translation steps performed; see Figure 1 (for Arabic and Russian, all steps except for cognitive debriefing were performed; for Bulgarian, all instruments underwent at least the first harmonization; for Czech, only forward translations were carried out); LV = linguistic validation; GOSE = Glasgow Outcome Scale—Extended; GOSE-Q = Glasgow Outcome Scale—Extended questionnaire version; GOAT = Galveston Orientation Amnesia Test; GAD-7 = Generalized Anxiety Disorder 7 Items Questionnaire; PHQ-9 = Patient Health Questionnaire 9; PCL-5 = Posttraumatic Stress Disorder Checklist; RPQ = Rivermead Post-Concussion Symptoms questionnaire; QOLIBRI = Quality of Life after Brain Injury Scale; QOLIBRI-OS = Quality of Life after Brain Injury—Overall Scale; SF-36v2 = Short Form Health Survey—Version 2; SF-12v2 = 12-Item Short Form Survey—Version 2; RAVLT = Rey Auditory Verbal Learning Test; TMT-A/B = Trail-Making Test A, B; CANTAB = Cambridge Neuropsychological Test Automated Battery; (1) RTI = reaction time, (2) SWM = spatial working memory, (3) PAL = paired associate learning, (4) RVP = rapid visual processing, (5) AST = attention switching task, (6) SOC = stockings of Cambridge.

TRANSLATION AND LINGUISTIC VALIDATION (LV) PROCESS

Phase 1 – Conceptual analyses of the original instrument

Conceptual analyses of the original instrument by the project coordinator, all language coordinators of the core team and two native/fluent target language speakers; in case of difficulties, collaboration with the instrument developer.

Phase 2 – Translations: forward translations, reconciled version and backward translation

For the primary instruments two independent translations, for the additional instruments one forward translation, into the target language, then reconciliation of the translations into one best version (**reconciled version I**); revision by the core team and the translating team in the target language; backward translation by a blinded native (or fluent) English speaker.

Phase 3 – Revision of the forward and backward translations

Revision of the forward translation(s), the reconciled version, and the backward translation by the core team; development of a **reconciled version II** together with the translating team in the target language.

Phase 4 – Cognitive debriefing

Assessment of the comprehensibility of all text elements (on the syntactical, semantic, idiomatic, and cultural adequacy); transcription and translation of the results of the cognitive debriefing interviews into English by the translating centers in the target countries for central review by the core team.

Phase 5 – Review of cognitive debriefing

Integration of the cognitive debriefing results by the core team in a **reconciled version III**, provision of this version to the translating team in the target language countries; a **reconciled version IV** is produced and revised by the core team resulting in a **reconciled version V**.

Phase 6 – International harmonization

A **pre-final version** is provided by the core team, and the translating team in the target language; discussion and revision with at least three adaptations to a **final international harmonization**, which were finally proofread by CENTER-TBI study members.

Phase 7 – Final version

Production of the **final version**.

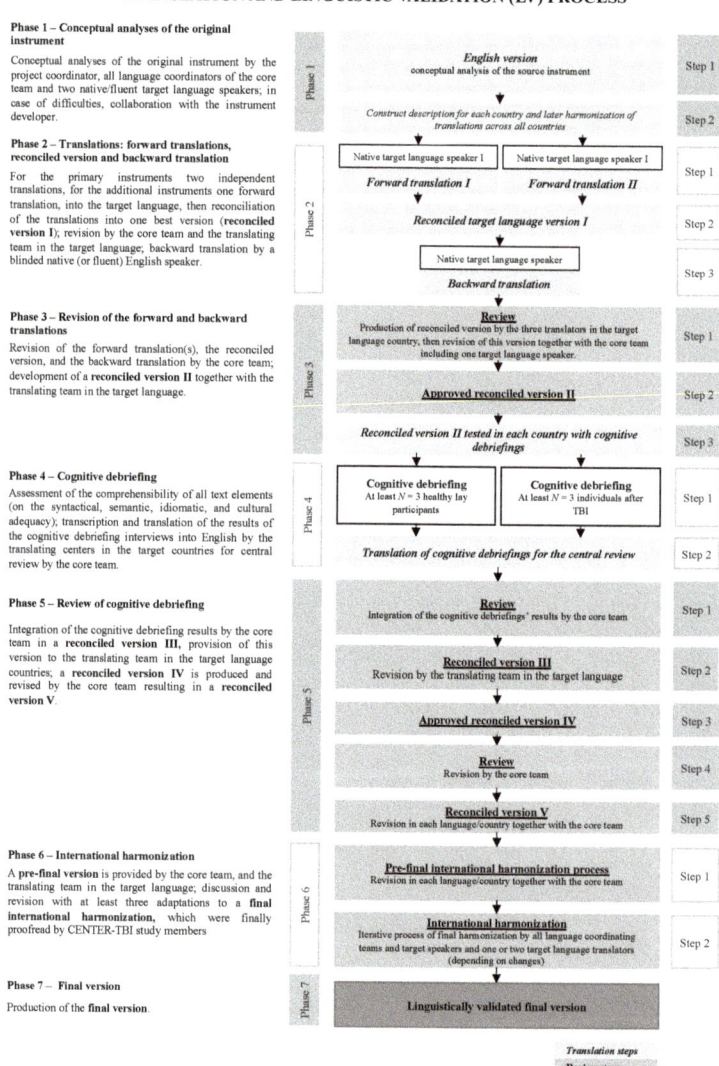

Figure 1. Translation and linguistic validation process.

The translations and linguistic validations of all instruments were coordinated by the core team of the University Medical Center Göttingen (UMG), consisting of one project coordinator and seven language coordinators, who led one to three translation teams in the participating countries. The core team included individuals whose language proficiency covered all required languages. In addition, the core team included at least one native speaker of each target language who was also fluent in English and who was responsible for that language. The core team and the translation teams in the participating countries comprised physicians, psychologists, teachers, linguists, nurses, occupational therapists, certified translators, administrative personnel, teachers, etc., who were experienced either in TBI research or clinical practice, outcome measurements, and/or translation.

We used a linguistic validation procedure that was guided by the recommendations of the MAPI Research Trust [24,25], adapted to the conditions of CENTER-TBI. As for various reasons (e.g., some centers dropped out of the study), some translations could not follow the entire process, we distinguish between *translation, linguistic validation* (without cognitive debriefings), and *full linguistic validation* (including cognitive debriefings). The outcome instruments were divided into two groups: (1) the core instruments (GOSE, QOLIBRI-OS, and SF-12v2) complemented by the additionally prioritized instruments (i.e., GOSE-Q, PCL-5, and QOLIBRI) and (2) the other instruments (GOAT, GAD-7, PHQ-9, RPQ, SF-36v2, RAVLT, TMT-A, B, and CANTAB). The procedure differed slightly for the two groups (see Phase 2).

2.3.1. Phase 1—Conceptual Analysis of the Original Instrument

A concept list was devised as a basis for the translations, enumerating difficulties encountered during the prescreening of the instruments, to ensure that every translator was familiar with the constructs used in the instruments (i.e., for the GOSE, GOSE-Q, GOAT, PCL-5, RPQ, QOLIBRI/QOLIBRI-OS, and RAVLT). This list included explanations concerning the translation of English idioms, words with multiple meanings, symptoms, and their intensity. For example, the item "As a result of your injury are there now problems in how you get on with friends or relatives?" from the GOSE-Q was explained by noting that in this context "get on" means "get along with". The item "Being 'superalert' or watchful or on guard" from the PCL-5 was explained as meaning very or extremely attentive. Moreover, translators were instructed to translate the Likert response scales considering the hierarchical order of the answers (e.g., from "not at all" to "extremely") and their equidistance, etc. Concerning the PerfOs, some of the examples are presented here. For the RAVLT, translators were encouraged to use culturally adapted translations for the word "church". Furthermore, this memory test includes homonyms, for which explanations were given, e.g., earth—the planet; turkey—the animal; orange—the fruit, etc. To further facilitate the comparability of the different RAVLT language versions, translators were asked to use a frequency list of words for each language (e.g., http://corpus.rae.es/lfrecuencias.html (accessed on 16 April 2021) for Spanish) to ensure that words with comparable frequencies were used. These strategies were adopted to support the comparability of the different language versions.

The explanatory concept list was discussed with all translation teams in the target languages/countries. In case of conceptual problems, the authors of the instruments were contacted.

2.3.2. Phase 2—Translation: Forward Translations, Reconciled Version, and Backward Translation

All the original instruments were available at least in English. For the GAD-7 and PHQ-9, translations and validations had already been published in (most of) the target languages and were freely available (https://www.phqscreeners.com (accessed on 16 April 2021)). Licenses for the use of the SF-36v2, SF-12v2 were obtained from Optum [52]. Thus, the GAD-7, PHQ-9, and SF-36v2/-12v2 were administered as such. For the GOSE, GOSE-Q, PCL-5, QOLIBRI, and QOLIBRI-OS, two independent forward translations were performed into several target languages by native speakers. The respective translations were reconciled into one version by the translation team in the target language. These reconciled versions were then revised and adapted by the core team, in agreement with the target language translation team. A native English speaker who was not familiar with the original English instrument translated the harmonized forward translation back into English.

All other instruments (i.e., GAD-7, PHQ-9, RPQ, RAVLT, TMT-A,B, and CANTAB subtests) underwent a single forward translation, due to limited resources. The test materials for the PerfO instruments comprise examples, visual and auditory materials which were—where appropriate—also subjected to the translation procedure. The other steps described above were the same for all instruments. See Figure 1 for an overview.

2.3.3. Phase 3—Revision of the Forward and Backward Translations

A review of the original instrument, the forward translation(s), the reconciled version, and the backward translation was carried out by the core team. Reconciled versions were then agreed upon together with the translation teams in the target language countries.

2.3.4. Phase 4—Cognitive Debriefing

These interviews, referred to as cognitive debriefings, are based on detailed structured questions whereby all answers are recorded. In the structured interview, participants were asked to share their thoughts about the meaning of each word, phrase, and item, and to comment on their comprehension of the respective instrument. The goal of a cognitive debriefing is to determine whether participants understand the text in the same way as it is intended in the original version of the instrument and whether its translation is culturally appropriate. These cognitive debriefings were performed in three to five individuals after TBI. Before this, three to five healthy individuals participated in the cognitive debriefings to anticipate and modify possible semantic, syntactical, idiomatic/pragmatic, and cultural issues early in the process. Clinicians were interviewed for the ClinROs.

The results were transcribed and translated into English by the translation teams. When linguistic and cultural problems were identified, the translations were further modified. The GOSE, the GOSE-Q, PCL-5, QOLIBRI, and QOLIBRI-OS underwent cognitive debriefings, which resulted in a *full linguistic validation*. No cognitive debriefings were performed for the other instruments (*linguistic validation*).

2.3.5. Phase 5—Review of Cognitive Debriefing

The results of the cognitive debriefings were reviewed in the target languages by the core and the translation teams: if there were linguistic and/or cultural issues, alternative wording suggested by the lay people and patients interviewed (or clinicians, in case of clinical ratings) was integrated into an updated version of the instrument.

2.3.6. Phase 6—International Harmonization

Final harmonization was performed by the core team for all the instruments. Furthermore, telephone or video conferences were held with the target language translation centers. In these, all concepts, such as cultural and linguistic equivalence, and all formal aspects were again discussed in detail, and if necessary appropriate adjustments were made. These versions were proofread by informed native speakers (investigators, participants, and management committee [MC] members of the CENTER-TBI study) for final adjustments.

2.3.7. Step 7—Final Version

Based on the revisions and results of the international harmonization, a final version of each of the instruments was produced.

2.4. Evaluation of Translations

The comparability of the translations was assessed by numerically coding any semantic, cultural, idiomatic/pragmatic, and syntactic/grammatical differences, first comparing the original instrument version with the first harmonized version and then comparing this with the internationally harmonized final version. This coding procedure was designed to examine whether the translations captured the original instruments as closely as possible. The semantic level included all changes and problems related to the meaning of words and use of vocabulary. Cultural differences reflected the cultural relevance of the translations in the respective target languages. Idiomatic/pragmatic issues dealt with the translation of English idioms into the target language, for example. Finally, the syntactic/ grammatical level included, e.g., sentence structure, punctuation, etc. To quantify the changes, we assessed the differences in the instructions, items, and response categories of the instruments at these four levels. The number of differences is expressed as a percentage (i.e., number of differences relative to the total number of text elements in question). This number varies from 0% (no differences at all) to a maximum of 900% (multiple differences). Values above 100% indicate multiple modifications in one text element (e.g., nine coded differences in one instruction are expressed as 900%). The same modification in the same item text is considered once (e.g., the use of the courtesy pronoun in ten items of an instrument is counted as one modification). To summarize the results, we have provided an average percentage of changes across the languages for each instrument. To avoid the influence of outliers (e.g., extensive number of changes in a few languages), mean and median percentages of coded differences are reported.

Additionally, we have reported issues identified in the cognitive debriefings using comprehension rates. These were calculated by taking the number of individuals who participated in the cognitive debriefings, who had no problems understanding the instructions, items, and responses, and who had no concerns regarding the phrasing and the cultural conformance, and dividing this number by the overall number of interviewees. Mean comprehension rates were evaluated using quartiles, a commonly used measure in health sciences providing information about the center and the spread of the data. A rate of 100% indicates full comprehension, values above 75% were considered good, values ranging from 25% to 75% acceptable, and values below 25% indicated poor understanding. The results of the cognitive debriefings and reports on the translational and linguistic validation issues and solutions informed further revisions and harmonization of the instruments.

To assess these issues, the following questions were asked about the instructions, each item, and the respective response categories:

1. Did you have difficulties understanding this instruction/the question/the response options?
2. What did you understand this to mean?
3. Is it relevant for your situation?
4. Are the response options clear and consistent with the question?
5. If anything was misleading or unclear, how would you reword it?

3. Results

In total, 237 translations and 211 linguistic validations were carried out in up to 20 languages, including 14 translations and 12 linguistic validations of one ClinRO, 20 translations and 18 linguistic validations of its questionnaire version, 20 translations and 18 linguistic validations of the clinical amnesia test, 63 translations and 55 linguistic validations of the six PRO instruments, and 120 translations and 108 linguistic validations of the PerfO instruments (see Table 4).

Table 4. Translations, *linguistic* and *full linguistic* validations for the instruments administered in the CENTER-TBI study.

Instrument	Translations		Linguistic Validations		Full Linguistic Validations (Including Cognitive Debriefings)	
	N	%	N	%	N	%
ClinRO, its questionnaire version, and a clinical amnesia test	54	100%	48	89%	26	54%
GOSE	14	100%	12	86%	10	83%
GOSE-Q	20	100%	18	90%	16	89%
GOAT	20	100%	18	90%	-	-
PROMs	63	100%	55	87%	31	56%
GAD-7	2	100%	2	100%	-	-
PHQ-9	1	100%	1	100%	-	-
PCL-5	19	100%	17	89%	15	88%
RPQ	17	100%	15	88%	-	-
QOLIBRI	12	100%	10	83%	8	80%
QOLIBRI-OS	12	100%	10	83%	8	80%

Table 4. Cont.

Instrument	Translations		Linguistic Validations		Full Linguistic Validations (Including Cognitive Debriefings)	
	N	%	N	%	N	%
PerfOs	120	100%	108	90%	-	-
CANTAB	83	100%	74	89%	-	-
RAVLT	20	100%	18	90%	-	-
TMT-A, B	17	100%	16	94%	-	-
Total	**237**	**100%**	**211**	**89%**	**57**	**27%**

Note: N = number of translations or linguistic validations, % = percentage, "-" = no translation or linguistic validation performed. Translations = overall number and percentage of performed translations; linguistic validation = overall number of performed linguistic validations and percentage in relation to all established translations; *full linguistic validations* include cognitive debriefings, *linguistic validations* do not; here, the overall number of *full linguistic validations* performed and percentage in relation to all performed *linguistic validations* is reported. Bold are for better readability.

3.1. Forward and Backward Translations, Comparison between the Original Version and the First Harmonization (Phases 2 and 3)

The forward and backward translations were performed for all outcome instruments. Some GOSE-Q translations conducted for the European multi-center Eurotherm study [53] were used as the forward translation (Dutch, German, French, Hungarian, Italian, Lithuanian, Russian, and Spanish). All instruments were then back-translated. Already existing and published translations of the Dutch and French GOSE, and the French translations of the QOLIBRI/QOLIBRI-OS were edited according to the comments of the translators and revised in an iterative process during the international harmonization (Phase 6).

The comparison between the original English versions and the first harmonization mainly revealed differences at the semantic level, followed by idiomatic and cultural issues (see Table 5). Considering both the mean and median percentage of differences, most changes were observed for the RPQ, followed by the GOSE-Q, GOSE, PCL-5, and the RAVLT.

Table 5. Average (mean and median) number of differences between the original English version and the first harmonized version.

Measure	Text Elements	No.	Average Number of Changes							
			Mean				Median			
			S	C	I/P	S/G	S	C	I/P	S/G
ClinRO, Its Questionnaire Version, and a Clinical Amnesia Test										
GOSE (10 translations)	In	11	47	3%	5%	9%	46%	0%	5%	0%
	I	19	24%	2%	4%	7%	17%	0%	0%	5%
	R	15	17%	1%	5%	2%	13%	0%	0%	0%
GOSE-Q (16 translations)	In	2	97%	22%	20%	23%	50%	0%	0%	0%
	I	14	18%	8%	7%	6%	14%	7%	4%	3%
	R	42	9%	1%	3%	3%	2%	0%	1%	0%
GOAT (16 translations)	In	8	13%	2%	8%	10%	6%	0%	0%	0%
	I	13	11%	4%	5%	3%	8%	0%	0%	0%
	R	-	-	-	-	-	-	-	-	-
PROMs *										
GAD-7 (2 translations)	In	1	0%	50%	0%	0%	0%	50%	0%	0%
	I	7	0%	0%	0%	0%	0%	0%	0%	0%
	R	5	0%	0%	0%	0%	0%	0%	0%	0%
PHQ-9 (1 translation)	In	1	0%	100%	0%	0%	0%	100%	0%	0%
	I	10	0%	10%	0%	0%	0%	10%	0%	0%
	R	5	0%	0%	0%	0%	0%	0%	0%	0%

Table 5. Cont.

| Measure | Text Elements | No. | Average Number of Changes ||||||||
| | | | Mean |||| Median ||||
			S	C	I/P	S/G	S	C	I/P	S/G
PCL-5 (15 translations)	In	1	60%	20%	0%	20%	0%	0%	0%	0%
	I	21	19%	2%	8%	7%	14%	0%	0%	5%
	R	5	12%	0%	3%	0%	0%	0%	0%	0%
RPQ (13 translations)	In	1	146%	46%	31%	46%	146%	0%	0%	0%
	I	17	10%	2%	1%	3%	6%	0%	0%	0%
	R	5	14%	0%	2%	3%	20%	0%	0%	0%
QOLIBRI (8 translations)	In	7	22%	7%	11%	25%	18%	0%	5%	29%
	I	37	10%	1%	4%	6%	5%	0%	5%	7%
	R	5	3%	0%	0%	0%	0%	0%	0%	0%
QOLIBRI-OS (8 translations)	In	1	50%	50%	25%	75%	0%	0%	0%	88%
	I	6	8%	0%	4%	2%	4%	0%	0%	0%
	R	5	3%	0%	3%	0%	0%	0%	0%	0%
PerfO *										
RAVLT (16 translations)	In	5	71%	13%	11%	33%	60%	0%	0%	0%
	I	45	7%	0%	1%	0%	6%	0%	0%	0%
	R	-	-	-	-	-	-	-	-	-
TMT A/B (14 translations)	In	6	58%	11%	17%	12%	42%	17%	8%	14%
	I	38	1%	0%	0%	0%	0%	0%	0%	0%
	R	-	-	-	-	-	-	-	-	-

Note: No. = Number of text elements; In = Instructions: average number of modifications between the original English version and the first harmonization (average in %, i.e., number of differences in relation to the total number of the respective text elements divided by the number of translations); I = Items: modifications in items; R = Response categories: modifications (if applicable, otherwise "-"); S/G = Syntactic/Grammatical level; C = Cultural level; I/P = Idiomatic/Pragmatic; ClinRO = clinician-reported outcome instrument; PROMs = patient-reported outcome measures; PerfOs = performance-based outcome instruments; GOSE = Glasgow Outcome Scale—Extended; instructions of the GOSE include introduction (1), commentary on the questions (9), and scoring (1); GOSE-Q = Glasgow Outcome Scale—Extended questionnaire version; instructions include introduction and header (1) and explanatory example for the item 9; different types of responses (dichotomous yes/no and polytomous item-related responses) result in 42 elements; GOAT = Galveston Orientation Amnesia Test (no response categories); GAD-7 = Generalized Anxiety Disorder 7 Items Questionnaire; PHQ-9 = Patient Health Questionnaire 9 Items; PCL-5 = Posttraumatic Stress Disorder Checklist; RPQ = Rivermead Post-Concussion Symptoms questionnaire; QOLIBRI = Quality of Life after Brain Injury Scale; instructions to the two parts (2) and five subscales (5); QOLIBRI-OS = Quality of Life after Brain Injury—Scale; RAVLT = Rey Auditory Verbal Learning Test; here, words are treated as items (5 × 15 = 45) (no response categories); instructions: introduction (1), explanations on the three trials (3), and the summary table for evaluation of the test result (1); TMT-A/B = Trail-Making Test A, B; in the TMT-A/B, letters and numbers are treated as items, there are no response categories; instructions of the TMT-A, B include introduction (1), explanation on the trial A (1) and trial B (1), trial B test (1), scoring (1), and hands check (1); CANTAB = Cambridge Neuropsychological Test Automated Battery. Cognitive debriefings and international harmonization of the Arabic, Russian, Bulgarian, and the Czech translations were not carried out and are therefore not reported. * Excluded from analyses, as translations of the SF-36v2/-12v were obtained from Optum. CANTAB analyses are not presented here, because in the meantime only updated versions from Cambridge Cognition can be used. Therefore, these are not available on the CENTER-TBI website.

At *the semantic level*, specifically, the term "(head, brain) injury" underwent semantic changes across many languages. Frequently, "injury" was translated as "trauma" which seemed more appropriate in the respective language contexts. Further semantic changes concerned the choice of words, with the aim of capturing the original instruments as closely as possible.

At the *idiomatic/pragmatic level*, the differences between translations comprised adaptations of English idioms and special phrases. For example, the question "How are you satisfied with your ability to get out and about" from the QOLIBRI had to be explained, as the idiom "get out and about" is phrased differently in many languages.

The *cultural level* included the use of specific pronominal forms, gender-appropriate language, and the translation of specific terms lacking or seldom used in the culture of the target language. Here, two tendencies were observed: (1) more informal gender-neutral translations (especially in Northern European languages) and (2) more formal gender-sensitive translations in other European languages and Hebrew. In addition, as already expected after devising the conceptual list, differences occurred in the translation of the explanatory text of the GOSE-Q, which included an example of "playing bingo" among other leisure activities. Since playing bingo is uncommon as a leisure activity in many countries, many translating teams used a culturally more appropriate example such as "going out to a restaurant". For a detailed overview, see Supplementary Materials Table S1 online.

3.2. Cognitive Debriefings and Quality of Translations (Phases 4 and 5)

Overall, the average comprehension rates of the participants interviewed for each instrument were above 90% for items and response categories and greater than or equal to 85% for the instructions (see Table 6). Some translations with lower comprehension rates (e.g., the Swedish GOSE/GOSE-Q, the instructions of the Slovakian GOSE-Q, the instructions and responses of the French GOSE-Q, the instructions of the French PCL-5, and the responses of the Slovakian QOLIBRI) required further revisions, which were carried out in the next harmonization step. However, all comprehension rates were at least within an acceptable range (25% to 75%) or above ($\geq$75%), except for the instructions of the Swedish version of the GOSE and the French version of the GOSE-Q, where all participants commented on the wording, which was corrected.

The translational challenges determined in the cognitive debriefings for the ClinRO, its questionnaire version, the PROMs on a linguistic (semantic, syntactic, and idiomatic), and cultural level are summarized in Table 7, together with their solutions.

Linguistic and cultural differences can occur not only in the translation of PROMs but also in the translation of PerfO instruments. The RAVLT can serve as an example of the complexity of the translational and linguistic validation process. A good example of some cultural differences is the word "church", which is used less often in countries where religious backgrounds other than Christianity are predominant. As a solution, the use of the terms "mosque", "synagogue", "temple", or "church" was implemented for these translations. It was also noticed that one to two-syllable nouns were usually used in the English version of the RAVLT, which is not the case in all languages. In the Lithuanian, Russian, and Hungarian languages, for example, nouns generally have two or more syllables, as reflected by the translated nouns. Since the number of syllables per word may influence verbal memory, such language-specific characteristics need to be considered for further multinational translation procedures concerning verbal memory.

3.3. Harmonization and Final Versions (Phases 6 and 7)

The harmonized versions underwent further revisions, depending on the complexity and conceptual clarity of the instrument, the quality of the translations, and results of the cognitive debriefings. When different opinions arose among the team members involved in the final national and international harmonization, a consensus was sought resulting in the most appropriate translations. Instrument developers were only contacted when problems could not be solved, which only happened twice (for the GOAT and PCL-5). These versions were reviewed by informed native speakers (members of the CENTER-TBI study) in the different languages for final adjustments.

Table 8 provides an overview of the changes in coding the semantic, cultural, idiomatic/pragmatic, and syntactic/grammatical differences and issues between the first harmonization and the final versions administered in the study. Most differences concerned semantic and syntactic/grammatical changes. The changes contained improvements of inappropriate translations, consistent use of gender-appropriate language, and grammatical issues (e.g., use of commas and spelling). Most of the issues involved the use of synonyms or words that were initially translated literally from English into the target language but that were not suitable in the context of this language.

Table 6. Average comprehension rates per language and outcome instrument in the cognitive debriefings.

No.	Language	GOSE N	GOSE IN	GOSE I	GOSE R	GOSE-Q N	GOSE-Q IN	GOSE-Q I	GOSE-Q R	PCL-5 N	PCL-5 IN	PCL-5 I	PCL-5 R	QOLIBRI N	QOLIBRI IN	QOLIBRI I	QOLIBRI R	QOLIBRI-OS N	QOLIBRI-OS IN	QOLIBRI-OS I	QOLIBRI-OS R
1	Arabic (for Israel)	-	-	-	-	-	-	-	-	-	-	-	-	-	-	-	-	-	-	-	-
2	Bosnian/Croatian/Serbian	3	100%	100%	100%	6	83%	98%	88%	6	83%	85%	83%	6	67%	92%	100%	6	67%	81%	100%
3	Bulgarian	-	-	-	-	-	-	-	-	-	-	-	-	-	-	-	-	-	-	-	-
4	Czech	*	*	*	*	-	-	-	-	-	-	-	-	-	-	-	-	-	-	-	-
5	Danish	*	*	*	*	6	100%	100%	100%	6	100%	100%	100%	*	*	*	*	*	*	*	*
6	Dutch	*	*	*	*	3	100%	93%	95%	3	100%	95%	100%	*	*	*	*	*	*	*	*
7	Finnish	*	*	*	*	6	100%	98%	100%	6	100%	99%	100%	*	*	*	*	*	*	*	*
8	French	*	*	*	*	4	0%	93%	74%	3	33%	92%	98%	*	*	*	*	*	*	*	*
9	German	*	*	*	*	3	67%	100%	100%	3	100%	80%	100%	*	*	*	*	*	*	*	*
10	Hebrew	2	100%	100%	100%	4	100%	100%	100%	4	100%	100%	100%	4	88%	96%	100%	4	100%	100%	100%
11	Hungarian	2	100%	89%	100%	6	100%	100%	100%	6	100%	96%	100%	6	100%	100%	100%	6	100%	83%	83%
12	Italian	6	100%	91%	100%	6	100%	100%	100%	6	100%	100%	100%	*	*	*	*	*	*	*	*
13	Latvian	10	100%	100%	100%	10	100%	100%	100%	10	100%	100%	100%	10	100%	100%	100%	10	100%	100%	100%
14	Lithuanian	6	100%	100%	100%	6	100%	100%	100%	6	100%	100%	100%	6	100%	100%	100%	6	100%	86%	100%
15	Norwegian	*	*	*	*	*	100%	99%	87%	*	*	*	*	*	*	*	*	*	*	*	*
16	Romanian	3	100%	100%	100%	6	100%	100%	90%	6	100%	100%	100%	6	100%	100%	81%	6	100%	100%	100%
17	Russian (for Israel)	-	-	-	-	-	-	-	-	-	-	-	-	-	-	-	-	-	-	-	-
18	Slovakian	3	100%	86%	97%	6	67%	98%	100%	6	100%	94%	90%	6	92%	98%	100%	6	83%	100%	33%
19	Spanish	3	67%	99%	92%	6	67%	88%	90%	6	100%	81%	100%	10	100%	97%	100%	10	90%	83%	100%
20	Swedish	3	0%	96%	93%	6	83%	70%	76%	6	83%	92%	100%	*	*	*	*	*	*	*	*
	Average	4	87%	96%	98%	5	85%	96%	94%	6	93%	94%	98%	7	93%	98%	98%	7	93%	92%	90%

Note: IN = instructions; I = items, R = item responses; — = no cognitive debriefing performed; * = already existing validated instruments not requiring cognitive debriefing. For the GOSE, mostly clinical personnel were interviewed. Average = the overall average number of participants. Translations are available for the following languages, but no cognitive debriefings: Arabic, Bulgarian, Czech, and Russian. N = number of cognitive debriefings performed, and average comprehension rates per instrument. Bold is for better readability.

Table 7. Translational issues.

Instrument	Language	Type of Issue	Text Element	Description of the Problems by Target Language Translators	Solution [1]
GOSE	Italian	Linguistic	Instruction/heading: Date of **injury**	Difficulties with translation of "**injury**" vs. "**trauma**"	Term "**trauma**" selected
GOSE-Q	Finnish	Cultural	Item 7 (response 2): Looking after family	"**Looking after family**" seems to be rather untypical for the Finnish society/culture (exception: maternity or paternity leave, homemaker)	Response extended by "**e.g., maternity or paternity leave**"
	Hebrew	Cultural	Item 9 (examples for social and leisure activities): going out to a pub or club, visiting friends, going to the cinema or **bingo**, going out for a walk, attending a football match, taking part in sport.	Playing **bingo** is rather untypical for Hebrew society/culture	Term "**bingo**" replaced by "**going out to a restaurant**"
	Norwegian	Cultural	Item 9 (examples for social and leisure activities): going out to a **pub** or club, visiting friends, going to the cinema or bingo, going out for a walk, attending a football match, taking part in sport.	Going to **pubs** is rather untypical for Norwegian society/culture	Term "**pub**" replaced by "**café**"
	Swedish	Linguistic	Item 12: As a result of your injury are there now problems in how you get on with friends or relatives? (response 1): **Things** are still much the same	The term "**things**" cannot be used in Swedish in that way	Term "**relationships**" related to the question selected
PCL-5	Danish, Latvian, Croatian/ Bosnian/ Serbian	Linguistic	Item 21: When you responded to the questions in this questionnaire, were your answers in reference to the stressful experience which caused your **traumatic brain injury**?	Difficulties with translation of the term "**injury**" ("**injury**" vs. "**trauma**", "**head injury**", or "**accident**")	The closest meaning to the term "**brain injury**" was selected in each language
	Arabic	Linguistic	Item 17: Being "superalert" or watchful or **on guard**?	Difficulties with translation of "**on guard**"	Corrected translation of "**on guard**" was implemented
RPQ	Finnish	Linguistic/Cultural	Introduction: We would like to know if **you** now suffer any of the symptoms given below. Because many of these symptoms occur normally, we would like **you** to compare **yourself** now with before the accident.	Comment on the translation of the term "**you**" (using pronominal courtesy form would be more appropriate)	**Pronominal courtesy form** was implemented
QOLIBRI	Romanian	Linguistic	Part E, item 5: **Overall**, how bothered are you by the effects of your brain injury?	Difficulties with translation of "**overall**" vs. "**in general**"	Term "**overall**" replaced by "**in general**"
		Linguistic	All items	No female forms of verbs were available	Female and male forms implemented
GOAT	Finnish	Cultural	Item 2a: Where are you now (**city**)?	"Finland is mostly rural, there are a lot of municipalities without towns"	Term "**city**" replaced by "**place**"

Note: [1] The solution was provided after discussion between the patients, the healthy individuals, the core team and the translation teams in the target languages. Bold is for better readability.

Table 8. Average (mean and median) number of differences between the first harmonized and the final internationally harmonized translations.

Measure	Text Elements	No.	Mean S	Mean C	Mean I/P	Mean S/G	Median S	Median C	Median I/P	Median S/G	Examples
ClinRO, its questionnaire version, and a clinical amnesia rating											
GOSE (10 translations)	In	11	31%	2%	10%	20%	18%	0%	9%	9%	S: Use of synonyms to find the closest possible, but not a literal, translation, e.g., "injury" vs. "trauma", "they" vs. "he/she". C: Use of courtesy (West, Middle, East, and Southern European languages) vs. informal (especially Northern European languages) pronominal form and gender-appropriate language (only emerged during harmonization in some translations). I/P: Use of appropriate expressions common for the target languages, e.g., "as it appears". S/G: Use of appropriate sentence structures and grammar suitable for the target languages, e.g., word order and spelling.
	I	19	22%	2%	1%	15%	21%	0%	0%	13%	
	R	15	9%	1%	1%	5%	7%	0%	0%	6%	
GOSE-Q (16 translations)	In	2	107%	9%	7%	23%	50%	0%	0%	0%	S: Use of synonyms to find the closest possible, but not a literal, translation, e.g., "injury" vs. "trauma". C: Use of courtesy (West, Middle, East, and Southern European languages) vs. informal (especially Northern European languages) pronominal form and gender-appropriate language; use of examples suitable for the target language countries, e.g., "playing bingo" vs. "going out to restaurant" (only emerged during harmonization in some translations). I/P: Use of appropriate translations of phrases "at least half as often" and "less than half as often". S/G: Use of appropriate sentence structures, e.g., word order.
	I	14	11%	1%	0%	10%	4%	0%	0%	7%	
	R	42	7%	6%	1%	3%	2%	0%	0%	2%	
GOAT (16 translations)	In	8	10%	6%	3%	10%	0%	0%	0%	0%	S: Use of synonyms to find the closest possible, but not a literal, translation, e.g., "injury" vs. "trauma" or "accident". C: Use of courtesy (West, Middle, East, and Southern European languages) vs. informal (especially Northern European languages) pronominal form and gender-appropriate language (only emerged during harmonization in some translations); use of time formats most common to the target language countries, e.g., "am/pm" seem to be uncommon in most languages/countries. I/P: Use of appropriate expressions common to the target languages in everyday use, e.g., "Where are you now?". S/G: Use of appropriate sentence structures and grammar suitable for the target languages, e.g., word order and spelling.
	I	13	16%	0%	7%	9%	8%	0%	0%	0%	
	R	-	-	-	-	-	-	-	-	-	

Table 8. Cont.

Measure	Text Elements	No.	Average Number of Changes									Examples
			Mean				Median					
			S	C	I/P	S/G	S	C	I/P	S/G		
PROMs *												
GAD-7 (2 translations)	In	1	0%	50%	0%	0%	0%	50%	0%	0%		S: - C: Use of courtesy pronominal form and gender-appropriate language (only emerged during harmonization in some translations). I/P: - S/G: Use of appropriate sentence structures and grammar suitable for the target languages, e.g., comma placement and spelling.
	I	7	0%	0%	0%	0%	0%	0%	0%	0%		
	R	5	0%	0%	0%	14%	0%	0%	0%	14%		
PHQ-9 (1 translation)	In	1	0%	0%	0%	0%	0%	0%	0%	0%		S: - C: - I/P: - S/G: Use of appropriate sentence structures and grammar suitable for the target languages, e.g., comma placement and spelling.
	I	10	0%	0%	0%	20%	0%	0%	0%	20%		
	R	5	0%	0%	0%	0%	0%	0%	0%	0%		
PCL-5 (15 translations)	In	1	100%	7%	7%	47%	0%	0%	0%	0%		S: Use of synonyms to find the closest possible, but not a literal, translation, e.g., "stressful" or "disturbing" experience. C: Use of courtesy pronominal form and gender-appropriate language (only emerged during harmonization in some translations). I/P: Use of appropriate expressions common to the target languages in everyday use, e.g., "Being 'superalert' or watchful or on guard". S/G: Use of appropriate tense, sentence structures and grammar suitable for the target languages, e.g., translating of verbs in present continuous (e.g., "being", "having", and "feeling").
	I	21	26%	1%	4%	14%	19%	0%	0%	14%		
	R	5	11%	0%	1%	7%	0%	0%	0%	0%		
RPQ (13 translations)	In	1	123%	23%	23%	77%	0%	0%	0%	77%		S: Use of synonyms to find the closest possible, but not a literal, translation of the terms, e.g., "injury" vs. "trauma", appropriate translation of "poor concentrations" or "forgetfulness". C: Use of courtesy pronominal form (only emerged during harmonization in some translations). I/P: Use of appropriate expressions, e.g., in translating response category "no more of a problem (than before)". S/G: Use of appropriate sentence structures, tense, and grammar suitable for the target languages, e.g., translating of verbs in present continuous (e.g., "being" and "feeling").
	I	17	6%	1%	3%	4%	6%	0%	0%	4%		
	R	5	9%	0%	3%	6%	0%	0%	0%	0%		

Table 8. Cont.

Measure	Text Elements	No.	Average Number of Changes					Median				Examples
			Mean									
			S	C	I/P	S/G	S	C	I/P	S/G		
QOLIBRI (8 translations)	In	7	14%	2%	0%	7%	14%	0%	0%	0%	S: Use of synonyms to find the closest possible, but not a literal, translation of the terms, e.g., "brain injury" vs. "trauma", "How satisfied are you..." and "How bothered are you...".
	I	37	10%	0%	1%	5%	9%	0%	0%	5%	C: Use of courtesy pronominal form and gender-appropriate language (only emerged during harmonization in some translations).
	R	5	20%	0%	0%	13%	10%	0%	0%	0%	I/P: Use of appropriate expressions, e.g., to be "in charge of your own life". S/G: Use of appropriate sentence structures and grammar suitable for the target languages, e.g., comma placement and spelling.
QOLIBRI-OS (8 translations)	In	1	25%	13%	38%	38%	0%	0%	0%	0%	S: Use of synonyms to find the closest possible, but not a literal, translation of the terms, e.g., "brain injury" vs. "trauma", "future prospects" vs. "plans for the future".
	I	6	13%	4%	2%	4%	6%	0%	0%	0%	C: Use of courtesy pronominal form and gender-appropriate language (only emerged during harmonization in some translations).
	R	5	5%	0%	3%	3%	0%	0%	0%	0%	I/P: Use of appropriate expressions common in everyday use, e.g., "don't hesitate to ask for help". S/G: Use of appropriate sentence structures and grammar suitable for the target languages, e.g., comma placement and spelling.
PerfO *												
RAVLT (16 translations)	In	5	81%	8%	9%	41%	30%	0%	0%	40%	S: Use of synonyms to find the closest possible, but not a literal, translation of the instructions.
	I	45	3%	0%	2%	1%	3%	0%	0%	0%	C: Use of courtesy pronominal form and gender-appropriate language (only emerged during harmonization in some translations); use of language- and/or culture-specific terms (e.g., "church" vs. "synagogue").
	R	-	-	-	-	-	-	-	-	-	I/P: Selection of suitable words more frequently used in everyday life, e.g., "tool" or "cake". S/G: Use of appropriate sentence structures and grammar suitable for the target languages, e.g., comma placement and spelling especially in the instructions.

Table 8. *Cont.*

Measure	Text Elements	No.	Average Number of Changes								Examples
			Mean				Median				
			S	C	I/P	S/G	S	C	I/P	S/G	
TMT A/B (14 translations)	In	6	14%	2%	5%	19%	0%	0%	0%	0%	S: Use of synonyms to find the closest possible, but not a literal, translation of the instructions, e.g., "participant" or "examiner". C: Use of courtesy pronominal form and gender-appropriate language (only emerged during harmonization in some translations). I/P: Selection of suitable words more frequently used in everyday life, e.g., to be "sure about" something. S/G: Use of appropriate sentence structures and grammar suitable for the target languages, e.g., comma placement and spelling, especially in the instructions.
	I	38	0%	0%	0%	0%	0%	0%	0%	0%	
	R	-	-	-	-	-	-	-	-	-	

Note: No. = No. of text elements; In = average modifications between the first harmonization and the final version in instructions (average in %, i.e., number of differences relative to the total number of the respective text elements divided by the number of translations); I = modifications in items; R = modifications in response categories (if applicable, otherwise "-"); S = syntactic level; C = cultural level; I/P = idiomatic/pragmatic level; S/G = syntactical/grammatical level; ClinRO = clinician-reported outcome instrument; PROM = patient-reported outcome measures; PerfO = performance-based outcome instruments; GOSE = Glasgow Outcome Scale—Extended; instructions of the GOSE include introduction (1), commentary on the questions (9), and scoring (1); GOSE-Q = Glasgow Outcome Scale—Extended questionnaire version; instructions of the GOSE-Q include introduction and header (1) and explanatory example for the item 9; different types of responses (dichotomous yes/no, including extensions for GOSE scoring) and polytomous item-related responses result in 42 elements; GOAT = Galveston Orientation Amnesia Test; the GOAT has no response categories; GAD-7 = Generalized Anxiety Disorder 7 Items Questionnaire; PHQ-9 = Patient Health Questionnaire 9; PCL-5 = Posttraumatic Stress Disorder Checklist; RPQ = Rivermead Post-Concussion Symptoms questionnaire; QOLIBRI = Quality of Life after Brain Injury Scale; instructions of the QOLIBRI include introduction to the two parts (2) and five subsections (5); QOLIBRI-OS = Quality of Life after Brain Injury—Overall Scale; RAVLT = Rey Auditory Verbal Learning Test; in the RAVLT, words are treated as items (5 × 15 = 45), there are no response categories; instructions of the RAVLT include introduction (1), explanations on the three trials (3), and the summary table for evaluation of the test result (1); TMT-A/B = Trail-Making Test A, B; in the TMT-A/B, letters and numbers are treated as items, there are no response categories; instructions of the TMT-A, B include introduction (1), explanation on the trial A (1) and trial B (1), trial B test (1), scoring (1), hands check (1); CANTAB = Cambridge Neuropsychological Test Automated Battery. * Excluded from analysis as translations of the SF-36v2/-12v were obtained from Optum. CANTAB analyses are not presented here as in the meantime only updated versions from Cambridge Cognition can be used. Therefore, these are not available on the CENTER-TBI website. Cognitive debriefings and international harmonization of the Arabic, Russian, Bulgarian, and the Czech translations were not carried out and are thus not reported.

Considering the average (i.e., the mean) relative number of coded differences, the instruments involving the most changes were the RPQ, followed by the GOSE-Q and the PCL-5. However, the main changes in the RPQ, and in the PCL-5 occurred only in a few languages (Swedish, German, Danish, and Bosnian/Croatian/Serbian), which is reflected in the average percentages. Based on the median, most changes were performed during the harmonization of the GOSE-Q, followed by the RAVLT and the GOSE. For a detailed overview, see Supplementary Materials Table S2 online.

In sum, these efforts resulted in linguistically validated translations into up to 20 languages of one ClinRO instrument, its questionnaire version, one clinical amnesia test, six PROMs, and three PerfO instruments, including six CANTAB subtests.

4. Discussion

The translations of the 17 outcome measures into up to 20 languages and the linguistic validations in up to 18 languages were achieved with input from over 150 international collaborators. These translated instruments provide a basis for reliable and valid future TBI outcome research and clinical practice, thereby facilitating data collection and comparisons across 18 countries in Europe and Israel. Translated and linguistically validated versions of the instruments used in the study are accessible in the public domain on the website of CENTER-TBI (https://www.center-tbi.eu/ (accessed on 16 April 2021)).

Recommendations: The following recommendations resulting from our linguistic validation work may be helpful for future international projects in the field of TBI and related areas.

First, it is important to work with translators with linguistic expertise, as well as expertise in the field of TBI, in addition to being native or fluent in English. In contrast to the MAPI guidelines [25], we only seldom resorted to certified professional translators as the professional translations had to be revised much more extensively in our study than the others. Furthermore, similar to Swaine-Verdier et al. (2004) [28], we also attempted—whenever possible—to integrate at least one person with a background in linguistics, teaching, or administration in the translation process. These vocational groups were assumed to be especially sensitized to the everyday use of language, comparable to the language of the individuals later answering the instruments [28]. In addition, regardless of the type of outcome measure (PROM, ClinRO, clinical amnesia test, or PerfO), it is important to consider the linguistic concepts and cultural background of each country, including the use of gender-appropriate language, courtesy, or informal pronominal forms, and specific idiomatic and pragmatic terms. Instruments with items using different and/or item-specific response formats and more detailed instructions do require more work compared with instruments consisting only of a few items with a standard Likert response scale. The translation and linguistic validation of clinical rating scales, such as the GOSE, were particularly time-consuming and complex. Detailed standardized training of raters is also recommended for this type of clinical scale, to enhance the comparability of the ratings.

Second, besides the selection of translators, the integration of extensive international harmonization panels and the good to excellent psychometric properties of the translated and linguistically validated PROMs described in von Steinbuechel et al. [32], as well as in van Praag et al. [54] and in Plass et al. [55], underline the quality of our translations of the instruments based on the procedure applied. Furthermore, we found face-to-face or video conferences very helpful during this procedure to enhance coherence across all languages. Visiting some translating country centers that participated in the linguistic validation procedure in person also served to intensify and ameliorate the process.

Third, as an understanding of the importance, implications, and intense workload of linguistic validation procedures is still underrepresented in the field of TBI research, more resources should be allocated to this type of undertaking. For future international multidimensional outcome studies on TBI, we wish to provide a solid basis for linguistic validation and its funding.

Fourth, the issue of commercial ownership of instruments is one that public funding bodies such as the EU and the National Institutes of Health (NIH) should consider before designating instruments as recommended data elements. While the costs involved in using such commercial instruments may not be an insurmountable burden in high-income countries, they may be extremely challenging in low- and middle-income countries. The SF-12v2, SF-36v2, and the CANTAB are only available on a commercial basis. All translations of the QOLBRI and the QOLIBRI-OS instruments described in this manuscript are freely available for academic use from www.center-tbi.eu (accessed on 16 April 2021) and https://qolibrinet.com (accessed on 16 April 2021). In addition, translations of these instruments developed within the CENTER-TBI project (Arabic, Bulgarian, Bosnian/Croatian/Serbian, Hebrew, Hungarian, Latvian, Lithuanian, Romanian, Russian, Slovakian, and Spanish) are also free for commercial use. All other translations of these instruments that preceded the CENTER-TBI project are not covered by CENTER-TBI agreements; they are free for academic research, but not for commercial use. For further information and potential (commercial) use, please access https://qolibrinet.com (accessed on 16 April 2021).

Fifth, many of the outcome instruments are available in a wide range of versions, the existence of which is not obvious. Resources, therefore, need to be used to identify appropriate versions ensuring the comparability of data.

Sixth and final, as the translation and linguistic validation procedures were labor- and resource-intensive, they could only be accomplished thanks to the dedication and using the personal resources of contributing CENTER-TBI participants, investigators, and MC members.

Overall, the freely available ClinRO, its questionnaire version, a clinical amnesia test, PROMs, and PerfOs and the results of the present study provide many opportunities for future translations and linguistic validations in other languages. The psychometric validation of the PROMs [32] in different languages establishes a reliable basis for national, international, and multicenter studies in the field of TBI.

Limitations. The translation and linguistic validation procedure described in the present study mainly followed the recommendations of MAPI [25] and ISPOR [26,27], with some adaptations in terms of the conceptual analyses, selection of translators, and the number of translations and cognitive debriefings. In contrast to these recommendations, we only contacted developers for the conceptual analysis of the original instruments when difficulties occurred with the concept description or if difficulties arose during the harmonization. Translators did not need to provide a language certificate but needed to be native speakers, fluent in English, experienced in the care of patients in the field of TBI, and preferably in outcome assessment. The effectiveness of this type of selection of professionals was also reflected in the good to excellent psychometric quality of the translations [53–55]. As the labor-intensive procedures required a pragmatic approach with an efficient use of limited resources, only one formal forward translation was carried out for the non-core or not additionally prioritized instruments (i.e., GOAT, GAD-7, PHQ-9, RPQ, TMT-A, B, RAVLT, and CANTAB).

However, we tried to compensate for potential deficits by means of intense iterative reviews, revisions, and international harmonization. Concerning the cognitive debriefings performed, we interviewed at least two clinicians, three-to-five laypersons, and three to five TBI patients, instead of the minimum five described by MAPI [25], which was an effective way of coping with the shortage in some countries (centers) of TBI patients willing to participate in the cognitive debriefings.

Finally, we decided to delay publication until the data and results of psychometric analyses of the translated instruments were available [32], which required completion of enrolment and six-month outcome assessment (2018) and subsequent data curation and analysis (2020 to 2021).

Future perspectives. Future research should perform cognitive debriefings and international harmonization of the Arabic, Russian, Bulgarian, and Czech translations, which have not been carried out. In the next step, the psychometric characteristics and measurement invariance of the concepts used in the different instruments should be a topic for future research [56–58].

5. Conclusions

Linguistically validated translations in up to 20 languages were produced for one ClinRO (GOSE) and its questionnaire version (GOSE-Q), one clinical amnesia test (GOAT), six PROMs (GAD-7, PHQ-9, PCL-5, RPQ, QOLIBRI, QOLIBRI-OS), and three PerfO instruments (RAVLT, TMT-A,B) and the CANTAB with six separate subtests for individuals after TBI. The translations of the outcome instruments, in so far as they are in the public domain, are available on the CENTER-TBI homepage (https://www.center-tbi.eu/, accessed on 16 April 2021).

The description of the linguistic validation process of these instruments may provide the basis for future linguistic and psychometric validations for national and multinational cross-cultural TBI outcome studies. The availability of these instruments with good to excellent psychometric properties in the field of TBI [32] in the most widely spoken languages in Europe and Israel may facilitate and improve outcome research and clinical evaluation of individuals after TBI in the future.

Supplementary Materials: The following are available online at https://www.mdpi.com/article/10.3390/jcm10132863/s1, Table S1: Comparisons between the original English versions and the first draft translations of one ClinRO, its questionnaire version, a clinical amnesia test, PROMs, and PerfO instruments, Table S2: Comparisons between the first draft translations and the final target language versions of one ClinRO, its questionnaire version, a clinical amnesia test, PROMs, and PerfO instruments.

Author Contributions: Conceptualization, N.v.S., U.K., A.C. and M.Z.; data curation, N.v.S.; formal analysis, U.K., A.C., F.B., A.M.P., K.C., I.M. and M.Z.; funding acquisition, N.v.S., S.P., A.I.R.M. and D.M.; methodology, N.v.S. and M.Z.; project administration, N.v.S.; resources, N.v.S.; supervision, N.v.S.; validation, N.v.S.; visualization, A.C., F.B. and M.Z.; writing—original draft, N.v.S., K.R., U.K., A.C. and M.Z.; writing—review and editing, N.v.S., K.R., U.K., Y.-J.W., A.C., A.M.P. K.C., I.M., F.B., S.P., L.W., E.W.S., A.I.R.M., D.M and M.Z. All authors have read and agreed to the published version of the manuscript.

Funding: CENTER-TBI was supported by the European Union 7th Framework programme (EC grant 602150). Additional funding was obtained from the Hannelore Kohl Stiftung (Germany), from OneMind (USA), and from Integra LifeSciences Corporation (USA). The funders of the study had no role in study design, data collection, data analysis, data interpretation, or writing of the report.

Institutional Review Board Statement: The CENTER-TBI study (EC grant 602150) was conducted in accordance with all relevant laws of the European Union (EU), if directly applicable or of direct effect, and all relevant laws of the country where the recruiting sites were located. Informed consent by the patients and/or the legal representative/next of kin was obtained, accordingly to the local legislations, for all patients recruited in the Core Dataset of CENTER-TBI and documented in the electronic case report form (e-CRF). For the full list of sites, ethical committees, and ethical approval details, see the official CENTER-TBI website (https://www.center-tbi.eu/project/ethical-approval, accessed on 16 April 2021).

Informed Consent Statement: Informed consent was obtained from all subjects involved in the study.

Data Availability Statement: All relevant data are available upon request from CENTER-TBI, and the authors are not legally allowed to share it publicly. The authors confirm that they received no special access privileges to the data. CENTER-TBI is committed to data sharing and in particular to responsible further use of the data. Hereto, we have a data-sharing statement in place: https://www.center-tbi.eu/data/sharing, accessed on 16 April 2021. The CENTER-TBI Management Committee, in collaboration with the General Assembly, established the Data Sharing policy, and Publication and Authorship Guidelines to assure correct and appropriate use of the data as the dataset is hugely complex and requires help of experts from the Data Curation Team or Bio- Statistical Team for correct use. This means that we encourage researchers to contact the CENTER-TBI team for any research plans and the Data Curation Team for any help in appropriate use of the data, including sharing of scripts. Requests for data access can be submitted online: https://www.center-tbi.eu/data, accessed on 16 April 2021. The complete Manual for data access is also available online: https://www.center-tbi.eu/files/SOP-Manual-DAPR-20181101.pdf, accessed on 16 April 2021.

Acknowledgments: The authors would like to thank the language coordinators from the University Medical Center Göttingen, Institute for Medical Psychology and Medical Sociology, who coordinated and drove the translation processes, beside some of the authors: Henning Bohnsack, Sylvia von Mackensen, Sabine Mayne, Beate Rother, and Nadine Sasse. The authors would also like to cordially thank all of those whose permission to acknowledge them we received who contributed to the translations, numerous revisions, cognitive debriefings and harmonizations, and the linguistic validation group. Unfortunately, we were unable to reach around 40 former collaborators. We would like to sincerely thank the entire linguistic validation group for all contributions. Additionally, among several others, we would like to express our sincere gratitude to Elisabeth Ginnerup-Nielsen, Johanna Nurmi, Aurore Mabilat, David Piterman, Judit Molnár, Barbara Danti, Liene Karaukle, Anastasia Olympiou, Andreea Gregore, Lucia Rahackova, Pedro Alejandro Rodriguez-Nunez, and Alena Lange, who contributed to the completion of the comparative analyses of the translations in the shortest possible time.

Conflicts of Interest: The authors declare no conflict of interest. The funders had no role in the design of the study; in the collection, analyses, or interpretation of data; in the writing of the manuscript; or in the decision to publish the results.

Appendix A. Linguistic Validation Group

Name	Affiliation
Abu Shkara Ramiz	Department of Neurosurgery, Hadassah-Hebrew University Medical Center, Jerusalem, Israel
Alshafai Nabeel	Neurosurgical Academy, Toronto, Canada
Andelic Nada	Department of Physical Medicine and Rehabilitation, Oslo University Hospital, Oslo, Norway and Faculty of Medicine, Institute of Health and Society, Research Centre for Habilitation and Rehabilitation Models and Services (CHARM), University of Oslo, Oslo, Norway
Azouvi Philippe	Physical and Rehabilitation Medicine, Hospital Raymond Poincaré, Garches, France
Bachvarova Maya	Institute for Medical Psychology and Medical Sociology, University Medical Center Göttingen, Göttingen, Germany
Bakx Wilbert	Department of brain injury, Adelante, Adult rehabilitation, Hoensbroek, The Netherlands
Bar Sapir Peleg	no affiliation
Björkdahl Ann	Ersta Sköndal Bräcke University College, Institute of Social Science, campus Bräcke, Gothenburg, Sweden
Branca Enrica	Institute for Medical Psychology and Medical Sociology, University Medical Center Göttingen, Göttingen, Germany
Brazinova Alexandra	Faculty of Medicine, Comenius University, Bratislava, Slovak Republic
Chatelle Camille	Louvain Bionics, Université catholique de Louvain, Ottignies-Louvain-la-Neuve, Belgium
Dahyot-Fizelier Claire	Department of Anesthesia and Intensive Care, University Hospital of Poitiers, INSERM U1070, University of Poitiers, Poitiers, France
Del Bianco Silvia	Neurointensive Care Unit, San Gerardo Hospital Monza, Monza, Italy
Furmanov Alex	Neurosurgery ICU, Hadassah Hebrew University Medical Center, Jerusalem, Israel
Godbolt Alison	University Department of Rehabilitation Medicine Stockholm, Danderyd Hospital, Sweden
Gürlich Robert	General University Hospital Kralovske Vinohrady, Prague, Czech Republic
Hedenäs Anna	University Department of Rehabilitation Medicine, Danderyd Hospital, Acquired Brain Injury Unit, Daycare, Stockholm, Sweden
Hoang Stéphane	Institute for Medical Psychology and Medical Sociology, University Medical Center Göttingen, Göttingen, Germany

Name	Affiliation
Kanuscak Martin	Institute for Medical Psychology and Medical Sociology, University Medical Center Göttingen, Göttingen, Germany
Karan Mladen	Department of Neurosurgery, Haukeland University Hospital, Bergen, Norway
Kondziella Daniel	Department of Neurology, Rigshospitalet, Copenhagen University Hospital, Copenhagen, Denmark
Koskinen Sanna	Department of Psychology and Logopedics, University of Helsinki, Helsinki, Finnland
Laleva Maria	Department of Neurosurgery, University Hospital Pirogov, Sofia, Bulgaria
Levi Leon	Rambam Healthcare Campus, Haifa, Israel
Liebertau Pia	Klinik IV, Klinikum Osnabrück, Germany, and Institut für Ethik und Geschichte der Medizin, University Medical Center Göttingen, Göttingen, Germany
Lundgaard Soberg Helene	Department of Physical Medicine and Rehabilitation, Oslo University Hospital, Oslo, Norway
Martino Costanza	Dipartimento Chirurgico e Grandi Traumi, Ospedale M. Bufalini, Cesena, Italy
Menovsky Tomas	Department of Neurosurgery, Antwerp University Hospital, Antwerp, Belgium
Milinkovic Sladana	Clinical Center of Vojvodina, Novi Sad, Serbia
Mondello Stefania	Department of Biomedical and Dental Sciences and Morphofunctional Imaging, University of Messina, Italy
Nelson David	Department of Physiology and Pharmacology, Karolinska Universitetssjukhus, Solna, Sweden
Oistensen Holthe Oyvor	Department of Physical Medicine and Rehabilitation, Oslo University Hospital, Oslo, Norway
Pestovskaya Natalia	Burdenko National Medical Research Center of Neurosurgery (NN Burdenko NMRCN), Moscow, Russia
Pfeiffer Anna	Institute for Medical Psychology and Medical Sociology, University Medical Center Göttingen, Göttingen, Germany
Popescu Codruta	Department of Practical Abilities, Human Science, University of Medicine and Pharmacy Iuliu Hatieganu, Cluj-Napoca, Romania
Potapov Aleksandr	Burdenko National Medical Research Center of Neurosurgery (NN Burdenko NMRCN), Moscow, Russia
Poulsen Ingrid	Department of Neurorehabilitation, TBI Unit, Rigshospitalet, Denmark and Research Unit Nursing and Health Care, Health, Aarhus University, Denmark
Radoi Andreea	Clinical Research Office at BarcelonaBeta Brain Research Center, Barcelona, Spain
Ragauskas Arminas	Health Telematics Science Institute, Kaunas University of Technology, Kaunas, Lithuania
Ramin Irina	Institute for Medical Psychology and Medical Sociology, University Medical Center Göttingen, Göttingen, Germany
Ramin Petr	Institute for Medical Psychology and Medical Sociology, University Medical Center Göttingen, Göttingen, Germany
Ramin Stanislav	Institute for Medical Psychology and Medical Sociology, University Medical Center Göttingen, Göttingen, Germany
Reggi Valeria	University of Brescia, Brescia, Italy and University of Bologna, Bologna, Italy
Reith Florence	Department of Neurosurgery, Sir Charles Gairdner Hospital, Perth, WA, Australia
Ribbers Gerard	Department of Rehabilitation Medicine, Erasmus MC, University Medical Center Rotterdam, Rotterdam, the Netherlands
Rocka Saulius	Clinic of Neurology and Neurosurgery, Vilnius University, Vilnius, Lithuania
Rosenlund Sorensen Christina	Department of Neurosurgery, Odense University Hospital, Odense, Denmark
Rosenthal Guy	Department of Neurosurgery, Hadassah-Hebrew University Medical Center, Jerusalem, Israel
Sahuquillo Juan	Department of Neurosurgery, Vall d'Hebron University Hospital, Barcelona, Spain

Name	Affiliation
Schäfer Kaja J.	Department of Pediatrics, Klinikum Bremerhaven-Reinkenheide gGmbH, Bremerhaven, Germany
Schou Rico	Neuroanesthesiology and -Intensive Care, University Hospital of Odense, Odense, Denmark
Siponkoski Sini-Tuulu	Cognitive Brain Research Unit, Department of Psychology and Logopedics, University of Helsinki, Helsinki, Finnland
Skandsen Toril	Institute of Neuromedicine and Movement sciences Norwegian University of Science and Technology Specialist in Physical and Rehabilitation Medicine St. Olavs Hospital, Trondheim University Hospital, Norway
Skoett Skare BruunMarie	Danish Dementia Research Centre, Department of Neurology, Rigshospitalet, University of Copenhagen, Denmark
Skowroneck Lukas	Department of Languages, Literature and Communication, University of Utrecht, Utrecht, the Netherlands
Sokkanen Sanna E.	South Karelia Social and Health Care District, University of Jyväskylä, Jyväskylä, Finnland
Sonne E. Morten	Centre of Head and Orthopaedics, Department of Anaesthesiology, Copenhagen University Hospital, Rigshospitalet, Copenhagen, Denmark
Steinbusch Catherine	Adelante Rehabilitation Centre Valkenburg, Valkenburg, the Netherlands
Stocchetti Nino	Dipartimento Fisiopatologia e Trapianti, Fondazione IRCCS Cà Granda Ospedale Maggiore Policlinico, Milan, Italy
Tamir Idit	Neurosurgery Department, Rabin Medical Center Petach Tikva, Petach Tikva, Israel
Tenovuo Olli	Turku Brain Injury Centre, University of Turku and Turku University Hospital, Turku, Finnland
Teunissen Charlotte	Vrije Universiteit Amsterdam, Amsterdam, The Netherlands
Theodorou Konstantina	Institute for Medical Psychology and Medical Sociology, University Medical Center Göttingen, Göttingen, Germany
Turcsányi Ditta	English and Hungarian as a Foreign Language Teacher
Valeinis Egils	Neurosurgery Clinic, Pauls Stradins Clinical University Hospital, Riga, Latvia
Van der MerschNils	Université Libre de Bruxelles, Bruxelles, Belgium
van Laake-Geelen Charlotte	Adelante Centre of Expertise in Rehabilitation and Audiology, Hoensbroek, The Netherlands
Van Praag Dominique	Department of Psychology, Antwerp University Hospital, Edegem and University of Antwerp, Antwerp, Belgium
Vargiolu Alessia	School of Medicine and Surgery, University of Milano—Bicocca, Milan, Italy
Velinov Nikolay	Department of Neurosurgery for Adults, Clinics of Neurosurgery, University Hospital Pirogov, Novi Sad, Serbia
Vilcinis Rimantas	Department of Neurosurgery, Hospital of Lithuanian University of Health Sciences, Kaunas, Lithuania
Vulekovic Petar	Clinic of Neurosurgery, Clinical Center of Vojvodina, Novi Sad, Serbia

Appendix B. Instruments Administered in the CENTER-TBI Study

Appendix B.1. Clinician-Reported Outcome Assessments (ClinRO), Its Clinical Version and a Clinical Amnesia Test

Glasgow Outcome Scale Extended (GOSE-Interview) [37]. This clinical rating evaluates patients' functional status and level of disability. The GOSE consists of 19 items with both dichotomous and polytomous responses measuring different domains (consciousness, independence at home and outside home, work, social and leisure activities, family and friendships, return to normal life, and epilepsy). Functional outcome is rated by a clinician on an eight-point scale (1 = dead, 2 = vegetative state, 3/4 = lower/upper severe disability, 5/6 = lower/upper moderate disability, and 7/8 = lower/upper good recovery).

Glasgow Outcome Scale Extended—Questionnaire version (GOSE-Q) [38]. This questionnaire addresses similar aspects to the GOSE interview in a format that a patient can answer with or without help, or a caretaker can complete. The GOSE-Q consists of 14 items with different response formats (from "yes"/"no" to specifically item-related rating scales and response categories). In the CENTER-TBI study, the GOSE-Q was used for data collection via mail or during a visit. The allocation to the respective functional status categories according to the GOSE definition was performed centrally.

Galveston Orientation Amnesia Test (GOAT) [39]. This standardized evaluation based on patient responses assesses whether an individual suffers from post-traumatic amnesia (PTA). It comprises ten items measuring orientation, memory for the first event that the participant can recall after the injury (anterograde amnesia), and memory for the last event that the participant can recall from before the injury (retrograde amnesia). The instrument is administered by clinical personnel.

Appendix B.2. Patient-Reported Outcome Measures (PROMs)

Generalized Anxiety Disorder 7 (GAD-7) [40]. With seven items, this self-report tool assesses symptoms of generalized anxiety disorder with a recall period of the past two weeks. The GAD-7 applies a four-point Likert scale (from 0 "not at all" to 3 "nearly every day").

Patient Health Questionnaire 9 (PHQ-9) [41]. This short self-report instrument captures presence and severity of major depression using nine items based on the Diagnostic and Statistical Manual of Mental Disorders, 4th edition (DSM-IV) [59], criteria with a recall period of the past two weeks.

Posttraumatic Stress Disorder Checklist (PCL-5) [42]. This self-report scale evaluates 20 posttraumatic stress disorder (PTSD) symptoms with a recall period of one week at the two-week assessment and a recall period of a month for later assessments. The rating is based on the Diagnostic and Statistical Manual of Mental Disorders, 5th edition (DSM-5) [60] and applies a five-point Likert scale (from 0 "not at all" to 4 "extremely").

Rivermead Post-Concussion Symptoms Questionnaire (RPQ) [43]. This self-report questionnaire measures 16 post-concussion symptoms after TBI applying a five-point Likert scale (from 0 "not experienced at all" to 4 = "a severe problem"). Individuals rate how much they suffered from the following symptoms over the last 24 h compared with their condition before the injury: headaches, dizziness, nausea and/or vomiting, noise sensitivity, sleep disturbance, fatigue, irritability, depression, frustration, forgetfulness and poor memory, poor concentration, slow thinking, blurred vision, light sensitivity, double vision, and restlessness. Two additional open questions assess further difficulties experienced after TBI which should be rated on the same scale as other symptoms.

Quality of Life after Brain Injury Scale (QOLIBRI) [44,45]. This is a disease-specific instrument for individuals after TBI, assessing HRQOL using 37 items on a five-point Likert scale (from 0 "not at all" to 4 "very"). Based on these items, the following six domains are evaluated: cognition, self, daily life and autonomy, social relationships, emotions, and physical problems.

Quality of Life after Brain Injury—Overall Scale (QOLIBRI-OS) [46]. The QOLIBRI-OS is a short screener of disease-specific HRQOL after TBI. It comprises six items, which measure physical conditions, cognition, emotions, daily life and autonomy, social relationships, and current and future prospects, respectively. The QOLIBRI-OS applies a five-point Likert scale (from 0 "not at all" to 4 "very").

Additionally, two generic PROMs assessing the subjective health status—the 36-item Short Form Health Survey—Version 2 (SF-36v2) [47] and the 12-item Short Form Survey—Version 2 (SF-12v2) [48]—were administered in the CENTER-TBI study. Both measures had already been translated into the target languages and had to be purchased from Optum [52] for one-time use.

Appendix B.3. Performance-Based Outcome Instruments (PerfO)

Cambridge Neuropsychological Test Automated Battery (CANTAB) [49]. The CANTAB is a computer-based, mainly language-independent test battery well suited for administration in multinational settings. The license to use this battery is made available by Cambridge Cognition [61]. Although the CANTAB is language-independent and is administered by trained personnel, participants should receive standardized information on the test procedure. The instructions are provided for each of six subtests and contain explanations and examples for each task (e.g., instructions for practice trials, hints for keyboard usage, prompts, etc.). To ensure the validity of the GOAT translations, this information should be equivalent across the languages. Therefore, the test instructions of the following six CANTAB tests, selected for the application in the CENTER-TBI study, needed to be translated into most languages:

1. Reaction Time (RTI)—The RTI is designed to measure motor and mental response speed, movement time, reaction time, response accuracy, and impulsivity.
2. Spatial Working Memory (SWM)—This test measures the subject's ability to remember spatial information and requires retention and manipulation of visual-spatial information, working memory, and executive functions.
3. Paired Associate Learning (PAL)—This test assesses conditional learning and episodic visual memory and is primarily sensitive to processes associated with the medial temporal lobe.
4. Rapid Visual Processing (RVP)—The RVP captures visual sustained attention, being sensitive to dysfunctions in the parietal and frontal lobe brain areas.
5. Attention Switching Task (AST)—As a measure of cued attentional set-shifting this test captures executive functioning and cognitive flexibility.
6. Stockings of Cambridge (SOC)—Spatial planning and spatial working memory are assessed with this measure of frontal-lobe functioning.

Rey Auditory Verbal Learning Test (RAVLT) [50]. This memory word list evaluates a range of memory functions, including verbal memory, shorter and longer retention of information and learning, and is administered by trained examiners. The instrument consists of two lists (A and B form) comprising 15 words, respectively. In total, there were four versions of the RAVLT, each with two different word lists. Three versions of two RAVLT word lists were administered in the CENTER-TBI study (lists 1 to 3 in 2-week, 3-month, and 6-month outcome assessments, respectively, and lists 3 to 1 at 6-, 12-, and 24-month outcome assessments, respectively).

Trail-Making Test A, B (TMT-A, B) [51]. This test measures executive functions, such as visual attention, speed, and mental flexibility, and consists of two parts (A+B). The TMT-A consists of 25 circles filled with numbers (1 to 25), which are to be connected in ascending order (from 1 to 2, from 2 to 3, etc.). The TMT-B includes both numbers (1 to 13) and letters (A to L), which are to be connected in ascending order from a letter to a number (i.e., from 1 to A, from A to 2, from 2 to B, etc.). In both tests, the time is measured, and the result is reported in seconds.

References

1. Maas, A.I.R.; Menon, D.K.; Adelson, P.D.; Andelic, N.; Bell, M.J.; Belli, A.; Bragge, P.; Brazinova, A.; Büki, A.; Chesnut, R.M.; et al. Traumatic Brain Injury: Integrated Approaches to Improve Prevention, Clinical Care, and Research. *Lancet Neurol.* **2017**, *16*, 987–1048. [CrossRef]
2. Menon, D.K.; Schwab, K.; Wright, D.W.; Maas, A.I. Position Statement: Definition of Traumatic Brain Injury. *Arch. Phys. Med. Rehabil.* **2010**, *91*, 1637–1640. [CrossRef]
3. Donders, J.; Oh, Y.I.; Gable, J. Self- and Informant Ratings of Executive Functioning After Mild Traumatic Brain Injury. *J. Head Trauma Rehabil.* **2015**, *30*, E30–E39. [CrossRef]
4. Ouellet, M.-C.; Beaulieu-Bonneau, S.; Morin, C.M. Sleep-Wake Disturbances after Traumatic Brain Injury. *Lancet Neurol.* **2015**, *14*, 746–757. [CrossRef]
5. Mcallister, T.W.; Flashman, L.A.; Sparling, M.B.; Saykin, A.J. Working Memory Deficits after Traumatic Brain Injury: Catecholaminergic Mechanisms and Prospects for Treatment—A Review. *Brain Inj.* **2004**, *18*, 331–350. [CrossRef]

6. Hamm, R.J.; Pike, B.R.; O'Dell, D.M.; Lyeth, B.G.; Jenkins, L.W. The Rotarod Test: An Evaluation of Its Effectiveness in Assessing Motor Deficits Following Traumatic Brain Injury. *J. Neurotrauma* **1994**, *11*, 187–196. [CrossRef] [PubMed]
7. Victor, T.L.; Boone, K.B.; Kulick, A.D. Assessing noncredible sensory, motor, and executive function, and test battery performance in mild traumatic brain injury cases. In *Mild Traumatic Brain Injury: Symptom Validity Assessment and Malingering*; Springer Publishing Company: New York, NY, USA, 2013; pp. 269–301. ISBN 978-0-8261-0915-6.
8. Rabinowitz, A.R.; Levin, H.S. Cognitive Sequelae of Traumatic Brain Injury. *Psychiatr. Clin. N. Am.* **2014**, *37*, 1–11. [CrossRef]
9. Piolino, P.; Desgranges, B.; Manning, L.; North, P.; Jokic, C.; Eustache, F. Autobiographical Memory, the Sense of Recollection and Executive Functions After Severe Traumatic Brain Injury. *Cortex* **2007**, *43*, 176–195. [CrossRef]
10. Ponsford, J.; Draper, K.; Schönberger, M. Functional Outcome 10 Years after Traumatic Brain Injury: Its Relationship with Demographic, Injury Severity, and Cognitive and Emotional Status. *J. Int. Neuropsychol. Soc.* **2008**, *14*. [CrossRef] [PubMed]
11. Bombardier, C.H. Rates of Major Depressive Disorder and Clinical Outcomes Following Traumatic Brain Injury. *JAMA* **2010**, *303*, 1938. [CrossRef]
12. Rauen, K.; Reichelt, L.; Probst, P.; Schäpers, B.; Müller, F.; Jahn, K.; Plesnila, N. Quality of Life up to 10 Years after Traumatic Brain Injury: A Cross-Sectional Analysis. *Health Qual Life Outcomes* **2020**, *18*, 166. [CrossRef]
13. Polinder, S.; Haagsma, J.A.; Van Klaveren, D.; Steyerberg, E.W.; Van Beeck, E.F. Health-Related Quality of Life after TBI: A Systematic Review of Study Design, Instruments, Measurement Properties, and Outcome. *Popul. Health Metrics* **2015**, *13*, 4. [CrossRef] [PubMed]
14. Von Steinbuechel, N.; Richter, S.; Morawetz, C.; Riemsma, R. Assessment of Subjective Health and Health-Related Quality of Life in Persons with Acquired or Degenerative Brain Injury. *Curr. Opin. Neurol.* **2005**, *18*, 681–691. [CrossRef] [PubMed]
15. Smith, D.H.; Johnson, V.E.; Stewart, W. Chronic Neuropathologies of Single and Repetitive TBI: Substrates of Dementia? *Nat. Rev. Neurol.* **2013**, *9*, 211–221. [CrossRef]
16. Nelson, L.D.; Ranson, J.; Ferguson, A.R.; Giacino, J.; Okonkwo, D.O.; Valadka, A.B.; Manley, G.T.; McCrea, M.A. The TRACK-TBI Investigators Validating Multi-Dimensional Outcome Assessment Using the Traumatic Brain Injury Common Data Elements: An Analysis of the TRACK-TBI Pilot Study Sample. *J. Neurotrauma* **2017**, *34*, 3158–3172. [CrossRef]
17. Alonso, J.; Bartlett, S.J.; Rose, M.; Aaronson, N.K.; Chaplin, J.E.; Efficace, F.; Leplège, A.; Lu, A.; Tulsky, D.S.; Raat, H.; et al. The Case for an International Patient-Reported Outcomes Measurement Information System (PROMIS®) Initiative. *Health Qual Life Outcomes* **2013**, *11*, 210. [CrossRef]
18. Thomson, H.J.; Winters, Z.E.; Brandberg, Y.; Didier, F.; Blazeby, J.M.; Mills, J. The Early Development Phases of a European Organisation for Research and Treatment of Cancer (EORTC) Module to Assess Patient Reported Outcomes (PROs) in Women Undergoing Breast Reconstruction. *Eur. J. Cancer* **2013**, *49*, 1018–1026. [CrossRef]
19. Bodien, Y.G.; McCrea, M.; Dikmen, S.; Temkin, N.; Boase, K.; Machamer, J.; Taylor, S.R.; Sherer, M.; Levin, H.; Kramer, J.H.; et al. Optimizing Outcome Assessment in Multicenter TBI Trials: Perspectives From TRACK-TBI and the TBI Endpoints Development Initiative. *J. Head Trauma Rehabil.* **2018**, *33*, 147–157. [CrossRef]
20. Tulsky, D.S.; Kisala, P.A.; Victorson, D.; Carlozzi, N.; Bushnik, T.; Sherer, M.; Choi, S.W.; Heinemann, A.W.; Chiaravalloti, N.; Sander, A.M.; et al. TBI-QOL: Development and calibration of item banks to measure patient reported outcomes following traumatic brain injury. *J. Head Trauma Rehabil.* **2016**, *31*, 40. [CrossRef] [PubMed]
21. U.S. Food & Drug Administration Drug Development Tool (DDT) Glossary 2017. Available online: https://www.fda.gov/drugs/drug-development-tool-ddt-qualification-programs/ddt-glossary (accessed on 1 February 2021).
22. Hunt, S.; Bhopal, R. Self reports in research with non-English speakers. *BMJ* **2003**, *327*, 352–353. [CrossRef]
23. Beaton, D.E.; Bombardier, C.; Guillemin, F.; Ferraz, M.B. Guidelines for the Process of Cross-Cultural Adaptation of Self-Report Measures. *Spine* **2000**, *25*, 3186–3191. [CrossRef]
24. Acquadro, C.; Conway, K.; Hareendran, A.; Aaronson, N. Literature Review of Methods to Translate Health-Related Quality of Life Questionnaires for Use in Multinational Clinical Trials. *Value Health* **2008**, *11*, 509–521. [CrossRef]
25. Acquadro, C. *Linguistic Validation Manual for Health Outcome Assessments*; MAPI Research Institute: Lyon, France, 2012.
26. Wild, D.; Grove, A.; Martin, M.; Eremenco, S.; McElroy, S.; Verjee-Lorenz, A.; Erikson, P. Principles of Good Practice for the Translation and Cultural Adaptation Process for Patient-Reported Outcomes (PRO) Measures: Report of the ISPOR Task Force for Translation and Cultural Adaptation. *Value Health* **2005**, *8*, 94–104. [CrossRef]
27. Wild, D.; Eremenco, S.; Mear, I.; Martin, M.; Houchin, C.; Gawlicki, M.; Hareendran, A.; Wiklund, I.; Chong, L.Y.; Von Maltzahn, R.; et al. Multinational Trials—Recommendations on the Translations Required, Approaches to Using the Same Language in Different Countries, and the Approaches to Support Pooling the Data: The ISPOR Patient-Reported Outcomes Translation and Linguistic Validation Good Research Practices Task Force Report. *Value Health* **2009**, *12*, 430–440. [CrossRef] [PubMed]
28. Swaine-Verdier, A.; Doward, L.C.; Hagell, P.; Thorsen, H.; McKenna, S.P. Adapting Quality of Life Instruments. *Value Health* **2004**, *7*, S27–S30. [CrossRef]
29. Perneger, T.V.; Leplège, A.; Etter, J.-F. Cross-Cultural Adaptation of a Psychometric Instrument. *J. Clin. Epidemiol.* **1999**, *52*, 1037–1046. [CrossRef]
30. McKown, S.; Acquadro, C.; Anfray, C.; Arnold, B.; Eremenco, S.; Giroudet, C.; Martin, M.; Weiss, D. Good practices for the translation, cultural adaptation, and linguistic validation of clinician-reported outcome, observer-reported outcome, and performance outcome measures. *J. Patient Rep. Outcomes* **2020**, *4*, 89. [CrossRef]

31. Fyndanis, V.; Lind, M.; Varlokosta, S.; Kambanaros, M.; Soroli, E.; Ceder, K.; Grohmann, K.K.; Rofes, A.; Simonsen, H.G.; Bjekic, J.; et al. Cross-linguistic adaptations of The Comprehensive Aphasia Test: Challenges and solutions. *Clin. Linguistics Phon.* **2017**, *31*, 697–710. [CrossRef] [PubMed]
32. Von Steinbuechel, N.; Rauen, K.; Bockhop, F.; Covic, A.; Krenz, U.; Plass, A.M.; Cunitz, K.; Polinder, S.; Wilson, L.; Steyerberg, E.W.; et al. Psychometric characteristics of the patient-reported outcome measures applied in the CENTER-TBI study. *J. Clin. Med.* **2021**, *10*, 2396. [CrossRef]
33. Maas, A.I.R.; Menon, D.K.; Steyerberg, E.W.; Citerio, G.; Lecky, F.; Manley, G.T.; Hill, S.; Legrand, V.; Sorgner, A. Collaborative European NeuroTrauma Effectiveness Research in Traumatic Brain Injury (CENTER-TBI): A Prospective Longitudinal Observational Study. *Neurosurgery* **2015**, *76*, 67–80. [CrossRef]
34. Steyerberg, E.W.; Wiegers, E.; Sewalt, C.; Buki, A.; Citerio, G.; De Keyser, V.; Ercole, A.; Kunzmann, K.; Lanyon, L.; Lecky, F.; et al. Case-Mix, Care Pathways, and Outcomes in Patients with Traumatic Brain Injury in CENTER-TBI: A European Prospective, Multicentre, Longitudinal, Cohort Study. *Lancet Neurol.* **2019**, *18*, 923–934. [CrossRef]
35. NINDS Common Data Elements. Available online: http://www.commondataelements.ninds.nih.gov/ (accessed on 1 February 2021).
36. Wilde, E.A.; Whiteneck, G.G.; Bogner, J.; Bushnik, T.; Cifu, D.X.; Dikmen, S.; French, L.; Giacino, J.T.; Hart, T.; Malec, J.F.; et al. Recommendations for the Use of Common Outcome Measures in Traumatic Brain Injury Research. *Arch. Phys. Med. Rehabil.* **2010**, *91*, 1650–1660.e17. [CrossRef]
37. Wilson, J.T.L.; Pettigrew, L.E.L.; Teasdale, G. Structured Interviews for the Glasgow Outcome Scale and the Extended Glasgow Outcome Scale: Guidelines for Their Use. *J. Neurotrauma* **1998**, *15*, 573–585. [CrossRef]
38. Wilson, L.; Edwards, P.; Fiddes, H.; Stewart, E.; Teasdale, G.M. Reliability of Postal Questionnaires for the Glasgow Outcome Scale. *J. Neurotrauma* **2002**, *19*, 999–1005. [CrossRef]
39. Levin, H.S.; O'donnell, V.M.; Grossman, R.G. The Galveston Orientation and Amnesia Test: A Practical Scale to Assess Cognition after Head Injury. *J. Nerv. Ment. Dis.* **1979**, *167*, 675–684. [CrossRef]
40. Spitzer, R.L.; Kroenke, K.; Williams, J.B.W.; Löwe, B. A Brief Measure for Assessing Generalized Anxiety Disorder: The GAD-7. *Arch. Intern. Med.* **2006**, *166*, 1092–1097. [CrossRef]
41. Kroenke, K.; Spitzer, R.L. The PHQ-9: A New Depression Diagnostic and Severity Measure. *Psychiatr. Ann.* **2002**, *32*, 509–515. [CrossRef]
42. Blevins, C.A.; Weathers, F.W.; Davis, M.T.; Witte, T.K.; Domino, J.L. The Posttraumatic Stress Disorder Checklist for DSM-5 (PCL-5): Development and Initial Psychometric Evaluation. *J. Trauma. Stress* **2015**, *28*, 489–498. [CrossRef]
43. King, N.S.; Crawford, S.; Wenden, F.J.; Moss, N.E.; Wade, D.T. The Rivermead Post Concussion Symptoms Questionnaire: A Measure of Symptoms Commonly Experienced after Head Injury and Its Reliability. *J. Neurol.* **1995**, *242*, 587–592. [CrossRef]
44. Von Steinbuechel, N.; Wilson, L.; Gibbons, H.; Hawthorne, G.; Höfer, S.; Schmidt, S.; Bullinger, M.; Maas, A.; Neugebauer, E.; Powell, J.; et al. Quality of Life after Brain Injury (QOLIBRI): Scale Development and Metric Properties. *J. Neurotrauma* **2010**, *27*, 1167–1185. [CrossRef]
45. Von Steinbuechel, N.; Wilson, L.; Gibbons, H.; Hawthorne, G.; Höfer, S.; Schmidt, S.; Bullinger, M.; Maas, A.; Neugebauer, E.; Powell, J.; et al. Quality of Life after Brain Injury (QOLIBRI): Scale Validity and Correlates of Quality of Life. *J. Neurotrauma* **2010**, *27*, 1157–1165. [CrossRef]
46. Von Steinbuechel, N.; Wilson, L.; Gibbons, H.; Muehlan, H.; Schmidt, H.; Schmidt, S.; Sasse, N.; Koskinen, S.; Sarajuuri, J.; Höfer, S.; et al. QOLIBRI Overall Scale: A Brief Index of Health-Related Quality of Life after Traumatic Brain Injury. *J. Neurol. Neurosurg. Psychiatry* **2012**, *83*, 1041–1047. [CrossRef] [PubMed]
47. Maruish, M.E.; Maruish, M.; Kosinski, M.; Bjorner, J.B.; Gandek, B.; Turner-Bowker, D.M.; Ware, J.E. *User's Manual for the SF-36v2 Health Survey*, 3rd ed.; Quality Metric Incorporated: Lincoln, RI, USA, 2011.
48. Ware, J.E.; Kosinski, M.; Turner-Bowker, D.M.; Gandek, B. *User's Manual for the SF12v2 Health Survey*; Quality Metric Incorporated: Lincoln, RI, USA, 2009.
49. Strauss, E.; Sherman, E.M.; Spreen, O. CANTAB. In *A Compendium of Neuropsychological Tests—Administration, Norms, and Commentary*; Oxford University Press: New York, NY, USA, 2006; pp. 415–424.
50. Strauss, E.; Sherman, E.M.; Spreen, O. Rey-Oesterrieth Auditory Verbal Leraning Test (RAVLT). In *A Compendium of Neuropsychological Tests—Administration, Norms, and Commentary*; Oxford University Press: New York, NY, USA, 2006; pp. 776–811.
51. Strauss, E.; Sherman, E.M.; Spreen, O. Trail Making Test (TMT). In *A Compendium of Neuropsychological Tests—Administration, Norms, and Commentary*; Oxford University Press: New York, NY, USA, 2006; pp. 655–678.
52. Optum The Optum®SF-36v2®Health Survey. Available online: https://www.optum.com/solutions/life-sciences/answer-research/patient-insights/sf-health-surveys/sf-36v2-health-survey.html (accessed on 1 February 2021).
53. Andrews, P.J.; Sinclair, H.L.; Battison, C.G.; Polderman, K.H.; Citerio, G.; Mascia, L.; Harris, B.A.; Murray, G.D.; Stocchetti, N.; Menon, D.K.; et al. European Society of Intensive Care Medicine Study of Therapeutic Hypothermia (32–35 °C) for Intracranial Pressure Reduction after Traumatic Brain Injury (the Eurotherm3235Trial). *Trials* **2011**, *12*, 8. [CrossRef]
54. Van Praag, D.L.G.; Fardzadeh, H.E.; Covic, A.; Maas, A.I.R.; Von Steinbüchel, N. Preliminary Validation of the Dutch Version of the Posttraumatic Stress Disorder Checklist for DSM-5 (PCL-5) after Traumatic Brain Injury in a Civilian Population. *PLoS ONE* **2020**, *15*, e0231857. [CrossRef]

55. Plass, A.M.; Van Praag, D.; Covic, A.; Gorbunova, A.; Real, R.; Von Steinbüchel, N. The Psychometric Validation of the Dutch Version of the Rivermead Post-Concussion Symptoms Questionnaire (RPQ) after Traumatic Brain Injury (TBI). *PLoS ONE* **2019**, *14*, e0210138. [CrossRef] [PubMed]
56. Teymoori, A.; Real, R.; Gorbunova, A.; Haghish, E.F.; Andelic, N.; Wilson, L.; Asendorf, T.; Menon, D.; Von Steinbüchel, N. Measurement Invariance of Assessments of Depression (PHQ-9) and Anxiety (GAD-7) across Sex, Strata and Linguistic Backgrounds in a European-Wide Sample of Patients after Traumatic Brain Injury. *J. Affect. Disord.* **2020**, *262*, 278–285. [CrossRef] [PubMed]
57. Gorbunova, A.; Zeldovich, M.; Voormolen, D.C.; Krenz, U.; Polinder, S.; Haagsma, J.A.; Hagmayer, Y.; Covic, A.; Real, R.G.L.; Asendorf, T.; et al. Reference Values of the QOLIBRI from General Population Samples in the United Kingdom and The Netherlands. *JCM* **2020**, *9*, 2100. [CrossRef]
58. Wu, Y.-J.; Rauen, K.; Zeldovich, M.; Voormolen, D.C.; Gorbunova, A.; Covic, A.; Cunitz, K.; Plass, A.M.; Polinder, S.; Haagsma, J.A.; et al. Reference Values and Psychometric Properties of the Quality of Life after Traumatic Brain Injury Overall Scale in Italy, the Netherlands, and the United Kingdom. *Value Health* **2021**.
59. American Psychiatric Association. *Diagnostic And Statistical Manual of Mental Disorders: DSM-IV*, 4th ed.; American Psychiatric Association: Washington, DC, USA, 1994; ISBN 0-89042-064-5.
60. American Psychiatric Association. *Diagnostic and Statistical Manual of Mental Disorders: DSM-5*, 5th ed.; American Psychiatric Publishing: Washington, DC, USA, 2013; ISBN 978-0-89042-555-8.
61. Cambridge Cognition CANTAB® [Cognitive Assessment Software]. Available online: https://www.cambridgecognition.com/cantab/ (accessed on 1 February 2021).

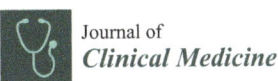

Article

Association of Flow Rate of Prehospital Oxygen Administration and Clinical Outcomes in Severe Traumatic Brain Injury

Won Pyo Hong [1,2], Ki Jeong Hong [1,3,4,*], Sang Do Shin [1,3,4], Kyoung Jun Song [1,3,5], Tae Han Kim [1,3,5], Jeong Ho Park [1,3,4], Young Sun Ro [1,3,4], Seung Chul Lee [1,6,7], Chu Hyun Kim [8] and Joo Jeong [1,3,4]

1 Laboratory of Emergency Medical Services, Biomedical Research Institute, Seoul National University Hospital, Seoul 03080, Korea; pyotang@gmail.com (W.P.H.); shinsangdo@gmail.com (S.D.S.); skci-va@gmail.com (K.J.S.); adoong2001@gmail.com (T.H.K.); timthe@gmail.com (J.H.P.); Ro.youngsun@gmail.com (Y.S.R.); scl0126@hanmail.net (S.C.L.); yukijeje@gmail.com (J.J.)
2 119 EMS Division, The Korean National Fire Agency, Sejong City 30128, Korea
3 Department of Emergency Medicine, College of Medicine, Seoul National University, Seoul 03080, Korea
4 Department of Emergency Medicine, Seoul National University Hospital, Seoul 03080, Korea
5 Department of Emergency Medicine, Boramae Medical Center, Seoul Metropolitan Government—Seoul National University, Seoul 07061, Korea
6 Graduate School, Dongguk University, Goyang-si 10326, Korea
7 Department of Emergency medicine, Emergency Medical Center, Dongguk University, Ilsan Hospital, Goyang-si 10326, Korea
8 Department of Emergency Medicine, Inje University College of Medicine, Seoul Paik Hospital, Seoul 04551, Korea; juliannnn@hanmail.net
* Correspondence: emkjhong@gmail.com

Abstract: The goal of this study was to investigate the association of prehospital oxygen administration flow with clinical outcome in severe traumatic brain injury (TBI) patients. This was a cross-sectional observational study using an emergency medical services-assessed severe trauma database in South Korea. The sample included adult patients with severe blunt TBI without hypoxia who were treated by EMS providers in 2013 and 2015. Main exposure was prehospital oxygen administration flow rate (no oxygen, low-flow 1~5, mid-flow 6~14, high-flow 15 L/min). Primary outcome was in-hospital mortality. A total of 1842 patients with severe TBI were included. The number of patients with no oxygen, low-flow oxygen, mid-flow oxygen, high-flow oxygen was 244, 573, 607, and 418, respectively. Mortality of each group was 34.8%, 32.3%, 39.9%, and 41.1%, respectively. Compared with the no-oxygen group, adjusted odds (95% CI) for mortality in the low-, mid-, and high-flow oxygen groups were 0.86 (0.62–1.20), 1.15 (0.83–1.60), and 1.21 (0.83–1.73), respectively. In the interaction analysis, low-flow oxygen showed lower mortality when prehospital saturation was 94–98% (adjusted odds ratio (AOR): 0.80 (0.67–0.95)) and ≥99% (AOR: 0.69 (0.53–0.91)). High-flow oxygen showed higher mortality when prehospital oxygen saturation was ≥99% (AOR: 1.33 (1.01~1.74)). Prehospital low-flow oxygen administration was associated with lower in-hospital mortality compared with the no-oxygen group. High-flow administration showed higher mortality.

Keywords: traumatic brain injury; prehospital; oxygenation; hypoxia; hyperoxia; emergency medical services

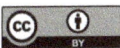

1. Introduction

Traumatic brain injury (TBI) is a major health and socioeconomic problem throughout the world [1]. About 5.48 million people are estimated to suffer from severe TBI each year (73 cases per 100,000 people), and the economic and social impact of TBI is considerable due to the direct and indirect costs of treatment, rehabilitation, and permanent sequelae. The World Health Organization reported the TBI global incidence is rising and was predicted to surpass many diseases as a major cause of death and disability by the year 2020 [2,3].

Prehospital hypoxia less than 90% of saturation was associated with higher mortality in previous studies, and Guidelines for the Management of Severe Traumatic Brain Injury recommends that hypoxia (partial pressure of oxygen in arterial blood (PaO2) < 60 mmHg or peripheral oxygen saturation (SpO2) < 90%) should be avoided, but there is no therapeutic range of oxygen saturation [4–6]. The Prehospital Trauma Life Support manual suggests that oxygen delivery should be provided based on the patient's breathing frequency, and this tends to encourage the use of a high fraction of inspired oxygen, which results in the common use of high-flow (15 L/min) oxygen administration [7].

However, recent studies, especially in intensive care unit settings, report that not only hypoxia but hyperoxia was associated with poor outcomes [8–11]. Oxidative stress with consequent impairment of endogenous antioxidant defense mechanisms plays a significant role in the secondary events leading to neuronal death [12].

Recent study of TBI management recommends an optimal PaO2 of more than 60 mmHg and less than 200 mmHg [13]. There are no guidelines on oxygen saturation level for optimal care in the prehospital setting, and possible effects of hyperoxia from high-flow oxygenation can easily be neglected. Prehospital high-flow oxygen administration is likely not associated with poor outcome because of short transportation time. It is uncertain, however, whether high-flow oxygen administration during emergency medical services (EMS) treatment is associated with poor outcomes from TBI.

The purpose of this study was to determine the association of prehospital oxygen administration flow rate on hospital mortality and neurological outcomes in severe TBI patients without hypoxia. We hypothesized that excessive oxygenation would adversely affect survival in patients with severe TBI without hypoxia.

2. Materials and Methods

2.1. Study Design

This was a cross-sectional observational study using a database from the nationwide registry of EMS-assessed severe trauma in Korea. This national severe trauma database was built from two data sources, including the EMS severe trauma registry recorded by EMS providers and hospital medical records collected by the Korea Disease Control and Prevention Agency. The study was reviewed and approved by the institutional review board of the study institution and informed consent was waived (Approval number: 1206-024-412).

2.2. Study Setting

The emergency medical services system in Korea is a single-tiered public service model by the government-run fire department. The service level of prehospital care is comparable with intermediate-level emergency medical technicians in the United States. Prehospital TBI protocol includes airway management and oxygen administration to the patient with hypoxia less than 94% of saturation (SpO2 < 94%) to avoid hypoxia, but there is no clear flow rate or method of oxygen administration or target saturation level. According to capacity and resources, emergency departments in Korea are divided into levels 1 to 3, and for the patients with severe trauma, and prehospital protocol recommends transferring patients with severe TBI to a level 1 or 2 emergency department for proper management.

2.3. Data Source

This study used the nationwide registry of the EMS-ST database built from the EMS severe trauma registry and hospital medical records. EMS providers used a field triage scheme consisting of four decision steps (physiologic, anatomic, mechanism of injury, and special considerations) to include patients with possible severe trauma [14], and the EMS severe trauma registry includes basic ambulance operation information and detailed prehospital monitoring and treatment information. Hospital medical records were collected by Korean CDC reviewers who received 26 h in an education course that included the coding for an abbreviated injury scale (AIS). The quality management committee, which consisted of emergency physicians, epidemiologists, statistical experts, and medical record review experts, held monthly meetings for quality assurance.

2.4. Selection of Participants

The study population included all patients with severe TBI who were treated by EMS providers in 10 provinces between January and December 2013 and in 17 provinces (whole country) between January and December 2015. All patients with severe blunt TBI older than 15 years old were enrolled. Severe TBI was defined according to an AIS score of 3 or above for a head lesion. Patients who had cardiac arrest at the scene, unknown prehospital oxygen saturation, prehospital hypoxia less than 94% of oxygen saturation (SpO2 < 94%), and unknown prehospital blood pressure or who had unknown information on hospital outcomes were excluded.

2.5. Variables and Measurements

The main exposure of interest was prehospital oxygen flow by EMS providers. Patients without oxygen administration were considered as reference, and low-flow oxygen was defined as 1~5 L/min of oxygen administration, mid-flow oxygen as 6~14 L/min, and high-flow oxygen as 15 L/min, regardless of method of oxygen supply. High prehospital oxygen saturation status was defined as more than 99% of oxygen saturation (SpO2 $\geq$ 99%) after oxygen administration.

Collected variables were demographic factors (age, gender, place of residence, past medical history), injury-related factors (time of trauma, place of injury, mechanism of injury (blunt or not)), prehospital factors (EMS transportation time, prehospital vital sign, and prehospital treatment, including amount of oxygen administration and prehospital oxygen saturation after oxygen administration), and hospital factors (level of emergency department, Injury Severity Score), as well as patient outcome after admission if the patient was admitted, and Glasgow Outcome Scale at hospital discharge.

2.6. Outcome

The primary outcome of the study was in-hospital mortality, defined as death in the emergency department or during admission, resulting from the injury. The secondary outcome was morbidity of patients, which was defined as poor according to the Glasgow Outcome Scale from 3 to 5 at hospital discharge.

2.7. Statistical Analysis

Descriptive analyses were performed to examine the distributions of the study variables. Counts and proportions were used for categorical variables, and medians and interquartile ranges were used for continuous variables. Categorical variables were assessed with the chi-square test, and continuous variables were compared using Mann–Whitney U tests. The p-values were based on a two-sided significance level of 0.05.

Adjusted odds ratios (AORs) with 95% confidence intervals (CIs) for saturation status for the study outcomes were calculated using multivariable logistic regression analysis, with no oxygen administration as the reference. The model was adjusted for gender, age, and underlying comorbidity; season and weekday; mechanism, intent, and alcohol; response time interval, scene time interval, and transport time interval; patient alertness, presence of hypotension (systolic blood pressure below 90 mmHg in prehospital setting), and level of emergency department; and Injury Severity Score from 9 to 15, 16 to 24, and above 25.

To determine the effect of hyperoxia on the patient, this study developed an interaction model with an interaction term between prehospital oxygen flow and prehospital saturation status as the final multivariable logistic model for the study outcomes. All statistical analysis was performed using SAS software, version 9.4 (SAS Institute Inc., Cary, NC, USA).

3. Results

A total of 35,169 patients were enrolled in the EMS-ST database during 2013 and 2015. The number of severe blunt traumatic brain injuries was 7697. After excluding ineligible patients, the final study population consisted of 1842 patients (Figure 1). Of the 1842 patients, the number of patients with no oxygen, low-flow oxygen, mid-flow oxygen, and high-flow oxygen was 244 (13.2%), 573 (31.1%), 607 (32.9%) and 418 (22.7%), respectively; the in-hospital mortality rates were 34.8%, 32.3%, 39.9% and 41.1%, respectively. Basic patient demographics are shown in Table 1. Patients were older in the no-oxygen group (median age was 61 years old) compared with other groups (median age 46, 44, and 37, respectively). Patient's residence, mechanism of injury, patient's alertness, prehospital hypotension, prehospital advanced airway management, prehospital IV access, and prehospital transport time were associated with the flow rate of oxygen administration (Tables 1 and 2).

In the multivariable logistic regression analysis, low-flow oxygen administration was likely to have better in-hospital outcomes (AOR 0.86 (0.62–1.20) for in-hospital mortality and AOR 0.80 (0.57–1.10) for poor neurologic outcome) (Table 3.) High-flow oxygen administration was likely to have more mortality and poor neurologic outcome compared with the no-oxygen administration group (AOR 1.21 (0.83–1.73) for mortality and 1.15 (0.81–1.64) for poor neurological outcome).

In the interaction model, using prehospital oxygenation and prehospital saturation status, the low-flow oxygen group showed low in-hospital mortality and better neurologic outcome in both saturation groups. Adjusted odds ratio (AOR) (95% CI) for mortality was 0.80 (0.67–0.95) in the 94~98% group and 0.69 (0.53–0.91) in 99~100% group. High-flow oxygen administration showed poor in hospital outcome (AOR (95% CI) was 1.33 (1.01–1.74)) in patients with high prehospital saturation (SpO2 ≥ 99%), which was statistically significant ($p = 0.04$) (Table 4).

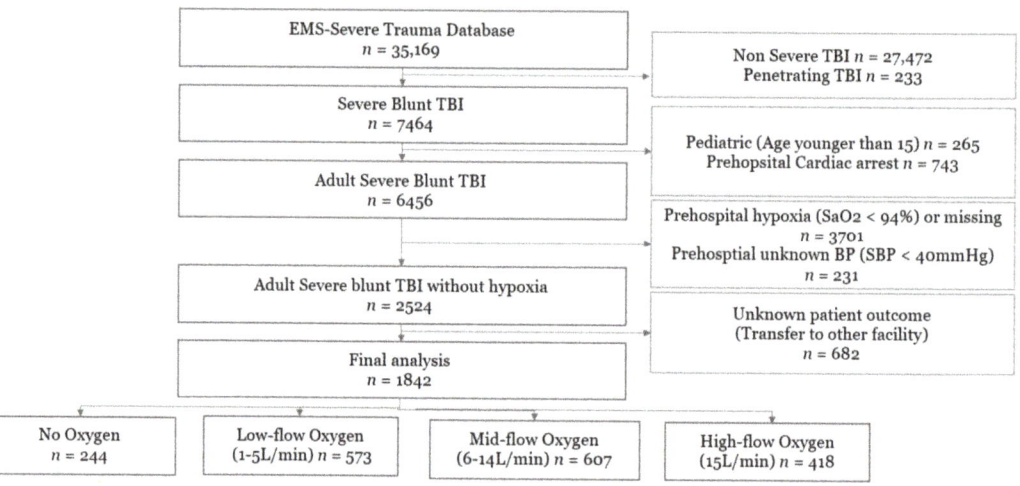

Figure 1. Inclusion of study population.

Table 1. Demographics of the study population.

		Total		No Oxygen		Flow Rate of Oxygen Administration						p-Value
						Low		Mid		High		
		n	%	n	%	n	%	n	%	n	%	
Total		1842	100	244	100	573	100	607	100	418	100	
Gender												0.16
	Male	1370	74.4	169	69.3	438	76.4	457	75.3	306	73.2	
	Female	472	25.6	75	30.7	135	23.6	150	24.7	112	26.8	
Age, years												<0.01
	15–64	1123	61.0	141	57.8	317	55.3	373	61.4	292	69.9	
	65–	719	39.0	103	42.2	256	44.7	234	38.6	126	30.1	
	Median (IQR)	58 (45–71)		61 (51–72)		46 (60–74)		44 (57–70)		37 (54–67)		

Table 1. Cont.

		Total		No Oxygen		Flow Rate of Oxygen Administration						p-Value
						Low		Mid		High		
		n	%	n	%	n	%	n	%	n	%	
Season												0.57
	Spring	461	25.0	61	25.0	142	24.8	148	24.4	110	26.3	
	Summer	476	25.8	65	26.6	144	25.1	154	25.4	113	27.0	
	Fall	503	27.3	71	29.1	148	25.8	164	27.0	120	28.7	
	Winter	402	21.8	47	19.3	139	24.3	141	23.2	75	17.9	
Weekday												0.66
	Monday	226	12.3	35	14.3	70	12.2	76	12.5	45	10.8	
	Tuesday	228	12.4	36	14.8	73	12.7	68	11.2	51	12.2	
	Wednesday	281	15.3	36	14.8	91	15.9	91	15.0	63	15.1	
	Thursday	294	16.0	43	17.6	85	14.8	92	15.2	74	17.7	
	Friday	262	14.2	21	8.6	80	14.0	92	15.2	69	16.5	
	Saturday	255	13.8	38	15.6	79	13.8	86	14.2	52	12.4	
	Sunday	296	16.1	35	14.3	95	16.6	102	16.8	64	15.3	
Metropolis area												<0.01
	Yes	756	41.0	61	25.0	260	45.4	254	41.8	181	43.3	
	No	1086	59.0	183	75.0	313	54.6	353	58.2	237	56.7	
Mechanism												<0.01
	Traffic accident	1056	57.3	121	49.6	303	52.9	367	60.5	265	63.4	
	Fall	741	40.2	116	47.5	258	45.0	228	37.6	139	33.3	
	Other blunt	45	2.4	7	2.9	12	2.1	12	2.0	14	3.3	
Intent												0.63
	Non-intentional	1755	95.3	234	95.9	547	95.5	583	96.0	391	93.5	
	Intentional	45	2.4	6	2.5	13	2.3	13	2.1	13	3.1	
	Unknown	42	2.3	4	1.6	13	2.3	11	1.8	14	3.3	
Alcohol consumption												0.09
	Non-alcohol	54	2.9	8	3.3	18	3.1	21	3.5	7	1.7	
	Alcohol	293	15.9	41	16.8	108	18.8	91	15.0	53	12.7	
	Unknown	1495	81.2	195	79.9	447	78.0	495	81.5	358	85.6	

Table 2. Pre-hospital and in-hospital clinical findings according to flow rate of oxygen administration.

	Total		No Oxygen		Flow Rate of Oxygen Administration						p-Value
					Low		Mid		High		
	n	%	n	%	n	%	n	%	n	%	
Total	1842	100	244	100	573	100	607	100.0	418	100	
Patient alertness											<0.01
Alert	284	15.4	65	26.6	122	21.3	64	10.5	33	7.9	
Verbal	416	22.6	88	36.1	155	27.1	122	20.1	51	12.2	
Pain	792	43.0	75	30.7	235	41.0	281	46.3	201	48.1	
Unresponsive	350	19.0	16	6.6	61	10.6	140	23.1	133	31.8	
Prehospital SBP											<0.01
<90 mmHg	110	6.0	6	2.5	23	4.0	41	6.8	40	9.6	
≥90 mmHg	1732	94.0	238	97.5	550	96.0	566	93.2	378	90.4	
Prehospital Saturation											0.07
94–98%	1054	57.2	132	54.1	354	61.8	336	55.4	232	55.5	
99–100%	788	42.8	112	45.9	219	38.2	271	44.6	186	44.5	
Prehospital advance airway											<0.01
No	1816	98.6	243	99.6	572	99.8	598	98.5	403	96.4	
Yes	26	1.4	1	0.4	1	0.2	9	1.5	15	3.6	

Table 2. Cont.

	Total		No Oxygen		Flow Rate of Oxygen Administration						p-Value
					Low		Mid		High		
	n	%	n	%	n	%	n	%	n	%	
Prehospital IV access											<0.01
No	1520	82.5	223	91.4	488	85.2	497	81.9	312	74.6	
Yes	322	17.5	21	8.6	85	14.8	110	18.1	106	25.4	
Response time interval (min)											0.01
0–3	149	8.1	21	8.6	47	8.2	49	8.1	32	7.7	
4–7	927	50.3	95	38.9	305	53.2	299	49.3	228	54.5	
8–11	418	22.7	67	27.5	127	22.2	131	21.6	93	22.2	
12–15	175	9.5	25	10.2	48	8.4	70	11.5	32	7.7	
16–	173	9.4	36	14.8	46	8.0	58	9.6	33	7.9	
Median (IQR)	7 (5–10)		8 (5–11.5)		7 (5–9)		7 (5–11)		7 (5–9)		
Scene time interval (min)											0.03
0–3	303	16.4	32	13.1	80	14.0	114	18.8	77	18.4	
4–7	949	51.5	113	46.3	309	53.9	317	52.2	210	50.2	
8–11	375	20.4	58	23.8	126	22.0	106	17.5	85	20.3	
12–15	128	6.9	27	11.1	34	5.9	37	6.1	30	7.2	
16–	87	4.7	14	5.7	24	4.2	33	5.4	16	3.8	
Median (IQR)	6 (4–9)		7 (4–10)		6 (4–8)		6 (4–8)		6 (4–9)		
Transport time interval (min)											<0.01
0–3	113	6.1	3	1.2	46	8.0	40	6.6	24	5.7	
4–7	480	26.1	33	13.5	170	29.7	148	24.4	129	30.9	
8–11	372	20.2	42	17.2	113	19.7	131	21.6	86	20.6	
12–15	250	13.6	31	12.7	63	11.0	98	16.1	58	13.9	
16–	627	34.0	135	55.3	181	31.6	190	31.3	121	28.9	
Median (IQR)	6 (4–9)		7 (4–10)		6 (4–8)		6 (4–8)		6 (4–9)		
Operation											<0.01
No	925	50.2	148	60.7	313	54.6	272	44.8	192	45.9	
Yes	917	49.8	96	39.3	260	45.4	335	55.2	226	54.1	
Brain Operation											<0.01
No	1213	65.9	186	76.2	386	67.4	374	61.6	267	<0.01	
Yes	629	34.1	58	23.8	187	32.6	233	38.4	151	36.1	
ICU admission											<0.01
No	346	18.8	67	27.5	117	20.4	99	16.3	63	15.1	
Yes	1496	81.2	177	72.5	456	79.6	508	83.7	355	84.9	
Ventilator apply											<0.01
No	930	50.5	169	69.3	340	59.3	266	43.8	155	<0.01	
Yes	912	49.5	75	30.7	233	40.7	341	56.2	263	62.9	
Co-morbidity											0.61
No	1658	90.0	220	90.2	508	88.7	552	90.9	378	90.4	
Yes	184	10.0	24	9.8	65	11.3	55	9.1	40	9.6	
Associated trauma other than head											<0.01
No	1291	70.1	192	78.7	433	75.6	402	66.2	<0.01	63.2	
Yes	551	29.9	52	21.3	140	24.4	205	33.8	154	36.8	
Injury Severity Score											<0.01
9–15	372	20.2	81	33.2	134	23.4	105	17.3	52	12.4	
16–25	692	37.6	95	38.9	194	33.9	220	36.2	183	43.8	
25–	778	42.2	68	27.9	245	42.8	282	46.5	183	43.8	
Survival to discharge											0.01
Survived	1158	62.9	159	65.2	388	67.7	365	60.1	246	58.9	
Expired	684	37.1	85	34.8	185	32.3	242	39.9	172	41.1	
Neurologic outcome measured by Glasgow outcome scale											<0.01
Good (1–2)	1127	61.2	152	62.3	381	66.5	356	58.6	238	<0.01	
Poor (3–5)	715	38.8	92	37.7	192	33.5	251	41.4	180	43.1	

Table 3. Pre-hospital and in-hospital clinical findings according to flow rate of oxygen administration.

	Total	Outcome		Unadjusted	Adjusted Model 1 *	Adjusted Model 2 **
	n	n	%	OR (95% CI)	OR (95% CI)	OR (95% CI)
Primary outcome: in-hospital mortality						
Total	1842	684	37.1			
Oxygen flow rate (L/min)						
No oxygen	244	85	34.8	1.00	1.00	1.00
Low-flow rate	573	185	32.3	0.89 (0.65–1.22)	0.88 (0.64–1.21)	0.86 (0.62–1.20)
Mid-flow rate	607	242	39.9	1.24 (0.91–1.69)	1.25 (0.92–1.70)	1.15 (0.83–1.60)
High-flow rate	418	172	41.1	1.31 (0.94–1.82)	1.33 (0.96–1.86)	1.21 (0.83–1.73)
Secondary outcome: poor neurologic outcome						
Total	1842	715	38.8			
Oxygen flow rate (L/min)						
No oxygen	244	92	37.7	1.00	1.00	1.00
Low-flow rate	573	192	33.5	0.83 (0.61–1.14)	0.82 (0.60–1.13)	0.80 (0.57–1.10)
Mid-flow rate	607	251	41.4	1.17 (0.86–1.58)	1.17 (0.86–1.59)	1.09 (0.78–1.50)
High-flow rate	418	180	43.1	1.25 (0.90–1.73)	1.27 (0.92–1.76)	1.15 (0.81–1.64)

* Model 1: Adjusted by gender, age, underlying co-morbidity; ** Model 2: Adjusted by gender, age, underlying co-morbidity, season, weekday, mechanism, intent, alcohol, response time interval, scene time interval, transport time interval, patient alertness, low blood pressure, abnormal respiration rate, intravenous fluid, prehospital oxygen saturation status or oxygen flow.

Table 4. Interaction analysis for clinical outcome according to oxygen flow rate by initial prehospital oxygen saturation level.

	Total	Outcome		Adjusted OR *
	n	n	%	OR * (95% CI)
Primary outcome: in-hospital mortality				
Saturation 94–98%				
No oxygen administration	132	48	36.4	1.00
Low-flow rate (1–5 L/min)	354	127	35.9	0.80 (0.67–0.95)
Mid-flow rate (6–14 L/min)	336	143	42.6	1.10 (0.94–1.29)
High-flow rate (15 L/min)	232	96	41.4	1.18 (0.98–1.42)
Saturation 99–100%				
No oxygen administration	112	37	33.0	1.00
Low-flow rate (1–5 L/min)	219	58	26.5	0.69 (0.53–0.91)
Mid-flow rate (6–14 L/min)	271	99	36.5	1.05 (0.83–1.34)
High-flow rate (15 L/min)	186	76	40.9	1.33 (1.01–1.74)
Secondary outcome: poor neurologic outcome				
Saturation 94–98%				
No oxygen administration	132	52	40.2	1.00
Low-flow rate (1–5 L/min)	354	132	37.3	0.78 (0.66–0.92)
Mid-flow rate (6–14 L/min)	336	149	44.3	1.09 (0.93–1.27)
High-flow rate (15 L/min)	232	103	44.4	1.17 (0.97–1.41)
Saturation 99–100%				
No oxygen administration	112	39	34.8	1.00
Low-flow rate (1–5 L/min)	219	60	27.4	0.69 (0.53–0.91)
Mid-flow rate (6–14 L/min)	271	102	37.6	1.05 (0.83–1.34)
High-flow rate (15 L/min)	186	77	41.4	1.29 (0.98–1.69)

* Adjusted by gender, age, underlying co-morbidity, season, weekday, mechanism, intent, alcohol, response time interval, scene time interval, transport time interval, patient alertness, low blood pressure, abnormal respiration rate, intravenous fluid, prehospital oxygen saturation status or oxygen flow.

4. Discussion

Prehospital administration of oxygen is widespread in our practice, but resuscitative oxygen administration frequently exceeds the physiological needs of patients with TBI and without TBI [7,15,16]. Although this is usually accepted to avoid hypoxia, toxicity of oxygen to the brain and other vital organs due to reactive oxygen species is well described [17–20], and 100% oxygen can cause cerebral vasoconstriction, reducing cerebral perfusion [21,22].

In our study, the low-flow oxygen group showed low in-hospital mortality and better neurologic outcome. AOR (95% CI) for mortality was 0.80 (0.67–0.95) in the 94~98% group and 0.69 (0.53–0.91) in the 99~100% group in the interaction model. This result implies that low-flow (1~5 L/min) oxygen administration could be helpful for the patients with severe TBI. Recent studies have reported that oxygen administration improves cerebral metabolism and decreases intracerebral pressure [23,24], and they recommend providing normo-baric hyperoxia in the treatment of patients with TBI, but other studies have reported contrary results [6], which needs further well-controlled study.

On the other hand, 186 patients (10.1%) received high-flow oxygen, even though their prehospital saturation was above 99%; mortality among them was highest (40.9%) among all groups. Brenner et al. reported that hyperoxia, which was defined as PaO2 higher than 200 mmHg, within the first 24 h of hospitalization is associated with worse short-term functional outcomes and higher mortality after TBI [13], but other studies showed no significant difference in in-hospital mortality among patients with hyperoxia (PaO2 > 300 mmHg) [25], and there was no association between maximum PaO2 in the first 24 h after admission and in-hospital mortality [26]. This study could not measure PaO2 due to the lack of a modality to measure it exactly in prehospital settings. Additionally, the hypothesis of this investigation was that a patient could have hyperoxia when oxygen saturation was above 99% after the administration of high-flow oxygen. In the interaction analysis, patients with high oxygen saturation after high-flow oxygen showed significantly poor outcomes (AOR 1.33 (95%CI: 1.01–1.74)), which implies that hyperoxia could be harmful.

Some authors reported that prehospital advanced airway techniques were related to poor outcomes in traumatic brain injury and that this was associated with prehospital hyperventilation, which was very common (60~70%); even the prehospital guideline recommends not to hyperventilate [27–30]. In this study setting, prehospital advanced airway techniques, including laryngeal mask airway and endotracheal intubation, were uncommon (1.4%) because cases with prehospital hypoxia less than 94% were excluded. When we analyzed that separately, it did not influence our result.

The primary goal of treatment for patients with TBI is to prevent secondary brain injury. This includes providing adequate oxygenation and circulation to perfuse the brain. Oxygen should be titrated not only to prevent hypoxia but also to prevent hyperoxia. Low-flow oxygen administration could be helpful to patients with severe TBI, and indiscriminate high-flow oxygen administration could be harmful to patients with severe TBI. A more specific prehospital oxygen administration guideline (therapeutic target range of oxygen saturation 94–98% and restriction of indiscriminate high-flow oxygen) should be applied. Moreover, further study, such as a randomized controlled study, should be conducted to elucidate a clear causal relationship.

Limitations

First, this was a cross-sectional observational study using a database from the nationwide registry of EMS-assessed severe trauma in Korea. Patients with severe TBI who visited the emergency department in their own vehicle could have been omitted from this registry. Second, the definition of hypoxia used in this study was the cutoff value of SpO2 94%, measured by pulse oximetry. The definition of hypoxia differed between the studies. Third, initiation time and duration of prehospital oxygen administration was not collected. Forth, additional physiologic parameters associated with outcome in TBI patients, such as PaO2, intracranial pressure, cerebral perfusion pressure, oxygen radicals, and cerebral metabolites, were not collected.

5. Conclusions

Prehospital low-flow oxygen administration was associated with low in-hospital mortality compared with the no-oxygen group in patients with severe traumatic brain injury, and high-flow oxygen administration showed higher mortality and could be harmful to patients with severe blunt traumatic brain injury. The proper therapeutic window for prehospital oxygenation may reduce the mortality rate of patients with severe TBI.

Author Contributions: Conceptualization, S.D.S. and K.J.S.; methodology, Y.S.R., T.H.K. and C.H.K.; software, W.P.H.; validation, Y.S.R., T.H.K. and C.H.K.; formal analysis, Y.S.R., T.H.K. and C.H.K.; investigation, W.P.H.; resources, J.H.P., J.J. and S.C.L.; data curation, J.H.P., J.J. and S.C.L.; writing—original draft preparation, W.P.H.; writing—review and editing, K.J.H.; visualization, W.P.H.; supervision, K.J.H.; project administration, K.J.H.; funding acquisition, none. All authors have read and agreed to the published version of the manuscript.

Funding: This research received no external funding.

Institutional Review Board Statement: The study was reviewed and approved by the institutional review board of the study institution (Approval number: 1206-024-412).

Informed Consent Statement: Patient consent was waived due to data collection from retrospective medical record review.

Data Availability Statement: Data was obtained from the Korea Disease Control and Prevention Agency and is available from the Korea Disease Control and Prevention Agency with the permission.

Acknowledgments: This study used the emergency medical services-based severe trauma database of the Korea Disease Control and Prevention Agency. Additionally, the use of the database for this study was approved by the Korea Disease Control and Prevention Agency.

Conflicts of Interest: The authors declare no conflict of interest.

References

1. Hyder, A.A.; Wunderlich, C.A.; Puvanachandra, P.; Gururaj, G.; Kobusingye, O.C. The impact of traumatic brain injuries: A global perspective. *NeuroRehabilitation* **2007**, *22*, 341–353. [CrossRef]
2. Iaccarino, C.; Carretta, A.; Nicolosi, F.; Morselli, C. Epidemiology of severe traumatic brain injury. *J. Neurosurg. Sci.* **2018**, *62*, 535–541. [CrossRef] [PubMed]
3. Kamal, V.K.; Agrawal, D.; Pandey, R.M. Epidemiology, clinical characteristics and outcomes of traumatic brain injury: Evidences from integrated level 1 trauma center in India. *J. Neurosci. Rural Pract.* **2016**, *7*, 515–525. [CrossRef]
4. *Head Injury: Triage, Assessment, Investigation and Early Management of Head Injury in Infants, Children and Adults*; NICE Guidance; NICE: London, UK, 2007.
5. Brain Trauma Foundation; American Association of Neurological Surgeons; Congress of Neurological Surgeons; Joint Section on Neurotrauma and Critical Care; AANS/CNS; Susan, L.B.; Randall, M.C.; Jamshid, G.; Flora, F.M.H.; Odette, A.H.; et al. Guidelines for the management of severe traumatic brain injury. I. Blood pressure and oxygenation. *J. Neurotrauma* **2007**, *24*, S7–S13.
6. Spaite, D.W.; Hu, C.; Bobrow, B.J.; Chikani, V.; Barnhart, B.; Gaither, J.B.; Denninghoff, K.R.; Anderson, P.D.; Keim, S.M.; Viscusi, C.; et al. The Effect of Combined Out-of-Hospital Hypotension and Hypoxia on Mortality in Major Traumatic Brain Injury. *Ann. Emerg. Med.* **2017**, *69*, 62–72. [CrossRef] [PubMed]
7. Wolfl, C.G.; Bouillon, B.; Lackner, C.K.; Wentzensen, A.; Gliwitzky, B.; Gross, B.; Brokmann, J.; Hauer, T. Prehospital Trauma Life Support (PHTLS): An interdisciplinary training in preclinical trauma care. *Unfallchirurg* **2008**, *111*, 688–694. [CrossRef] [PubMed]
8. Stolmeijer, R.; Bouma, H.R.; Zijlstra, J.G.; Drost-de Klerck, A.M.; Ter Maaten, J.C.; Ligtenberg, J.J.M. A Systematic Review of the Effects of Hyperoxia in Acutely Ill Patients: Should We Aim for Less? *BioMed Res. Int.* **2018**, *14*, 7841295. [CrossRef]
9. Taher, A.; Pilehvari, Z.; Poorolajal, J.; Aghajanloo, M. Effects of Normobaric Hyperoxia in Traumatic Brain Injury: A Randomized Controlled Clinical Trial. *Trauma Mon.* **2016**, *21*, e26772. [CrossRef] [PubMed]
10. Damiani, E.; Donati, A.; Girardis, M. Oxygen in the critically ill: Friend or foe? *Curr. Opin. Anaesthesiol.* **2018**, *31*, 129–135. [CrossRef]
11. Rincon, F.; Kang, J.; Vibbert, M.; Urtecho, J.; Athar, M.K.; Jallo, J. Significance of arterial hyperoxia and relationship with case fatality in traumatic brain injury: A multicentre cohort study. *J. Neurol. Neurosurg. Psychiatry* **2014**, *85*, 799–805. [CrossRef]
12. Frati, A.; Cerretani, D.; Fiaschi, A.I.; Frati, P.; Gatto, V.; Russa, R.L.; Pesce, A.; Pinchi, E.; Santurro, A.; Fraschetti, F.; et al. Diffuse Axonal Injury and Oxidative Stress: A Comprehensive Review. *Int. J. Mol. Sci.* **2017**, *18*, 2600. [CrossRef]
13. Brenner, M.; Stein, D.; Hu, P.; Kufera, J.; Wooford, M.; Scalea, T. Association between early hyperoxia and worse outcomes after traumatic brain injury. *Arch Surg.* **2012**, *147*, 1042–1046. [CrossRef]
14. Sasser, S.M.; Hunt, R.C.; Sullivent, E.E.; Wald, M.M.; Mitchko, J.; Jurkovich, G.J.; Henry, M.C.; Salomone, J.P.; Wang, S.C.; Galli, R.L.; et al. National Expert Panel on Field Triage, Centers for Disease Control and Prevention (CDC). Guidelines for field triage of injured patients. Recommendations of the National Expert Panel on Field Triage. *MMWR Recomm. Rep.* **2009**, *58*, 1–35.
15. Hopple, J. No clue about O(2): Teaching oxygen therapy to prehospital providers. *JEMS* **2011**, *36*, 26–29. [PubMed]

16. Cornet, A.D.; Kooter, A.J.; Peters, M.J.; Smulders, Y.M. Supplemental oxygen therapy in medical emergencies: More harm than benefit? *Arch Intern. Med.* **2012**, *172*, 289–290. [CrossRef]
17. Bostek, C.C. Oxygen toxicity: An introduction. *AANA J.* **1989**, *57*, 231–237.
18. Demchenko, I.T.; Welty-Wolf, K.E.; Allen, B.W.; Piantadosi, C.A. Similar but not the same: Normobaric and hyperbaric pulmonary oxygen toxicity, the role of nitric oxide. *Am. J. Physiol.- Lung Cell. Mol. Physiol.* **2007**, *293*, 229–238. [CrossRef] [PubMed]
19. Bitterman, N. CNS oxygen toxicity. *Undersea Hyperb. Med.* **2004**, *31*, 63–72.
20. Doppenberg, E.M.; Rice, M.R.; Di, X.; Young, H.F.; Woodward, J.J.; Bullock, R. Increased free radical production due to subdural hematoma in the rat: Effect of increased inspired oxygen fraction. *J. Neurotrauma* **1998**, *15*, 337–347. [CrossRef] [PubMed]
21. Rossi, S.; Stocchetti, N.; Longhi, L.; Balestreri, M.; Spagnoli, D.; Zanier, E.R.; Bellinzona, G. Brain oxygen tension, oxygen supply, and oxygen consumption during arterial hyperoxia in a model of progressive cerebral ischemia. *J. Neurotrauma* **2001**, *18*, 163–174. [CrossRef]
22. Bulte, D.P.; Chiarelli, P.A.; Wise, R.G.; Jezzard, P. Cerebral perfusion response to hyperoxia. *J. Cereb. Blood Flow Metab.* **2007**, *27*, 69–75. [CrossRef]
23. Tolias, C.M.; Reinert, M.; Seiler, R.; Gilman, C.; Scharf, A.; Bullock, M.R. Normobaric hyperoxia–induced improvement in cerebral metabolism and reduction in intracranial pressure in patients with severe head injury: A prospective historical cohort-matched study. *J. Neurosurg.* **2004**, *101*, 435–444. [CrossRef]
24. Diringer, M.N.; Aiyagari, V.; Zazulia, A.R.; Videen, T.O.; Powers, W.J. Effect of hyperoxia on cerebral metabolic rate for oxygen measured using positron emission tomography in patients with acute severe head injury. *J. Neurosurg.* **2007**, *106*, 526–529. [CrossRef] [PubMed]
25. Briain, D.Ó.; Nickson, C.; Pilcher, D.V.; Udy, A.A. Early Hyperoxia in Patients with Traumatic Brain Injury Admitted to Intensive Care in Australia and New Zealand: A Retrospective Multicenter Cohort Study. *Neurocrit. Care* **2018**, *29*, 443–451. [CrossRef] [PubMed]
26. Russell, D.W.; Janz, D.R.; Emerson, W.L.; May, A.K.; Bernard, G.R.; Zhao, Z.; Koyama, T.; Ware, L.B. Early exposure to hyperoxia and mortality in critically ill patients with severe traumatic injuries. *BMC Pulm. Med.* **2017**, *17*, 29. [CrossRef] [PubMed]
27. Branson, R.D.; Johannigman, J.A. Pre-hospital oxygen therapy. *Respir. Care* **2013**, *58*, 86–97. [CrossRef] [PubMed]
28. Goldberg, S.A.; Rojanasarntikul, D.; Jagoda, A. The prehospital management of traumatic brain injury. *Handb. Clin. Neurol.* **2015**, *127*, 367–378.
29. Thomas, S.H.; Orf, J.; Wedel, S.K.; Conn, A.K. Hyperventilation in traumatic brain injury patients: Inconsistency between consensus guidelines and clinical practice. *J. Trauma* **2002**, *52*, 47–52. [CrossRef]
30. Dumont, T.M.; Visioni, A.J.; Rughani, A.I.; Tranmer, B.I.; Crookes, B. Inappropriate prehospital ventilation in severe traumatic brain injury increases in-hospital mortality. *J. Neurotrauma* **2010**, *27*, 1233–1241. [CrossRef]

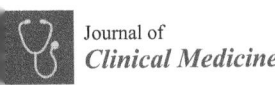

Article

Implementation of Computed Tomography Angiography (CTA) and Computed Tomography Perfusion (CTP) in Polish Guidelines for Determination of Cerebral Circulatory Arrest (CCA) during Brain Death/Death by Neurological Criteria (BD/DNC) Diagnosis Procedure

Romuald Bohatyrewicz [1], Joanna Pastuszka [1,*], Wojciech Walas [2], Katarzyna Chamier-Cieminska [3], Wojciech Poncyljusz [3], Wojciech Dabrowski [4], Joanna Wojczal [5], Piotr Luchowski [5], Maciej Guzinski [6], Elzbieta Jurkiewicz [7], Monika Bekiesinska-Figatowska [8], Radoslaw Owczuk [9], Jerzy Walecki [10], Olgierd Rowinski [11], Maciej Zukowski [12], Krzysztof Kusza [13], Mariusz Piechota [14], Andrzej Piotrowski [7], Marek Migdal [7], Marzena Zielinska [15] and Marcin Sawicki [3]

Citation: Bohatyrewicz, R.; Pastuszka, J.; Walas, W.; Chamier-Cieminska, K.; Poncyljusz, W.; Dabrowski, W.; Wojczal, J.; Luchowski, P.; Guzinski, M.; Jurkiewicz, E.; et al. Implementation of Computed Tomography Angiography (CTA) and Computed Tomography Perfusion (CTP) in Polish Guidelines for Determination of Cerebral Circulatory Arrest (CCA) during Brain Death/Death by Neurological Criteria (BD/DNC) Diagnosis Procedure. *J. Clin. Med.* **2021**, *10*, 4237. https://doi.org/10.3390/jcm10184237

Academic Editor: Rafael Badenes

Received: 15 July 2021
Accepted: 9 September 2021
Published: 18 September 2021

Publisher's Note: MDPI stays neutral with regard to jurisdictional claims in published maps and institutional affiliations.

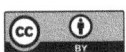

Copyright: © 2021 by the authors. Licensee MDPI, Basel, Switzerland. This article is an open access article distributed under the terms and conditions of the Creative Commons Attribution (CC BY) license (https://creativecommons.org/licenses/by/4.0/).

1. Department of Anesthesiology and Intensive Therapy, Pomeranian Medical University, 70-204 Szczecin, Poland; romuald.bohatyrewicz@pum.edu.pl
2. Pediatric and Neonatal Intensive Care Unit, Institute of Medical Science, University of Opole, 45-040 Opole, Poland; wojciechwalas@wp.pl
3. Department of Diagnostic Imaging and Interventional Radiology, Pomeranian Medical University, 70-204 Szczecin, Poland; kac.iiafix@gmail.com (K.C.-C.); wojciech.poncyljusz@pum.edu.pl (W.P.); msaw3108@gmail.com (M.S.)
4. Department of Anesthesiology and Intensive Care, University of Lublin, 20-059 Lublin, Poland; w.dabrowski5@gmail.com
5. Department of Neurology, Medical University of Lublin, 20-954 Lublin, Poland; jwojczal@poczta.onet.pl (J.W.); pluchowski@wp.pl (P.L.)
6. Department of General Radiology, Interventional Radiology and Neuroradiology, Wroclaw Medical University, 50-367 Wroclaw, Poland; guziol@wp.pl
7. Department of Diagnostic Imaging, The Children's Memorial Health Institute, 04-730 Warsaw, Poland; E.Jurkiewicz@IPCZD.PL (E.J.); a.piotrowski@ipczd.pl (A.P.); m.migdal@IPCZD.PL (M.M.)
8. Department of Diagnostic Imaging, Institute of Mother and Child, 01-211 Warsaw, Poland; monika.bekiesinska@imid.med.pl
9. Department of Anesthesiology and Intensive Therapy, Faculty of Medicine, Medical University of Gdansk, 80-210 Gdansk, Poland; r.owczuk@gumed.edu.pl
10. Diagnostic Radiology Department, Central Clinical Hospital of the Ministry of the Interior in Warsaw, 02-507 Warsaw, Poland; jerzywalecki@o2.pl
11. Department of Clinical Radiology, Medical University of Warsaw, 02-091 Warsaw, Poland; olgierd.rowinski@wum.edu.pl
12. Departament of Anesthesiology Intensive Care and Acute Poisoning, Pomeranian Medical University, 70-204 Szczecin, Poland; zukowski@pum.edu.pl
13. Department of Anaesthesiology and Intensive Therapy, Poznan University of Medical Sciences, 61-701 Poznan, Poland; k-kusza@wp.pl
14. Department of Anaesthesiology and Intensive Therapy, Centre for Artificial Extracorporeal Kidney and Liver Support, Dr W. Bieganski Regional Specialist Hospital, 91-347 Lodz, Poland; mariuszpiechota@poczta.onet.pl
15. Department of Anesthesiology and Intensive Therapy, Wroclaw Medical University, 50-367 Wroclaw, Poland; marzena.zielinska@umed.wroc.pl
* Correspondence: joanna.pastuszka@pum.edu.pl

Abstract: Background: Brain death/death by neurologic criteria (BD/DNC) guidelines are routinely analyzed, compared and updated in the majority of countries and are later implemented as national criteria. At the same time, extensive works have been conducted in order to unify clinical procedures and to validate and implement new technologies into a panel of ancillary tests. Recently evaluated computed tomography angiography and computed tomography perfusion (CTA/CTP) seem to be superior to traditionally used digital subtraction angiography (DSA), transcranial Doppler (TCD) and cerebral perfusion scintigraphy for diagnosis of cerebral circulatory arrest (CCA). In this narrative review, we would like to demonstrate scientific evidence supporting the implementation of CTA/CTP in Polish guidelines for BD/DNC diagnosis. Research and implementation process: In the first of our base studies concerning the potential usefulness of CTA/CTP for the confirmation of CCA during BD/DNC diagnosis procedures, we showed a sensitivity of 96.3% of CTA in a group of 82 patients. CTA was validated against DSA in this report. In the second study, CTA showed a sensitivity of 86% and CTP showed a sensitivity of 100% in a group of 50 patients. In this study, CTA and CTP were validated against clinical diagnosis of BD/DNC supported by TCD. Additionally, we propose our CCA criteria for CTP test, which are based on ascertainment of cerebral blood flow (CBF) < 10 mL/100 g/min and cerebral blood volume < 1 mL/100 g in regions of interest (ROIs) localized in all brain regions. Based on our research results, CTA/CTP methods were implemented in Polish BD/DNC criteria. To our knowledge, CTP was implemented for the first time in national guidelines. Conclusions: CTA and CTP-derived CTA might be in future the tests of choice for CCA diagnosis, proper and/or Doppler pretest might significantly increase sensitivity of CTA in CCA diagnosis procedures. Whole brain CTP might be decisive in some cases of inconclusive CTA. Implementation of CTA/CTP in the Polish BD/DNC diagnosis guidelines does not show any major obstacles. We believe that in next edition of "The World Brain Death Project" CTA and CTP will be recommended as ancillary tests of choice for CCA confirmation during BD/DNC diagnosis procedures.

Keywords: brain death; death by neurologic criteria; cerebral blood flow; CT angiography; CT perfusion

1. Background

In this narrative review, we present the evolution of Polish guidelines for brain death/death by neurologic criteria (BD/DNC) diagnosis and demonstrate scientific evidence supporting the implementation of computed tomography angiography (CTA) and computed tomography perfusion (CTP) for confirmation of cerebral circulatory arrest (CCA).

The first Polish BD/DNC criteria implemented in 1984 as whole-brain death criteria were similar to the so-called "Harvard brain death criteria" [1]. Later, these Polish criteria underwent a unique evolution: in 1990, they were converted into brainstem death criteria and, later, in 2007, they were reversed back to whole-brain death criteria [2], subsequently being amended in 2020 [3]. During this conversion, we reimplemented an opportunity for facultative usage of instrumental ancillary tests, including brain blood perfusion tests.

Currently, in Poland, although formally facultative, instrumental ancillary tests are used in the majority of BD/DNC diagnosis procedures. This is exactly the reverse of what is proposed in current international recommendations [4]. There are various reasons for this. Despite receiving the official support of health care authorities and three consecutive Popes, we have faced unclear or even negative statements from some religious commentors and selected Catholic media. The matter is sometimes complicated by political activities, which induce doctors' uncertainty and filling of a lack of legal safety. Polish physicians would feel more comfortable and safer if they could demonstrate the results of instrumental ancillary tests confirming BD diagnosis. Brain blood perfusion tests are considered to be the most evident from all sides of the discussion—physicians, relatives of the deceased and public opinion. It is obvious to everybody, regardless of the level of education, that non-perfused tissue must be dead.

There are three brain blood flow ancillary tests that, despite known disadvantages, have a long-established position in BD/DNC diagnosis:

1. Catheter digital subtraction angiography (DSA), selective or from the aortic arch;
2. Transcranial Doppler ultrasonography (TCD);
3. Cerebral perfusion scintigraphy.

Use of DSA, which is still considered to be a gold standard and reference method, is gradually decreasing [4]. It is invasive and requires procedural skills, time and availability of an angiography suite. It was reimplemented in Polish BD criteria in 2007 and was approved again in the amendment in 2020 [3]. TCD is completely noninvasive, its sensitivity exceeds 90% and the specificity is 100%. Despite its obvious advantages, TCD is not frequently used in Poland because it has to be performed with unique devices that, currently, are not widely available. Additionally, it is highly operator-dependent and requires certification of the performing physician. The last of the "traditional" cerebral perfusion tests, scintigraphy, is currently seldom available in the majority of Polish hospitals.

In this difficult situation, it has become of crucial importance to develop and introduce an ancillary test that would be less invasive than DSA, easily available, uncomplicated to perform and easy to interpret.

2. Early Research into Using CTA/CTP for Diagnosing BD/DNC in Poland

In 2005, we considered CTA and CTP to be the tests of choice for the future, which is consistent with the current opinion of Greer et al. [4]. Modern multi-slice CT scanners are fast enough to visualize vasculature and perfusion of the whole brain with a single intravenous injection of iodinated contrast medium and, finally, to confirm CCA. Both CTA and CTP, if performed with a calibrated intravenous contrast injection and precise scanning protocols, are operator-independent at the stage of performance and providing raw data.

The research team of the Department of Anesthesiology and Intensive Care together with co-workers from the Department of Diagnostic Imaging and Interventional Radiology of the Pomeranian Medical University in Szczecin have been involved in research programs and legislation since the implementation of the first Polish BD/DNC criteria published in 1984. In 2005–2007, Romuald Bohatyrewicz was a co-chairman and in 2015–2019, chairman, of the Ministry of Health's Task Force for review of these criteria.

In 2007, we suggested the possibility of implementing CTA as a new brain blood flow test, but this was not accepted by the rest of the Task Force members because of insufficient evidence in the literature and lack of experience in Poland. In this situation, we organized a national multi-center trial (N N403 171137), entitled "Evaluation of CT angiography and CT perfusion in brain death diagnosis", in a group of adult brain-dead patients, followed by a series of publications. The first of them, published in 2010 [5], confirmed the ability of CTA/CTP to diagnose CCA in our population of BD/DNC patients and our findings were compatible with data published by other authors at that time [6–10]. Unfortunately, our CTP findings could not be applied to CCA diagnosis because the generation of CT scanners used at that time in Poland could cover only a thin layer of the brain, about 30 mm thick.

During initial attempts to implement CTA for CCA diagnosis, there was no consensus regarding the evaluation criteria, which have evolved as research progressed [6–13]. The most popular scoring systems (10, 7, 4 points), shown in Figure 1, were based on analysis of the opacification of the following:

1. Pericallosal segments of the right and left anterior cerebral artery (ACA-A3);
2. Cortical segments of the right and left middle cerebral artery (MCA-M4);
3. Cortical segments of the right and left posterior cerebral artery (PCA-P2);
4. Basilar artery (BA);
5. Right and left internal cerebral vein (ICV);
6. Great cerebral vein (GCV)—the vein of Galen.

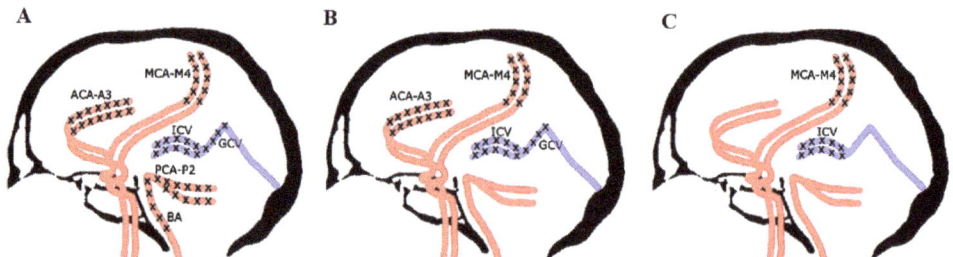

Figure 1. Various scales used for CCA diagnosis in CTA imaging: (**A**) 10-point scale, where positive result (score = 10) confirming CCA is stated when bilateral ACA-A3, MCA-M4, PCA-P2 and ICV and single GCV and BA are not opacified; (**B**) 7-point scale, where positive result (score = 7) confirming CCA is stated when bilateral ACA-A3, MCA-M4 and ICV and single GCV are not opacified; (**C**) 4-point scale, where positive result (score = 4) confirming CCA is stated when bilateral MCA-M4 and ICV are not opacified.

Initially, we analyzed CTA imaging in a group of 82 patients undergoing routine BD/DNC diagnosis with DSA included as a standard element of this procedure. CTA was completed first and was followed by DSA [14]. In this situation, CTA could be validated against DSA with a very short time interval between these two procedures, which is consistent with the recommendation for method validation recently published by Greer et al. [4]. The sensitivity reported in this study reached 96.3% according to the 4-point scale, 74.4% according to the 7-point scale and 67.1% according to the 10-point scale [14].

After meticulous analysis of these data, we finally accepted the 4-point scale proposed by the French guidelines for diagnosis of BD/DNC [15]. According to this 4-point scale, CCA may be confirmed if there is a bilateral absence of contrast filling of cortical segments of the middle cerebral arteries (MCA-M4) and internal cerebral veins (ICVs), as presented in Figure 1. Unilateral opacification of one or two cortical branches of the MCA does not preclude the diagnosis of CCA as long as the contrast does not fill the ICVs.

Additionally, we noticed (unpublished results) that if CTA tests were performed shortly after the appearance of brainstem areflexia, more widespread opacification of cerebral vessels, thus excluding CCA diagnosis, was recorded, which was also confirmed by the data published by Welschehold and Kerhuel [13,16]. The explanation for this phenomenon is quite simple: in this short period, the intracranial pressure (ICP) did not exceed the mean arterial pressure (MAP), leading to CCA. Premature CTA examinations lead to a dramatic decrease in test sensitivity, which is one of the sources of undeserved opinions about the poor utility of this method for CCA determination. Such cases are rather unlikely in Poland because our doctors prefer more conservative approaches and generally initiate diagnostic procedures after a longer observation period. Nevertheless, in the Polish guidelines [3], we recommended a minimal 6-h observation time before CTA/CTP examinations, which is identical to the French guidelines [15].

3. Comparison with the Other Instructions for CCA Confirmation by CTA Imaging

Recently Lewis et al. reviewed diagnostic requirements for ancillary testing for BD/DNC in 78 official national BD/DNC protocols and found that in 14 European countries CTA was included in to a panel of ancillary tests [17], but according to our knowledge this method was in detail described in national guidelines and relatively frequently used only in France, Germany and recently in Poland. French and Polish protocols and diagnostic criteria based on 4-point scale are similar while German protocol elaborated on the grounds of publication of Welschehold [13] is based on recognition of lack of opacification of 7 intracranial arteries in late arterial phase [18]. Comparison of these three diagnostic protocols is demonstrated in Table 1.

Table 1. Comparison of three frequently used European national guidelines for determination CCA with CTA during BD/DNC diagnosis procedures.

	Polish (2020 *)	French (2011 *)	German (2015 *)
Recommended delay after appearance of clinical signs of BD/DNC (h)	6	6 **	not specified
1. Non-contrast scanning used as a reference			
2. Early post-contrast scanning			
Contrast volume (mL)	80	2 mL/kg (max 120)	65
Scanning time	triggered by bolus-tracking in extracranial carotid arteries	20 s after start of contrast injection	not performed
Assessed vessel			
STA (bilaterally) ***	2	2	not performed
3. Late post-contrast scanning			
Scanning time	40 s after start of early post-contrast scanning	60 s after start of contrast injection	15 s after filling of extracranial carotid arteries detected with bolus-tracking
Evaluation scale	4-point	4-point	7-point late arterial
Assessed vessel			
STA (bilaterally) ***			2
MCA-M1 (bilaterally)			2
ACA-A1 (bilaterally)			2
BA			1
PCA-P1 (bilaterally)			2
MCA-M4 (bilaterally)	2	2	
ICV (bilaterally)	2	2	
Delay to next exam if the previous was inconclusive (h)	12	not specified	not specified

Notes: BD—brain death; STA—superficial temporal artery; ACA—anterior cerebral artery; A1—1st division of ACA; MCA—middle cerebral artery; M1—1st division of MCA; M4—4th division of MCA; PCA—posterior cerebral artery; P1—1st division of PCA; BA—basilar artery; ICV—internal cerebral vein. * year of implementation. ** time delay of 6 h can be shortened by performing transcranial Doppler ultrasound. *** assessment of filling of extracranial arteries like STA serves as a control of effective contrast administration to the head.

4. Sensitivity and Specificity of CTA in CCA Determination during BD/DNC Diagnosis Procedures

Test accuracy is defined by two important factors, sensitivity and specificity. The sensitivity of CTA and CTP in BD/DNC diagnostic procedures refers to their ability to correctly indicate BD/DNC in patients with true BD/DNC. In our studies, it would be the proportion of positive (confirmed) CCA in a group with confirmed BD/DNC diagnosis. Specificity would relate to the test's ability to correctly identify patients without the BD/DNC. In our case this would be the proportion of patients without recognized CCA (negative) in a group of patients who are not brain dead. In our studies evaluating CTA the reference was DSA while in those evaluating CTP we used clinical diagnosis as the reference. A test with a sensitivity of around 90% would be considered to have good diagnostic performance. Obviously, in this special clinical situation, the aim should be to achieve 100% specificity.

Assessment of accuracy of the test requires the established ground truth as a reference. However, in previous studies evaluating CTA and CTP in the BD/DNC diagnostic procedure different reference standards were used, e.g., clinical signs of BD/DNC (most commonly), DSA, perfusion scintigraphy or TCD. This is one of causes of significant divergence in reported sensitivities. Therefore, we agree with the authors of „World Brain Death Project" [4] that establishing unified reference for studies evaluating CTA and CTP in the BD/DNC diagnostic procedure is desirable.

According to information available in "World Brain Death Project" concerning blood perfusion tests, their sensitivity varies mainly in a range of 52–100% while declared specificity is close to 100% with remark included: "Specificity is assumed on basis of experimental data but should be interpreted with caution given the limitation of studies that reported only on clinically confirmed BD/DNC" [4]. We support this opinion.

We did not determine specificity of CTA/CTP examination during BD/DNC diagnostic procedures which in fact is one of the limitations of our studies. In the context of our research it would concern the frequency of false positive diagnoses of CCA, potentially supporting incorrect BD/DNC diagnosis. Such situation would be catastrophic in case of BD/DNC diagnosis in a patient with survival and recovery potential which is also highlighted in "World Brain Death Project". Fortunately, such theoretical situation is unlikely because all ancillary tests are only additional tools used in complex procedure of BD/DNC diagnosis process including assessment of devastating brain injury, analysis of preconditions and prerequisites and, finally, meticulous clinical examination [4]. In case of any doubts termination of BD/DNC diagnosis process is worldwide recommended. This happened in a few reported cases of patients demonstrating brainstem areflexia with persisted respiratory drive and CCA diagnosed by DSA [19,20]. However, no one of these patients survived, but such discrepancy between instrumental test and clinical findings might be highly confusing. This might be explained by the fact, that infratentorial space, especially medulla oblongata is surrounded by osseous and obscured by highly vascularized structures. In some cases, it may be supplied by the posterior inferior cerebellar artery atypically originating from extracranial segment of vertebral artery [19]. Vestigial blood supply sufficient to preserve at least minimal partial function of respiratory centre might remain undetected by any of blood flow tests. Considering this, specificity of 100% is not achievable in any one of the blood flow studies.

Nevertheless, specificity remains problematic during assessment of brain blood perfusion tests because patients non suspected but close to develop BD/DNC are rarely included in such studies. However, it would be possible to identify them in a group of patients hospitalized in centers where neurointerventional procedures are carried out on regular basis. We included such 5 participants in one of our publications [21]. We found only one publication by Welschehold et al. [13] elaborating prospectively the issue of CTA specificity during CCA diagnostic procedures. He performed CTA in 30 patients immediately after the first signs of loss of brainstem reflexes were noticed and a few hours later, after definitive legal determination of BD/DNC [13]. He found CCA in 3 out of 30 patients short after onset of brainstem areflexia but before legal determination of BD/DNC and interpreted them as false positives. All of these 3 patients were later legally declared brain dead. CCA appeared in this group in fact earlier than in remaining 27 cases and considering findings of these 3 patients as false positives, although formally justified, is slightly unfortunate.

Majority of questions concerning sensitivity and specificity of CTA/CTP tests as well as CCA dynamics will be answered by extensive prospective multicenter trial NCT0309851 initiated in 2017 by Chassé and Shankar in Canada. They planned enrollment of 333 participants, with high risk of BD/DNC, not in a course of BD/DNC diagnosis at that moment. The study is oriented for determination of CTA/CTP accuracy in BD/DNC procedures with special attention for diagnosis of brainstem hypoperfusion. We were discussing with Canadian Colleagues possible Polish multicenter participation in this study, but after meticulous analysis of the project we realized, that Polish Bioethical Committee would not accept invasive tests in patients who do not demonstrate complete brainstem areflexia as being not in the best interest of patients and in the same time useless for potential BD/DNC diagnosis. Therefore, finally, we did not join the trial.

5. Research Advancement with CTP in Poland

At the same time, we noticed that in rare cases of patients demonstrating BD/DNC symptoms, preserved trace opacification of intracranial arteries may be observed in DSA examination. This phenomenon is known as stasis filling, defined as delayed, weak and persistent opacification of the proximal cerebral arterial segments, without opacification of the cortical branches or venous outflow [22]. In these rare cases, CTP often shows residual cerebral blood flow (CBF) below 10 mL/100 g/min and a cerebral blood volume (CBV) below 1.0 mL/100 g. These values are the established thresholds for neuronal necrosis [23] and following this, they may be considered thresholds for global or regional CCA diagnosis [24,25].

Advanced research activity concerning CTP became possible after the advent of a new generation of CT scanners fast enough to visualize vasculature and perfusion of the whole brain with a single intravenous injection of iodinated contrast medium. At that time, we stopped performing CTA imaging and switched to reconstruction of CTA images from the CTP source images as timing-invariant (TI)-CTA. TI-CTA provides angiography by overlapping all time frames and displaying the maximum enhancement over time. This makes the technique time independent, which means that the maximum enhancement of a vessel is displayed independently of contrast arrival time. Therefore, TI-CTA is not sensitive to delayed arrival of the contrast material in cerebral vessels and, thus, should display any vessel present. This technique was previously described and shown to be reliable by Smit et al. [26].

CTP criteria for CCA during the BD/DNC diagnostic procedure were not published before; therefore, we elaborated our original instruction of assessment based on an analysis of the CBF and CBV in 1-cm^2 circular regions of interest (ROIs), including the midbrain (two ROIs), the pons (two ROIs) and the medulla oblongata (two ROIs) as well as the cerebellum (eight ROIs); cortical regions of the frontal (12 ROIs), parietal (12 ROIs), temporal (12 ROIs) and occipital lobes (eight ROIs); and the basal ganglia (eight ROIs), drawn bilaterally and placed on each 10-mm axial slice, as shown in Figure 2. We recognized CCA in CTP examination if the CBF value was below 10 mL/100 g/min and CBV was below 1.0 mL/100 g in all ROIs [25]. The most frequent combinations of CTA and CTP images are shown in Figure 3.

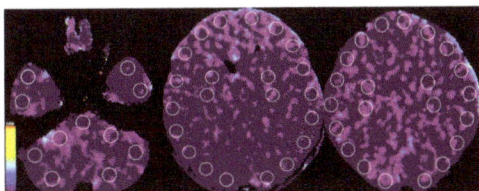

Figure 2. Criteria of CCA in CTP imaging. Axial sections of brain with marked positions of ROIs. Color scale illustrates range of CBF (mL/100 g/min). CBF < 10 mL/100 g/min confirms CCA.

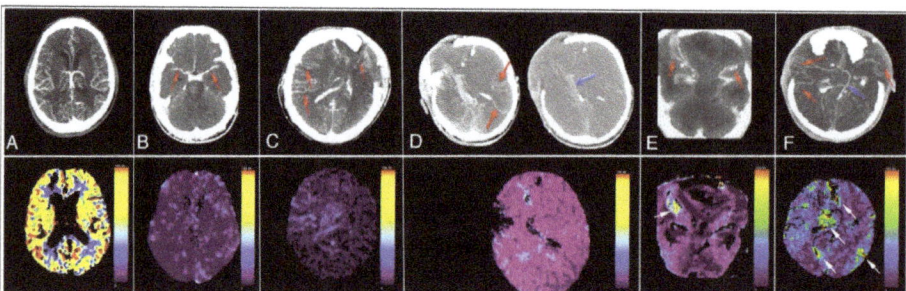

Figure 3. Different CTA (upper row) and CTP (lower row) patterns during CCA diagnosis procedures: (**A**) patient with suspected ischemic stroke with normal CTA and CTP; (**B**) patient with opacification limited to proximal segments of middle cerebral arteries MCA-M1 inCTA (red arrows) and CBF value < 10 mL/100 g/min in CTP; both techniques confirm CCA. (**C**) Patient with bilateral opacification of cortical arterial segments (MCA-M4; red arrows) in CTA, not consistent with CCA diagnosis and CBF value < 10 mL/100 g/min in CTP, which confirms CCA diagnosis; (**D**) patient with opacified MCA-M4 segments (red arrows) and opacified internal cerebral vein (blue arrow) in CTA, not consistent with CCA diagnosis and CBF value < 10 mL/100 g/min, which confirms CCA diagnosis; (**E**) patient with opacified MCA-M2/M3 segments (red arrows) in CTA, consistent with CCA diagnosis and isolated single sub-craniectomy area with CBF value > 10 mL/100 g/min (white arrow), also consistent with CCA diagnosis; (**F**) patient with opacified MCA-M4 segments (red arrows) and opacified internal cerebral vein (blue arrow) in CTA, not consistent with CCA diagnosis and multiple scattered areas with CBF value > 10 mL/100 g/min (white arrows), also inconsistent with CCA diagnosis. Color scales illustrate range of CBF (mL/100 g/min). CBF < 10 mL/100 g/min confirms CCA.

In the next step of our research program, we hypothesized that CTP would be a more sensitive approach than CTA in CCA diagnosis. To verify this, we conducted a study aiming to compare the sensitivities of CTP and CTA in recognizing CCA during BD/DNC diagnosis procedures. A group of 50 patients undergoing this diagnostic procedure were included in the study. All of them met the standard BD/DNC criteria based on confirmation of catastrophic brain injury, exclusion of confounders and confirmation of brainstem areflexia and apnea during two series of clinical examinations [25]. Additionally, TCD examination confirming CCA was completed in the majority of them; however, this information was not included in the publication.

In 43 out of 50 patients, CTA confirmed CCA, as demonstrated in Figure 3, patient B. In the remaining seven patients, CTA revealed opacification of M4 segments, ICVs or both, as shown in Figure 3, patients C and D. These CTA findings were inconsistent with CCA according to the 4-point scale. In all 50 patients, CBF was below 10 mL/100 g/min and CBV was below 1.0 mL/100 g, which confirmed CCA according to our criteria. In summary, in this publication, we reported a sensitivity of 86% and 100% for CTA and CTP, respectively. Additionally, these results confirmed our hypothesis that in borderline cases, when CTA is inconclusive, CTP may be a decisive method for CCA diagnosis. Later, after analysis of a few additional cases, we stated that in special situations in patients with clinical signs of BD, isolated areas of decompression may be preserved in the region of craniectomy or open fractures. These isolated areas may exhibit CBF and CBV values above the thresholds of 10 mL/100 g/min and 1 mL/100 g, respectively. This phenomenon does not exclude the diagnosis of CCA if the CBF and CBV values are below these thresholds in other ROIs, including those in the brainstem, as shown in Figure 3, patient E. Appearance of multiple areas with CBF and CBV above the threshold values is, according to our current opinion, inconsistent with CCA diagnosis, as shown in Figure 3, patient F.

Noteworthily, another research group led by Shankar [24,27] postulated a slightly different approach to the possible usefulness of CTP imaging in BD/DNC diagnostic procedures or withdrawal of life-sustaining therapy. They focused on demonstration of brain hypoperfusion limited to the brainstem area, which is, in fact, somehow parallel to brainstem areflexia and the brainstem death concept, suggesting "isolated brainstem death".

CTP in this situation does not necessarily confirm global CCA as it was demonstrated in our report [25]. It is highly questionable whether isolated brainstem death diagnosis confirmed by CTP imaging, but coexisting with preserved supratentorial perfusion and possibly persisted EEG activity, might justify BD/DNC diagnosis.

6. Implementation of CTA/CTP Examination into the Polish National Guidelines for BD/DNC

Based on our published research data [14,25] and unpublished observations, finally, we implemented CTA/CTP examination in the Polish national guidelines for BD/DNC diagnosis in patients over 12 years of age at the beginning of 2020 [3]. To our knowledge, this was the first implementation of CTP in official BD/DNC diagnosis guidelines. A diagram showing two alternative CT diagnostic approaches depending on the technical capabilities of the scanner, local tradition and the radiologist's competence is demonstrated in Figure 4.

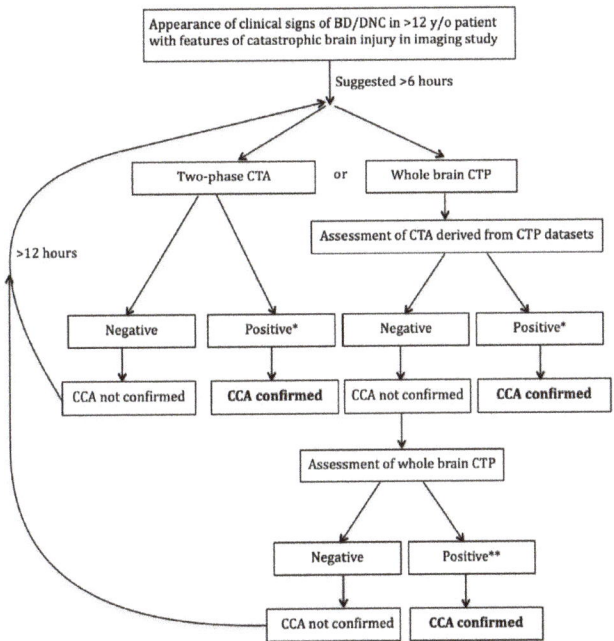

Figure 4. Schematic algorithm of application of CTA and CTP for CCA confirmation according to Polish national guidelines for BD/DNC diagnosis. Notes: * bilateral non-filling of cortical arteries (MCA-M4) and ICVs in late phase with normal filling of extracranial arteries in early phase; filling of one or two cortical arteries on the same side is permissible as long as the ICVs are not filled. ** CBF below 10 mL/100 g/min and CBV below 1.0 mL/100 g in all ROIs. Presence of small, isolated foci with CBF or CBV above these values are permissible in regions of local decompression due to craniectomy or open skull fracture. BD/DNC—brain death/death by neurologic criteria; CCA—cerebral circulatory arrest.

CTA/CTP examinations for BD/DNC diagnosis procedures were approved for patients > 12 years old, assuming that above this age, the skull is not pliable and the brain reaches morphological maturity. We presumed that the mechanisms of CCA might be similar in younger age groups, at least >2 years old without patent sutures or fontanels and in patients < 2 years old, according to our knowledge, it is unpredictable, as with the results of other traditional methods used for CCA diagnosis [4]. Therefore, in order to explore this issue, we recently invited all Polish and foreign pediatric intensive care units to participate in a multi-center study for the validation of CTA and CTP in determination of CCA during the BD/DNC diagnosis procedure in a pediatric population below 12 years of age [28].

Immediately after the introduction of CTA/CTP for CCA diagnosis into Polish guidelines, we started monitoring the usage of these methods all over the country. Unfortunately, this was extremely difficult due to the COVID-19 pandemic, but nevertheless, we did not notice any major problems. Sometimes, first attempts were invalid because of protocol violations. Furthermore, radiologists, especially in small hospitals, were reluctant to write a final conclusion on whether elaborated images fulfill or do not fulfill tabulated CCA criteria due to fear of making a misdiagnosis in such a specific clinical situation. Occasionally, we observed a premature CTA examination almost immediately after appearance of brainstem areflexia resulting in the presence of persisted opacification of M4 segments of the middle cerebral artery because the intracranial pressure still did not reach a value sufficient to completely block intracranial blood flow. Repeated examinations after 12 h usually confirmed CCA. Interestingly, we recognized expected and unexpected reasons for acceptance or refusal for implementation of these new technologies. In many middle-sized hospitals, in which DSA and any other brain blood perfusion studies were unavailable, CTA was relatively easily implemented as the only ancillary test facilitating and shortening of BD/DNC diagnostic process. Surprisingly, implementation process was slow in some of most advanced interventional radiology centers with permanent availability of diagnostic/interventional team. In such units, apart from strong adherence to diagnostic traditions, it was sometimes easier to organize DSA than CTA/CTP. Additionally, this was treated as a chance for training of residents in DSA procedures.

Implementation of CTP was more complicated. Not all CT scanners in Polish hospitals are able to perform whole-brain perfusion imaging. Moreover, even in well-equipped reference hospitals, usually only a few radiologists are experienced in CTP postprocessing and interpretation because in Poland, it is a relatively new technology introduced mainly in departments involved in neuroradiologic procedures. Furthermore, data postprocessing is extremely time-consuming. Due to these all difficulties, even in centers that implemented this technique in Poland, CTP examinations are usually performed within working hours and in the remainder of the week, CCA diagnosis is based on CTA.

7. Comparison with Recommendations Made in the World Brain Death Project

1. Recently Greer at al. published in JAMA great work elaborated by international group of experts, entitled "Determination of Brain Death/Death by Neurologic Criteria: The World Brain Death Project" consisting of introduction part and 17 supplements [4]. It summarizes current knowledge about various aspects of pathophysiology of brain injury leading, finally, to BD/DNC, all aspects of diagnostic procedures, possible organ procurement and, finally, future research agenda. The following is stated in it: "It is recommended that when ancillary testing is performed and demonstrates the presence of brain blood flow, BD/DNC cannot be declared at that time". This indirectly points out the necessity for the elaboration of precise diagnostic criteria for CTA/CTP after implementation of these new technologies for investigation of CCA, both in infratentorial and supratentorial spaces. Our research results and their interpretations are consistent with this point of view.
2. The following is stated in the "Determination of Brain Death/Death by Neurologic Criteria. The World Brain Death Project" publication: "It is recommended that when ancillary testing is performed and demonstrates the presence of brain blood flow, BD/DNC cannot be declared at that time" [4]. This indirectly points out the necessity for the elaboration of precise criteria for CTA/CTP after implementation of these new technologies for investigation of CCA, both in infratentorial and supratentorial spaces. Our research results and their interpretations are consistent with this point of view.

On the other hand, our positive opinion concerning the feasibility of CTA and CTP for CCA confirmation during BD/DNC diagnosis is discrepant with the opinion of Greer et al. [4], who stated that these methods require further consensus on the phases and timing of image acquisition, as well as consensus upon and validation of the interpretation criteria subsequently used. According to Greer, this also concerns validation in comparison to "gold-standard" BD/DNC cerebral perfusion tests such as DSA or radionuclide scintigraphy. To support our standpoint, we highlight that in our earlier publications CTA was validated against DSA [5,14,29] and in our later studies CTA/CTP were validated against clinical diagnosis supported by TCD [21,25].

In order to verify the reason of some kind of distrust of Greer at al. towards validity of CTA/CTP for CCA diagnosis we extensively analyzed Supplement 5 to "World Brain Death Project". This supplement deals with all ancillary tests used for BD/DNC with special attention directed towards brain blood perfusion tests, including CTA/CTP. We found information about "one report of false positive result" and because of its crucial importance we meticulously analyzed the source publication [30] where we found following facts:

1. Non contrast CT (Figure 1) in our opinion confirms severe edema in course of devastating brain injury indirectly indicating presence of severe intracranial hypertension,
2. CTA imaging pattern is typical for CCA (Figure 2); however, the authors declare it doubtful because of possible hypotension during the procedure which is an obvious diagnostic protocol violation and makes the examination not interpretative,
3. In TCD imaging (Figure 3) intracranial arteries might be not properly identified and flow spectra incorrectly interpreted:
    a. The typical flow spectrum in OA (ophthalmic artery) is usually different from the one showed in Figure 3. In transorbital window in TCD (transcranial Doppler) it should be higher resistive than presented on the depth 50–60 mm as OA is an artery of predominantly elastic type. Furthermore, presented flow was inconsistent with intracranial hypertension. Therefore, the flow described as the right OA perhaps does not represent true flow in OA. Regardless of these doubts the flow in OA is not a TCD criterion for CCA diagnosis. Therefore, the reason for demonstration of flow in a vessel identified as OA by default in order to support supposition of preserved cerebral perfusion remains doubtful.
    b. In patients with high intracranial pressure the flow spectra in cerebral arteries change in a very characteristic manner. The systolic phase of spectrum become very short (velocities are normal or diminished) and all diastolic velocities decline to baseline or near it. Such type of flow can persist for some time and usually leads to CCA, while in Figure 3, the flow spectrum in artery recognized by the authors as left middle cerebral artery (LMCA) is low resistant with gradual reduction of velocity during systole and diastole. This does not represent residual flow consistent with severe intracranial hypertension.

In summary, using of this publication as an argument suggesting inaccuracy of CTA in BD/DNC diagnostic procedures is questionable.

It is stated in 'The World Brain Death Project" that "there is still no consensus on the technical criteria for CT angiography as ancillary test and considerable variation on reported sensitivity in the diagnosis of BD/DNC". We agree with this opinion but, on the other hand, we believe that secondary analysis of available literature would help to remove some concerns. Large number of scales used and unclear information about time gap between the onset of brainstem areflexia and proceeding of CTA are highly confusing. However, if we restrict our attention to reports providing detailed information about time gap between the onset of brainstem areflexia and CTA, the data look more optimistic. Kerhuel using French criteria based on 4-point score showed that short time between clinical brain death and CTA leads to higher number of inconclusive results (low sensitivity) and postulated that time delay > 6 h provides sensitivity of 92% [16]. Similar tendency was reported by Welschehold [13]. This clearly points out that proper timing is a crucial factor determining CTA sensitivity regardless of protocol used and that minimal time delay should be recommended in international and national guidelines.

We would like to highlight that in Europe three detailed instructions are currently used, French [15] German [18] and Polish [3], based on earlier extensive research completed in these countries [6–8,10–14,21,22,25,28,29]. Interestingly, a proposition of earlier TCD was included in French instruction to minimize delay from the onset of brainstem areflexia to CTA and to avoid premature examination [15]. TCD, even uncertified or Duplex Doppler examination of both vertebral arteries and both internal carotid arteries in the extracranial segments may be performed to determine a proper time for CT tests We included this proposition in the recently initiated Polish trial concerning validation CTA for CCA diagnosis in the pediatric population [28]. In addition, we are planning to recommend Duplex Doppler as pretest before CTA in future amendment of Polish BD/DNC criteria. Summarizing our considerations concerning influence of time delay on CTA sensitivity, we presume that prospective great trial currently conducted by Chassé and Shankar in Canada will answer the majority of concerns.

Furthermore, we would like to comment on another inaccuracy we found in "World Brain Death Project", creating negative opinion about the validity of CTA/CTP in BD/DNC procedures and simultaneously about our research results concerning our first article published in 2010 [5]. In Table 4 of Supplement 5, the "Polish scale" was cited as a source of information, with a reported sensitivity of 41.7%. This was incorrect, because in this paper, we only demonstrated an observed opacification level of all vessels examined in a group of 24 patients with confirmed BD/DNC. We neither validated the results according to any scoring scale, nor reported any sensitivity in it. Therefore, the term "Polish scale", as well as the information about sensitivity of 41.7%, is not supported by presented data. Finally, we did not suggest the re-addition of anterior and posterior circulation assessments to the 4-point scale. However, if the data of this small group presented in Table 1 were analyzed using a 4-point scale, we would obtain a sensitivity of 100%.

The last inaccuracy on which we would like to comment concerns a source of Figure 4 visualizing "variation in methods of assessing brain blood flow on CTA, depending on choice of anatomical vasculature and time of imaging" which was of our authorship [14], but incorrectly presented as originating from the publication of the other authors. We tried to correct this erroneous information concerning our publications in a letter to editor, but unfortunately, it was not accepted because of "space limitations in the letters section".

8. Conclusions

Based on our experience, results of our investigations, extensive literature review and, finally, recent observations and confidential discussions with diagnostic teams we conclude:

1. CTA and CTP-derived CTA might be in future the tests of choice for CCA diagnosis due to increasing availability and relatively easy interpretation.
2. Proper timing based on time elapse after the appearance of brain stem areflexia and/or Doppler pretest might significantly reduce preterm examinations and significantly increase sensitivity of CTA in CCA diagnosis procedures.
3. Whole brain CTP might be decisive in some cases of inconclusive CTA.
4. The monitoring of the implementation of CTA/CTP according to recently amended Polish BD/DNC diagnosis guidelines does not show any major obstacles, occasionally appearing teaching troubles and excessively large sticking to traditional diagnostic schemes are gradually eliminated.
5. We strongly believe that in next edition of "The World Brain Death Project", CTA and CTP will be recommended as ancillary tests of choice for CCA diagnosis during BD/DNC diagnosis procedures. We strongly believe that in next edition of "The World Brain Death Project" CTA and CTP will be recommended as ancillary tests of choice for CCA confirmation during BD/DNC diagnosis procedures.

Author Contributions: Conceptualization, R.B., J.P., W.W., K.C.-C., W.P., W.D., J.W. (Joanna Wojczal), P.L., M.G., E.J., M.B.-F., R.O., J.W. (Jerzy Walecki), O.R., K.K., M.P., A.P., M.M., M.Z. (Marzena Zielinska), and M.S.; data curation, M.Z. (Maciej Zukowski). All authors have read and agreed to the published version of the manuscript.

Funding: This study was financed from the project of the Polish Ministry of Education and Science.

Conflicts of Interest: All authors declare that they have no conflict of interest.

References

1. Ad Hoc Committee of the Harvard Medical School to Examine the Definition of Brain Death. A definition of irreversible coma. Report of the ad hoc committee of the harvard medical school to examine the definition of brain death. *J. Am. Med. Assoc.* **1968**, *205*, 5694976.
2. Bohatyrewicz, R.; Zukowski, M.; Marzec-Lewenstein, E.; Biernawska, J.; Solek-Pastuszka, J.; Sienko, J.; Sulikowski, T.; Bohatyrewicz, A. Reversal to whole-brain death criteria after 15-year experience with brain stem death criteria in Poland. *Transplant. Proc.* **2009**, *41*, 2959–2960. [CrossRef]
3. Announcement of the Minister of Health from the 4th of December 2019 on the Method and Criteria for Establishing Permanent Irreversible Cessation of Brain Function. 2020. Available online: https://monitorpolski.gov.pl/M2020000007301.pdf (accessed on 11 June 2021).
4. Greer, D.M.; Shemie, S.D.; Lewis, A.; Torrance, S.; Varelas, P.; Goldenberg, F.D.; Bernat, J.L.; Souter, M.; Topcuoglu, M.A.; Alexandrov, A.W.; et al. Determination of brain death/death by neurologic criteria. *J. Am. Med. Assoc.* **2020**, *324*, 1078–1097. [CrossRef] [PubMed]
5. Bohatyrewicz, R.; Sawicki, M.; Walecka, A.; Walecki, J.; Rowinski, O.; Czajkowski, Z.; Krzysztalowski, A.; Solek-Pastuszka, J.; Zukowski, M.; Marzec-Lewenstein, E.; et al. Computed tomographic angiography and perfusion in the diagnosis of brain death. *Transplant. Proc.* **2010**, *42*, 3941–3946. [CrossRef] [PubMed]
6. Dupas, B.; Gayet-Delacroix, M.; Villers, D.; Antonioli, D.; Veccherini, M.F.; Soulillou, J.P. Diagnosis of brain death using two-phase spiral CT. *Am. J. Neuroradiol.* **1998**, *19*, 641–647. [PubMed]
7. Leclerc, X.; Taschner, C.A.; Vidal, A.; Strecker, G.; Savage, J.; Gauvrit, J.Y.; Pruvo, J.P. The role of spiral CT for the assessment of the intracranial circulation in suspected brain-death. *J. Neuroradiol.* **2006**, *33*, 90–95. [CrossRef] [PubMed]
8. Combes, J.-C.; Chomel, A.; Ricolfi, F.; D'Athis, P.; Freysz, M. Reliability of computed tomographic angiography in the diagnosis of brain death. *Transplant. Proc.* **2007**, *39*, 16–20. [CrossRef]
9. Escudero, D.; Otero, J.; Marqués, L.; Parra, A.; Gonzalo, J.A.; Albaiceta, G.M.; Cofiño, L.; Blanco, A.; Vega, P.; Murias, E.; et al. Diagnosing brain death by CT perfusion and multislice CT angiography. *Neurocrit. Care* **2009**, *11*, 261–271. [CrossRef]
10. Frampas, E.; Videcoq, M.; De Kerviler, E.; Ricolfi, F.; Kuoch, V.; Mourey, F.; Tenaillon, A.; Dupas, B. CT Angiography for brain death diagnosis. *Am. J. Neuroradiol.* **2009**, *30*, 1566–1570. [CrossRef]
11. Welschehold, S.; Boor, S.; Reuland, K.; Thömke, F.; Kerz, T.; Reuland, A.; Beyer, C.; Gartenschläger, M.; Wagner, W.; Giese, A.; et al. Technical aids in the diagnosis of brain death: A comparison of SEP, AEP, EEG, TCD and CT angiography. *Dtsch. Arztebl. Int.* **2012**, *109*, 624–630. [CrossRef]
12. Welschehold, S.; Kerz, T.; Boor, S.; Reuland, K.; Thömke, F.; Beyer, C.; Wagner, W.; Müller-Forell, W.; Giese, A. Detection of intracranial circulatory arrest in brain death using cranial CT-angiography. *Eur. J. Neurol.* **2013**, *20*, 173–179. [CrossRef] [PubMed]
13. Welschehold, S.; Kerz, T.; Boor, S.; Reuland, K.; Thömke, F.; Reuland, A.; Beyer, C.; Tschan, C.; Wagner, W.; Müller-Forell, W.; et al. Computed tomographic angiography as a useful adjunct in the diagnosis of brain death. *J. Trauma Acute Care Surg.* **2013**, *74*, 1279–1285. [CrossRef] [PubMed]
14. Sawicki, M.; Bohatyrewicz, R.; Safranow, K.; Walecka, A.; Walecki, J.; Rowinski, O.; Solek-Pastuszka, J.; Czajkowski, Z.; Guzinski, M.; Burzynska, M.; et al. Computed tomographic angiography criteria in the diagnosis of brain death—Comparison of sensitivity and interobserver reliability of different evaluation scales. *Neuroradiology* **2014**, *56*, 609–620. [CrossRef] [PubMed]
15. De Radiologie, S.F.; De Neuroradiologie, S.F.; De La Biomédecine, A. Recommandations sur les critères diagnostiques de la mort encéphalique par la technique d'angioscanner cérébral. *J. Neuroradiol.* **2011**, *38*, 36–39. [CrossRef] [PubMed]
16. Kerhuel, L.; Srairi, M.; Georget, G.; Bonneville, F.; Mrozek, S.; Mayeur, N.; Lonjaret, L.; Sacrista, S.; Hermant, N.; Marhar, F.; et al. The optimal time between clinical brain death diagnosis and confirmation using CT angiography: A retrospective study. *Minerva Anestesiol.* **2016**, *82*, 1180–1188. [PubMed]
17. Lewis, A.; Liebman, J.; Kreiger-Benson, E.; Kumpfbeck, A.; Bakkar, A.; Shemie, S.D.; Sung, G.; Torrance, S.; Greer, D. Ancillary Testing for Determination of Death by Neurologic Criteria Around the World. *Neurocrit. Care* **2020**, *34*, 473–484. [CrossRef]
18. Beschluss der Bundesärztekammer über die Richtlinie gemäß §16 Abs. 1 S. 1 Nr. 1 TPG für die Regeln zur Feststellung des Todes nach § 3 Abs. 1 S. 1 Nr. 2 TPG und die Verfahrensregeln zur Feststellung des endgültigen, nicht behebbaren Ausfalls der Gesamtfunktion des Großhirns, des Kleinhirns und des Hirnstamms nach § 3 Abs. 2 Nr. 2 TPG, Vierte Fortschreibung. *Deutsches Ärzteblatt*, 30 March 2015; 112(A-1256/B-1052/C-1024).
19. Wujtewicz, M.A.; Szarmach, A.; Chwojnicki, K.; Sawicki, M.; Owczuk, R. Subtotal Cerebral Circulatory Arrest with Preserved Breathing Activity: A Case Report. *Transplant. Proc.* **2016**, *48*, 282–284. [CrossRef] [PubMed]

20. Bohatyrewicz, R.; Walecka, A.; Bohatyrewicz, A.; Zukowski, M.; Kepinski, S.; Marzec-Lewenstein, E.; Sawicki, M.; Kordowski, J. Unusual movements, "spontaneous" breathing, and unclear cerebral vessels sonography in a brain-dead patient: A case report. *Transplant. Proc.* **2007**, *39*, 2707–2708. [CrossRef]
21. Sawicki, M.; Solek-Pastuszka, J.; Chamier-Cieminska, K.; Walecka, A.; Bohatyrewicz, R. Accuracy of Computed Tomographic Perfusion in Published: Diagnosis of Brain Death: A Prospective Cohort Study. *Med. Sci. Monit.* **2018**, *24*, 2777–2785. [CrossRef]
22. Sawicki, M.; Bohatyrewicz, R.; Safranow, K.; Walecka, A.; Walecki, J.; Rowinski, O.; Solek-Pastuszka, J.; Czajkowski, Z.; Marzec-Lewenstein, E.; Motyl, K.; et al. Dynamic evaluation of stasis filling phenomenon with computed tomography in diagnosis of brain death. *Neuroradiology* **2013**, *55*, 1061–1069. [CrossRef]
23. Astrup, J.; Siesjö, B.K.; Symon, L. Thresholds in cerebral ischemia—The ischemic penumbra. *Stroke* **1981**, *12*, 723–725. [CrossRef]
24. Shankar, J.; Vandorpe, R. CT Perfusion for Confirmation of Brain Death. *Am. J. Neuroradiol.* **2012**, *34*, 1175–1179. [CrossRef] [PubMed]
25. Sawicki, M.; Sołek-Pastuszka, J.; Chamier-Ciemińska, K.; Walecka, A.; Walecki, J.; Bohatyrewicz, R. Computed tomography perfusion is a useful adjunct to computed tomography angiography in the diagnosis of brain death. *Clin. Neuroradiol.* **2017**, *29*, 101–108. [CrossRef] [PubMed]
26. Smit, E.J.; Vonken, E.-J.; Van Der Schaaf, I.C.; Mendrik, A.M.; Dankbaar, J.W.; Horsch, A.D.; Van Seeters, T.; Van Ginneken, B.; Prokop, M. Timing-Invariant Reconstruction for Deriving High-Quality CT Angiographic Data from Cerebral CT Perfusion Data. *Radiology* **2012**, *263*, 216–225. [CrossRef] [PubMed]
27. Shankar, J.J.S.; Stewart-Perrin, B.; Quraishi, A.-U.-R.; Bata, I.; Vandorpe, R. Computed Tomography Perfusion Aids in the Prognostication of Comatose Postcardiac Arrest Patients. *Am. J. Cardiol.* **2018**, *121*, 874–878. [CrossRef] [PubMed]
28. Bohatyrewicz, R.; Solek-Pastuszka, J.; Sawicki, M. Invitation to participate in multi-center study for validation of cerebral computed tomography angiography (CTA) and computed tomography perfusion (CTP) in determination of cerebral circulatory arrest (CCA) during brain death/death by neurological criteria (BD/DNC) diagnosis procedure in pediatric population below 12 years of age. *Anaesthesiol. Intensiv. Ther.* **2021**, *53*, 97–102.
29. Sawicki, M.; Solek-Pastuszka, J.; Jurczyk, K.; Skrzywanek, P.; Guzinski, M.; Czajkowski, Z.; Manko, W.; Burzynska, M.; Safranow, K.; Poncyljusz, W.; et al. Original Protocol Using Computed Tomographic Angiography for Diagnosis of Brain Death: A Better Alternative to Standard Two-Phase Technique? *Ann. Transplant.* **2015**, *20*, 449–460.
30. Greer, D.M.; Strozyk, D.; Schwamm, L.H. False positive CT angiography in brain death. *Neurocrit. Care* **2009**, *11*, 272–275. [CrossRef] [PubMed]

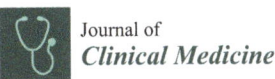

Article

Effects of the COVID-19 Pandemic on Treatment Efficiency for Traumatic Brain Injury in the Emergency Department: A Multicenter Study in Taiwan

Carlos Lam [1,2], Ju-Chuan Yen [3,4], Chia-Chieh Wu [1,2], Heng-Yu Lin [5] and Min-Huei Hsu [6,*]

1. Emergency Department, Wan Fang Hospital, Taipei Medical University, Taipei 11696, Taiwan; lsk@w.tmu.edu.tw (C.L.); setfreej@gmail.com (C.-C.W.)
2. Department of Emergency, School of Medicine, College of Medicine, Taipei Medical University, Taipei 11030, Taiwan
3. Department of Ophthalmology, Taipei City Hospital, Renai Branch, Taipei 10629, Taiwan; m701061@tmu.edu.tw
4. Graduate Institute of Biomedical Informatics, College of Medical Technology, Taipei Medical University, Taipei 11030, Taiwan
5. School of Medicine, College of Medicine, Taipei Medical University, Taipei 11030, Taiwan; b101105091@tmu.edu.tw
6. Graduate Institute of Data Science, College of Management, Taipei Medical University, Taipei 11030, Taiwan
* Correspondence: 701056@tmu.edu.tw; Tel.: +886-2-66382736 (ext. 1105)

Abstract: The coronavirus disease 2019 (COVID-19) pandemic has impacted emergency department (ED) practice, including the treatment of traumatic brain injury (TBI), which is commonly encountered in the ED. Our study aimed to evaluate TBI treatment efficiency in the ED during the COVID-19 pandemic. A retrospective observational study was conducted using the electronic medical records from three hospitals in metropolitan Taipei, Taiwan. The time from ED arrival to brain computed tomography (CT) and the time from ED arrival to surgical management were used as measures of treatment efficiency. TBI treatment efficiencies in the ED coinciding with a small-scale local COVID-19 outbreak in 2020 (P1) and large-scale community spread in 2021 (P2) were compared against the pre-pandemic efficiency recorded in 2019. The interval between ED arrival and brain CT was significantly shortened during P1 and P2 compared with the pre-pandemic interval, and no significant delay between ED arrival and surgical management was found, indicating increased treatment efficiency for TBI in the ED during the COVID-19 pandemic. Minimizing viral spread in the community and the hospital is vital to maintaining ED treatment efficiency and capacity. The ED should retain sufficient capacity to treat older patients with serious TBI during the COVID-19 pandemic.

Keywords: COVID-19 pandemic; treatment efficiency; traumatic brain injury; emergency department

Citation: Lam, C.; Yen, J.-C.; Wu, C.-C.; Lin, H.-Y.; Hsu, M.-H. Effects of the COVID-19 Pandemic on Treatment Efficiency for Traumatic Brain Injury in the Emergency Department: A Multicenter Study in Taiwan. *J. Clin. Med.* **2021**, *10*, 5314. https://doi.org/10.3390/jcm10225314

Academic Editor: Rafael Badenes

Received: 28 September 2021
Accepted: 9 November 2021
Published: 15 November 2021

Publisher's Note: MDPI stays neutral with regard to jurisdictional claims in published maps and institutional affiliations.

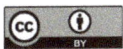

Copyright: © 2021 by the authors. Licensee MDPI, Basel, Switzerland. This article is an open access article distributed under the terms and conditions of the Creative Commons Attribution (CC BY) license (https://creativecommons.org/licenses/by/4.0/).

1. Introduction

Due to geographic proximity with China, hospitals in Taiwan rapidly prepared for the impending arrival of the coronavirus disease 2019 (COVID-19) infection soon after the outbreak was first reported in Wuhan, China, in 2019 [1]. Although the number of COVID-19 cases reported in European countries began to grow exponentially [2,3], the Taiwan Centers for Disease Control (CDC) implemented strict border control and infection control measures to prevent virus transmission [4]. Controlled access to medical facilities was enforced, and a screening station was established outside of the emergency department (ED) to secure hospitals [5]. The rapid response by the CDC and the cooperation by the population resulted in outstanding performance for controlling the COVID-19 pandemic in Taiwan in 2020 [6].

In contrast to many countries that suffered from healthcare system damage due to severe community and hospital spread of the virus, the hospitals in Taiwan were able to continuously provide regular services after the pandemic was declared in 2020. People's daily lives remained relatively unchanged until the barricade was broken through in 2021. A cluster of COVID-19 infections was identified in metropolitan Taipei in May 2021, and the infection rapidly spread across many communities on the island [7]. A ban against large gatherings and the semi-lockdown of cities were immediately implemented when the number of confirmed cases escalated from 1199 to 4917 over a two-week period, resulting in a substantial decrease in outdoor activities.

After the outbreak of community infection, the continuous emergence of COVID-19 pneumonia forced hospitals in Taiwan to restrict their daily workloads to ensure the sufficient availability of human resources in dedicated COVID-19 wards [8,9]. These highly contagious patients also profoundly disturbed the daily workflow in the ED [10].

A significant decrease in ED visits for injury was observed in many countries after the pandemic was declared [11–15]. Although no widespread transmission of COVID-19 infection was reported in Taiwan in 2020, a similar trend in decreased ED visits was reported in Taiwan [16,17]. The drop in ED visits for injury was even more profound following the detection of community spread in 2021. Traumatic brain injury (TBI) is one of the most common diseases treated in the ED, and nearly 80% of treated cases are classified as mild injuries. Although the number of TBI cases has steadily increased over time [18,19], the number of TBI cases in the ED declined significantly during the COVID-19 pandemic, which is known as the "coronavirus lockdown effect" [20]. A study in the United Kingdom showed that referrals for TBI decreased by 49.6% [21], and the decreases reported in India, the Netherlands, and Ireland were 60%, 36%, and 17.1%, respectively [20,22,23]. For TBI patients, a brain computed tomography (CT) scan is indispensable to detect the presence of brain hemorrhage. Previous studies showed that the average daily number of brain CT scans decreased during the pandemic. However, the proportion of cases with acute findings rose significantly [24]. A similar trend was reported for other injuries and diseases treated in the ED [14,25].

The restriction of the hospital's human resources in the operation room also impacted the treatment of the TBI during the pandemic. In addition, the processes implemented to determine COVID-19 infection status also delayed operations, which may have contributed to the increased mortality rate observed during the lockdown period [26,27]. The current consensus recommendation is that all medical personnel should wear appropriate protective equipment when performing surgery on patients with suspected COVID-19 infection [28,29]. These infection control precautions likely complicated the surgery procedures.

The emergence of the Delta variant indicated that the battle against the COVID-19 pandemic would be continuous. In Taiwan, only one wave of community spread was reported one year after the pandemic declaration, representing a course that differed from most other countries. Therefore, our study aimed to evaluate the impacts of the COVID-19 pandemic on the treatment efficiency of TBI in the ED. The pre-pandemic era was compared with a period of small-scale local infection during the early stages of the COVID-19 pandemic in 2020 and with the period marked by large-scale community spread that occurred after May 2021. The results of this study provide important information for the staff of EDs and neurosurgery departments and for hospital administration regarding the maintenance of efficiency and the appropriate management of TBI in the ED during the COVID-19 pandemic.

2. Materials and Methods

2.1. Data Source

A retrospective observational study was conducted using the Clinical Research Database (CRD) of the Taipei Medical University. The CRD contains the electronic medical records from the following three affiliated teaching hospitals: Taipei Medical University Hospital, Wan Fang Hospital, and Shuang Ho Hospital. These three hospitals are located in metropolitan Taipei and are accredited as advanced emergency responsibility hospitals that provide comprehensive care for major trauma patients.

We extracted data for ED visits, brain CT scans, and brain operations from the CRD between 1 January and 31 July 2019, 2020, and 2021. Identifiable information from these hospital data was encrypted to ensure patient confidentiality. The Institutional Review Board of Taipei Medical University approved this study (No.: N202106027).

2.2. Sample Selection

We selected all ED visits due to traumatic injury between 1 January and 31 July 2019, 2020, and 2021 and only included those associated with the International Classification of Diseases, Tenth Revision, Clinical Modification (ICD-10-CM) codes for trauma: S00–S99. TBI was identified by the ICD-10 codes S00–S09. Figure 1 presents the flow chart for sample selection.

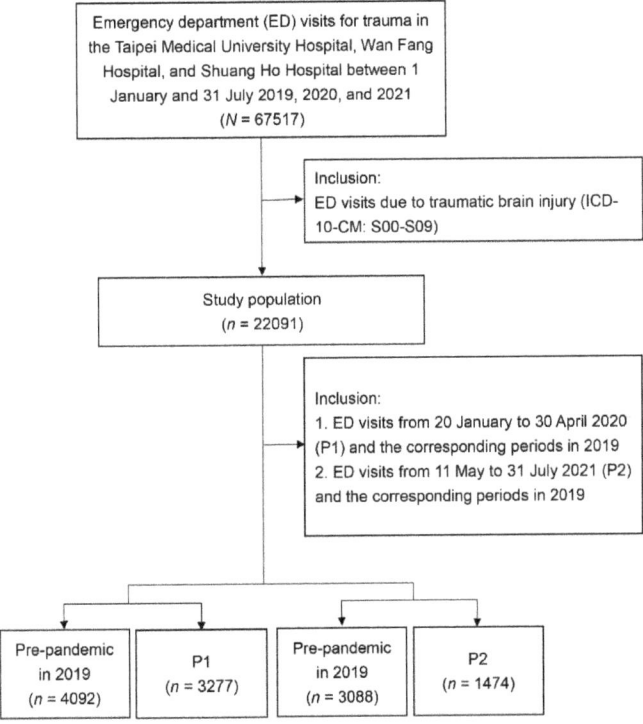

Figure 1. Sample selection procedure from the CRD of Taipei Medical University. CRD, Clinical Research Database; ED, emergency department; P1, 20 January to 30 April 2019; P2, 11 May to 31 July 2021. Pre-pandemic period refers to the same span from 2019.

All trauma-related ED visits at participating hospitals during the period associated with small-scale local infection from January 20 to 30 April 2020 (period one, P1) and the period associated with large-scale community spread from 11 May to 31 July 2021 (period two, P2) were included in our study. The treatment efficiencies for TBI in the ED during P1 and P2 were compared with corresponding periods in 2019 (pre-pandemic).

2.3. Measurement

Collected characteristics of the sample included sex, age, triage level, and TBI patterns. The triage level was categorized as critical (levels I and II), urgent (level III), and less urgent (levels IV and V). The TBI patterns included mild head injury (ICD-10-CM: S00, S01, S09, and S06.0) and serious head injury (ICD-10-CM: S06.1–S06.9).

The time from ED arrival to the completion of brain CT and the time from ED arrival to the start of brain operation were used as proxies to represent treatment efficiency for TBI. We only included brain operations coded as urgent in the ED and performed within 24 h after ED arrival.

2.4. Statistical Analysis

We first plotted weekly ED visits from 1 January to 31 July 2019, 2020, and 2021 to demonstrate the numbers of yearly ED visits due to trauma, TBI, mild head injury, and serious head injury. We also plotted the numbers and rates of brain CT scans and brain operations among TBI-related ED visits.

The sample characteristics, TBI patterns, numbers of brain CT scans, and numbers of operations during P1 and P2 were separately compared with their corresponding pre-pandemic values using the Chi-square and Wilcoxon rank-sum tests. Kaplan–Meier survival analysis was used to evaluate time-to-event data (time to brain CT), and differences were evaluated using a nonparametric log-rank test. A 2-sided p-value of <0.05 was considered statistically significant. All statistical analyses were performed using SAS version 9.4 (SAS Institute, Cary, NC, USA).

3. Results

The number of ED visits due to trauma and TBI each week decreased starting in late January 2020 and gradually increased after 30 April 2020. In 2021, the weekly number of ED visits due to trauma and TBI sharply dropped starting on 14 May (Figures 2 and 3). Mild head injuries were reduced during P1 and P2 compared with the pre-pandemic period (Figure 4). However, the drop in serious head injuries was insignificant in P1 (Figure 5). Although the number of brain CT scans performed for TBI decreased in P2, the rate of brain CTs rose sharply (Figure 6). The rate of brain operations also significantly increased in P2 (Figure 7).

The numbers of ED visits were 3277 during P1 and 4092 during the corresponding pre-pandemic period and 1474 during P2 and 3088 during the corresponding pre-pandemic period. The distribution of intracranial injuries (S06.0–S06.9) and neurosurgical procedures and their frequency in the pre-pandemic and pandemic periods are shown in the Supplementary Figure S1 and Table S1.

Table 1 shows a comparison between the proportions of TBI-related ED visits and TBI injury patterns before and after the COVID-19 pandemic. The proportion of TBI-related ED visits in P2 was significantly higher than that in the corresponding pre-pandemic period in 2019 (33.57% vs. 31.27%, $p = 0.007$). No significant difference was noted in the proportions of TBI-related visits between P1 and the pre-pandemic period. The proportion of mild head injury was significantly reduced during P2 compared with the respective pre-pandemic period in 2019 (83.22% vs. 87.01%, $p = 0.001$), whereas the proportions of serious head injury significantly increased in P2 compared with the respective pre-pandemic period (11.30% versus 5.79%, $p < 0.0001$). No such change was found in P1.

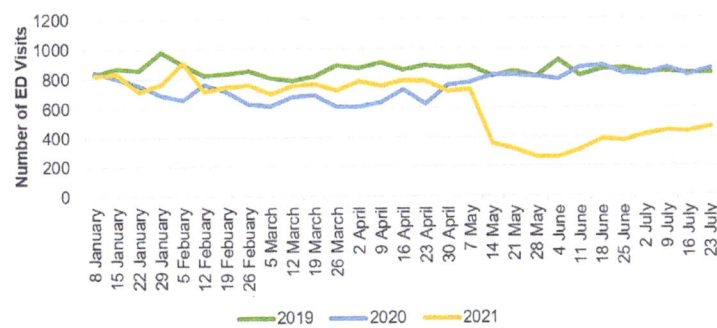

Figure 2. Weekly trauma-related ED visits from January to July 2019, 2020, and 2021. ED, emergency department.

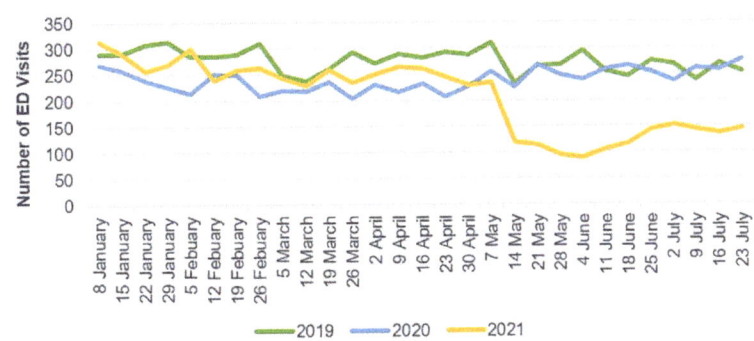

Figure 3. Weekly TBI-related ED visits from January to July 2019, 2020, and 2021. ED, emergency department; TBI, traumatic brain injury.

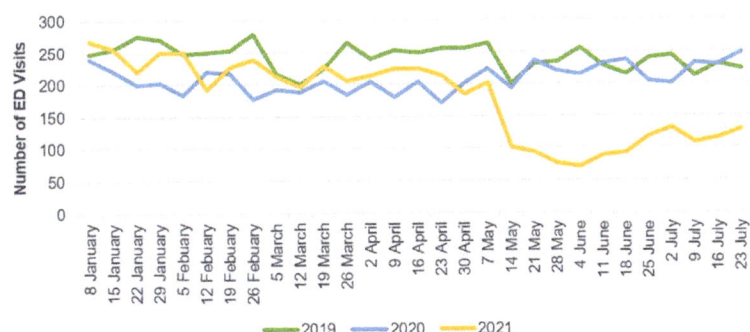

Figure 4. Weekly ED visits due to mild head injury from January to July 2019, 2020, and 2021. ED, emergency department.

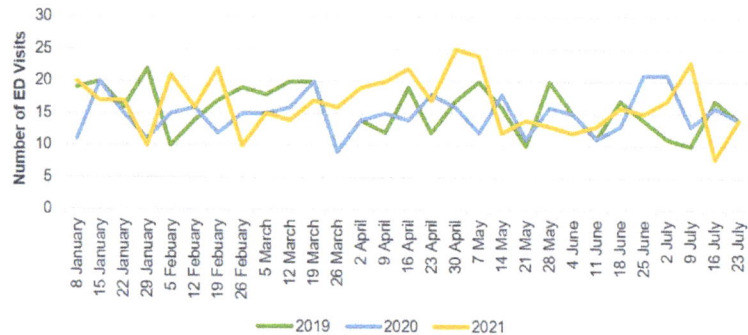

Figure 5. Weekly ED visits due to serious head injury from January to July 2019, 2020, and 2021. ED, emergency department.

Table 2 shows a comparison of the characteristics of TBI samples before and after the COVID-19 pandemic. The ages of patients who visited the ED for TBI during P1 and P2 were significantly older (P1: 44 years vs. 42 years, $p < 0.001$; P2: 54 years versus 42 years, $p < 0.0001$) than those during the respective pre-pandemic periods. A comparison of the triage levels also showed significant increases in critical TBI during P1 and P2 (P1: 13.61% vs. 11.93%, $p < 0.001$; P2: 22.59% vs. 11.82%, $p < 0.0001$).

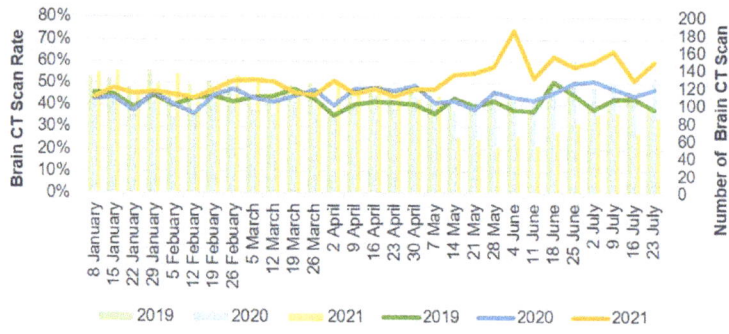

Figure 6. Brain CT scan rate for TBI in the ED from January to July 2019, 2020, and 2021. CT scan, computerized tomography scan; ED, emergency department; TBI, traumatic brain injury.

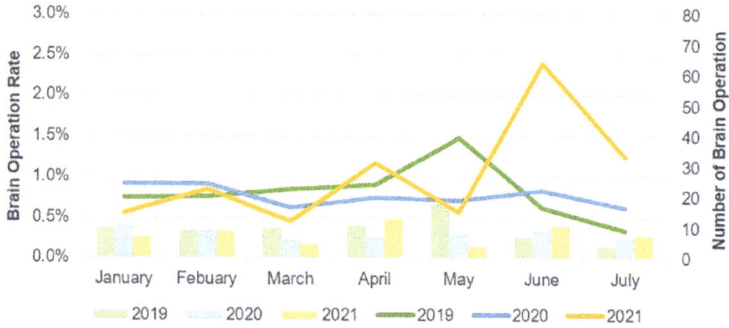

Figure 7. Brain operation rate for TBI in the ED from January to July 2019, 2020, and 2021. ED, emergency department; TBI, traumatic brain injury.

Table 3 shows a comparison between the treatment efficiencies for TBI-related ED visits before and after the COVID-19 pandemic. During P1 and P2, the times from ED arrival to brain CT were significantly shorter than for the respective pre-pandemic periods (P1: 22 min versus 30 min, $p < 0.0001$; P2: 21 min vs. 27 min, $p < 0.0001$). No significant change was observed in the time from ED arrival to brain operation for either P1 or P2 compared with the respective pre-pandemic period.

The Kaplan–Meier curves also showed significant differences in the time from ED arrival to brain CT between the COVID-19 pandemic era (stratified by P1 and P2) and the pre-COVID-19 pandemic era (Figure 8).

Table 1. Comparison of the proportions of TBI-related ED visits and injury patterns before and after the COVID-19 pandemic.

Variable	Pre-Pandemic Period Corresponding to P1		P1		p	Pre-Pandemic Period Corresponding to P2		P2		p
	n	%	n	%		n	%	n	%	
Trauma population										
TBI					0.472					0.007
No	8318	67.00	6523	66.55		6800	68.73	2925	66.43	
Yes	4096	33.00	3279	33.45		3094	31.27	1478	33.57	
TBI population										
Mild head injury					0.083					0.001
No	505	12.33	449	13.69		402	12.99	248	16.78	
Yes	3591	87.67	2830	86.31		2692	87.01	1230	83.22	
Serious head injury					0.089					<0.0001
No	3864	94.34	3062	93.38		2915	94.21	1311	88.70	
Yes	232	5.66	217	6.62		179	5.79	167	11.30	

TBI, traumatic brain injury; ED, emergency department; COVID-19, coronavirus disease 2019; P1, January to 30 April 2019; P2, 11 May to 31 July 2021. Pre-pandemic period refers to the same span from 2019.

Table 2. Comparison of the TBI sample characteristics before and after the COVID-19 pandemic.

Variable	Pre-Pandemic Period Corresponding to P1 (n = 4092)		P1 (n = 3277)		p	Pre-Pandemic Period Corresponding to P2 (n = 3088)		P2 (n = 1474)		p
	n	%	n	%		n	%	n	%	
Sex					0.403					0.117
Female	1808	44.18	1416	43.21		1417	45.89	640	43.42	
Male	2284	55.82	1861	56.79		1671	54.11	834	56.58	
Age (years), median (IQR)	42	(19–66)	44	(22–68)	<0.001	42	(19–66)	54	(29–73)	<0.0001
Age (years)					0.001					<0.0001
0–14	812	19.84	537	16.39		620	20.08	188	12.75	
15–24	522	12.76	397	12.11		409	13.24	128	8.68	
25–44	833	20.36	728	22.22		598	19.37	274	18.59	
45–64	857	20.94	683	20.84		632	20.47	347	23.54	
65+	1068	26.10	932	28.44		829	26.85	537	36.43	
Triage					<0.001					<0.0001
Critical (Levels I and II)	488	11.93	446	13.61		365	11.82	333	22.59	
Urgent (Level III)	3479	85.02	2772	84.59		2619	84.81	1120	75.98	
Less urgent (Levels IV and V)	125	3.05	59	1.80		104	3.37	21	1.42	

IQR, interquartile range. TBI, traumatic brain injury; COVID-19, coronavirus disease 2019; P1, January to 30 April 2019; P2, 11 May to 31 July 2021. Pre-pandemic period refers to the same span from 2019.

Table 3. Comparison of treatment efficiencies for TBI-related ED visits before and after the COVID-19 pandemic.

Variable	Pre-Pandemic Period Corresponding to P1 (n = 4092)		P1 (n = 3277)		p	Pre-Pandemic Period Corresponding to P2 (n = 3088)		P2 (n = 1474)		p
	n	%	n	%		n	%	n	%	
Brain CT scan					0.205					<0.0001
No	2379	58.14	1857	56.67		1803	58.39	619	41.99	
Yes	1713	41.86	1420	43.33		1285	41.61	855	58.01	
Time from ED arrival to brain CT scan (minute), median (IQR)	30	(20–45)	22	(14–35)	<0.0001	27	(18–42)	21	(13–34)	<0.0001
Brain operation					0.459					0.020
No	4057	99.14	3254	99.30		3066	99.29	1453	98.58	
Yes	35	0.86	23	0.70		22	0.71	21	1.42	
Time from ED arrival to brain operation (hour), median (IQR)	6	(3–15)	4	(2–6)	0.174	5	(3–8)	5	(3–7)	0.788

IQR, interquartile range. CT, computed tomography; TBI, traumatic brain injury; COVID-19, coronavirus disease 2019; P1, January to 30 April 2019; P2, 11 May to 31 July 2021. Pre-pandemic period refers to the same span from 2019.

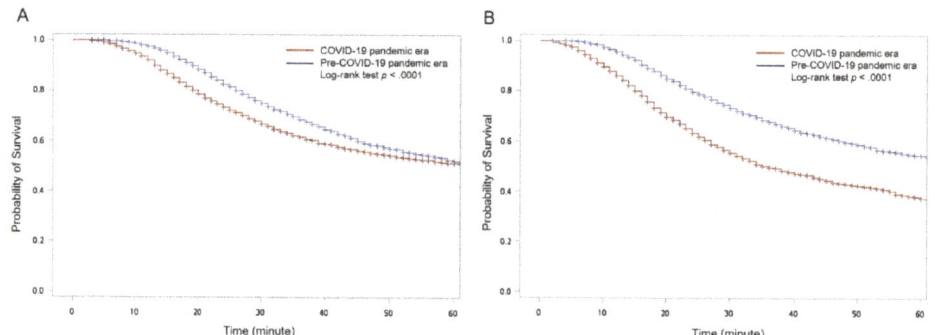

Figure 8. Kaplan–Meier curves with log-rank test for the time from emergency department (ED) arrival to brain computed tomography (CT) for traumatic brain injury (TBI)-related ED visits between the COVID-19 pandemic era and the pre-COVID-19 pandemic era during (**A**) P1 and (**B**) P2.

4. Discussion

At the beginning of the pandemic, in 2020, the number of TBI cases treated by the ED declined, consistent with reports from foreign countries [30,31]. This decrease has been attributed to a reduction in outdoor activities, which led to a decrease in road traffic injuries. A significant increase in the ages of TBI patients treated by the ED was observed because most of those injured due to household activities, such as accidental falls, are older adults. During this period, the reduction in outdoor activities was primarily the result of spontaneous changes in behavior in response to reports by the mass media. After a period during which no significant viral spread was reported, the population's activities eventually returned to pre-pandemic levels. Consistently, the TBI numbers reported for the second quarter of 2020 gradually returned to the levels reported before the outbreak.

The outbreak in May 2021 (P2) was associated with a completely different pattern, with a large-scale community infection that spread across many communities [32]. The relevant authorities immediately banned large gatherings and implemented a city-wide semi-lockdown strategy to stop the spread [7]. During P2, outdoor activities and commuting were severely restricted, which was associated with a sharp decrease in TBI numbers, and the increase in the average patient age during this period was more pronounced than that observed for P1, indicating that the outdoor activities among younger adults were almost completely stopped, resulting in an increase in the proportion of TBI cases among older adults.

The COVID-19 outbreak impacted TBI patterns in the ED, associated with a decrease in mild and serious head injuries treated during P1 and P2 compared with 2019. The decrease in P2 was more obvious compared with P1. These results showed the effects of the city-wide semi-lockdown strategy during the large-scale community spread of the virus. During P2, the relevant authorities banned large gatherings, including school and work. Since most road traffic injuries in Taiwan are mild injuries [33], the semi-lockdown strategy during P2 restricted commuting, resulting in a sharp decline in the number of mild head injuries treated in the ED.

Because the reduction in overall trauma cases was small during P1, no significant changes in TBI proportions were noted compared with the proportions in 2019. However, the overall number of trauma cases treated in the ED declined significantly during P2, resulting in an increase in the proportion of TBI cases. The reduced commuting in P2 increased the proportions of serious head injuries. Although no such change was shown in P1, the proportions of patients who arrived at the ED in critical condition (triage levels I and II) increased during both P1 and P2, and the proportion of critical cases reported during P2 was almost double that for 2019. Therefore, the ED should maintain sufficient capacity to treat critical patients.

The outbreak also impacted brain CT execution in the ED. The number of brain CT scans performed during P1 and P2 decreased compared with the number performed in 2019. However, the decrease in P2 was more obvious compared with P1. The lockdown strategy sharply reduced the occurrence of mild head injury in P2, causing a significant rise in the proportions of brain CT scans.

When the COVID-19 outbreak was first reported in December 2019, all hospitals in Taiwan responded immediately. Access control was used to prevent high-risk patients from entering the hospital, and patient visiting activities were also banned [7]. Outside of the ED, screening stations were established to divert patients into low-, medium-, and high-risk areas for treatment. All ED staff, including emergency medical technicians, routinely used personal protective equipment, such as face shields, surgical gowns, and N95 masks [34]. As a result of these measures, no spread of COVID-19 infection has been reported in hospitals and EDs. Brain CT scans ordered for low-risk patients were performed as before, and only local disinfection was required after the examination. Therefore, the majority of TBI cases in the ED were examined without delay. Due to the preservation of ED capacity and the decline in TBI numbers, the time interval between ED arrival and brain CT performance was significantly shortened during P1.

Due to the lack of community or hospital COVID-19 spread during P1, patients who entered the operating room from a low-risk area in the ED were only submitted to a COVID-19 antigen test. The operating room staff used the same personal protective equipment required by ED staff, and most brain operations were performed similarly to the pre-pandemic period. No significant delay between ED arrival and brain operation was noted during P1.

During P2, clusters of infections in several communities were serious, and deaths increased daily, causing large psychological and behavioral impacts on society. People substantially reduced hospital visits due to fear of contacting infected patients. The continuous presentation of patients with COVID-19 pneumonia resulted in a huge burden on human resources for hospitals as the medical staff was increasingly diverted to treat COVID-19 patients [35]. The proper protection of the ED workforce allowed for the maintenance of treatment capacity. The COVID-19 PCR test was extensively used to detecting asymptomatic infections. For patients who required surgery, a rapid respiratory panel was universally used to reduce waiting times. ED staff used N100 masks or powered air-purifying respirators due to the extremely high probability of viral transmission when treating infected patients. For those COVID-19 patients who required CT scans or surgery, all staff members in contact with the patients, including ED physicians and neurosurgeons, were required to use full protection, including an isolation suit. The field exposed to the patient was treated according to a thorough disinfection procedure using bleach and alcohol.

These infection prevention measures delayed treatment in the ED. However, due to the sharp decline in the number of TBI cases and the preservation of the ED's treatment capacity, the execution time for brain CT scans was significantly shortened, and the waiting time for brain operations did not increase. These results showed that the treatment efficiency for TBI in the ED increased during P2. During an outbreak of community spread, the proportions of TBI cases requiring brain CT and brain operations increased. Therefore, medical centers should maintain sufficient treatment capacity in the ED and neurosurgery departments to allow for the treatment of serious head injuries during COVID-19 outbreaks with community spread [20].

The multicenter approach strengthened the generalizability of our findings. However, community spread during P2 was concentrated in certain communities rather than evenly distributed. Therefore, the impacts of the pandemic on treatment efficiency were influenced by the locations of the hospitals. In addition, the study period only included the three months of the outbreak. During this period, the decrease in the total number of serious head injuries may bias the statistical results. Finally, the COVID-19 pandemic in Taiwan was well controlled. The number of patients infected by the virus was limited, and the health care system was not burdened to the same extent as in many other countries. Therefore, extrapolation of the results to other settings may be difficult.

5. Conclusions

The COVID-19 pandemic had a significant impact on the treatment efficiency for TBI in the ED. The impacts of preventing large gatherings and the city-wide semi-lockdown after a COVID-19 outbreak with community spread differed from impacts of self-initiated reductions in outdoor activities due to social panic during the early stages of the pandemic. Minimizing the spread of COVID-19 in the community and in hospitals and protecting ED capacity is vital to maintaining treatment efficiency for TBI. The proportion of older patients and the proportion of serious head injuries increase when overall numbers of TBI decline due to decreased participation in outdoor activities and commuting. Therefore, the ED and neurosurgery departments should retain sufficient capacity to treat these patients during a pandemic outbreak.

Supplementary Materials: The following are available online at https://www.mdpi.com/article/10.3390/jcm10225314/s1, Figure S1: The distribution of the intracranial injuries (S06.0–S06.9) between the COVID-19 pandemic era and the pre-COVID-19 pandemic era during (**A**) P1 and (**B**) P2, Table S1: The neurosurgical procedures and its frequency in the pre-pandemic and pandemic periods.

Author Contributions: Conceptualization, C.L. and M.-H.H.; data curation, C.-C.W. and M.-H.H.; formal analysis, C.-C.W. and M.-H.H.; funding acquisition, C.L. and M.-H.H.; investigation, H.-Y.L. and M.-H.H.; methodology, C.L. and M.-H.H.; project administration, M.-H.H.; resources, M.-H.H.; supervision, M.-H.H.; validation, C.L., J.-C.Y. and M.-H.H.; visualization, C.L. and M.-H.H.; writing—original draft, C.L., C.-C.W. and H.-Y.L.; writing—review and editing, J.-C.Y. and M.-H.H. All authors have read and agreed to the published version of the manuscript.

Funding: This research was jointly supported by grants from Taipei Medical University–Wan Fang Hospital (Grant number: 99TMU-WFH-15) and Taipei Medical University (Grant number: TMU108-AE1-B49).

Institutional Review Board Statement: The study was conducted according to the guidelines of the Declaration of Helsinki and approved by the Institutional Review Board of Taipei Medical University (No.: N202106027).

Informed Consent Statement: Due to the study's retrospective culture and the anonymous data, the need for informed consent was waived.

Data Availability Statement: The data that support the findings of this study are available from the corresponding author upon reasonable request.

Acknowledgments: The authors would like to thank Hsin-Ying Lin at Wan Fang Hospital, Taipei Medical University for her helpful comments to improve this manuscript.

Conflicts of Interest: The authors declare no conflict of interest.

References

1. Jian, S.W.; Kao, C.T.; Chang, Y.C.; Chen, P.F.; Liu, D.P. Risk assessment for COVID-19 pandemic in Taiwan. *Int. J. Infect. Dis.* **2021**, *104*, 746–751. [CrossRef] [PubMed]
2. COVID-19 Situation Reports #5—March 31 2020. Available online: https://www.ncfhcc.org/wp-content/uploads/2020/04/5_SitRep_Alliance-COVID_3.31.2020.pdf (accessed on 16 September 2021).
3. Weekly Epidemiological Update—14 September 2020. Available online: https://www.who.int/publications/m/item/weekly-epidemiological-update--14-september-2020 (accessed on 16 September 2021).
4. Crucial Policies for Combating COVID-19. Available online: https://covid19.mohw.gov.tw/en/mp-206.html (accessed on 16 September 2021).
5. Tan, T.W.; Tan, H.L.; Chang, M.N.; Lin, W.S.; Chang, C.M. Effectiveness of epidemic preventive policies and hospital strategies in combating COVID-19 outbreak in Taiwan. *Int. J. Environ. Res. Public Health* **2021**, *18*, 3456. [CrossRef]
6. Chang, Y.C. *Taiwanese Medical and Security Policy towards the COVID-19 Pandemic. A Best Practice*; European Intelligence Academy: Athens, Greece, 2021.
7. Press Releases—Taiwan Centers for Disease Control. Available online: https://www.cdc.gov.tw/En/Category/ListContent/tov1jahKUv8RGSbvmzLwFg?uaid=R1K7gSjoYa7Wojk54nW7fg (accessed on 21 September 2021).
8. Sen-Crowe, B.; Sutherland, M.; McKenney, M.; Elkbuli, A. A closer look into global hospital beds capacity and resource shortages during the COVID-19 pandemic. *J. Surg. Res.* **2021**, *260*, 56–63. [CrossRef] [PubMed]
9. Kokudo, N.; Sugiyama, H. Hospital capacity during the COVID-19 pandemic. *Glob. Health Med.* **2021**, *3*, 56–59. [CrossRef] [PubMed]
10. Chen, T.Y.; Lai, H.W.; Hou, I.L.; Lin, C.H.; Chen, M.K.; Chou, C.C.; Lin, Y.R. Buffer areas in emergency department to handle potential COVID-19 community infection in Taiwan. *Travel Med. Infect. Dis.* **2020**, *36*, 101635. [CrossRef]
11. Garcia, S.; Albaghdadi, M.S.; Meraj, P.M.; Schmidt, C.; Garberich, R.; Jaffer, F.A.; Dixon, S.; Rade, J.J.; Tannenbaum, M.; Chambers, J.; et al. Reduction in ST-segment elevation cardiac catheterization laboratory activations in the United States during COVID-19 pandemic. *J. Am. Coll. Cardiol.* **2020**, *75*, 2871–2872. [CrossRef]
12. Lazzerini, M.; Barbi, E.; Apicella, A.; Marchetti, F.; Cardinale, F.; Trobia, G. Delayed access or provision of care in Italy resulting from fear of COVID-19. *Lancet Child Adolesc. Health* **2020**, *4*, e10–e11. [CrossRef]
13. Santana, R.; Sousa, J.S.; Soares, P.; Lopes, S.; Boto, P.; Rocha, J.V. The demand for hospital emergency services: Trends during the first month of COVID-19 response. *Port. J. Public Health* **2020**, *38*, 30–36. [CrossRef]
14. Bres Bullrich, M.; Fridman, S.; Mandzia, J.L.; Mai, L.M.; Khaw, A.; Vargas Gonzalez, J.C.; Bagur, R.; Sposato, L.A. COVID-19: Stroke admissions, emergency department visits, and prevention clinic referrals. *Can. J. Neurol. Sci.* **2020**, *47*, 693–696. [CrossRef]
15. Choi, D.H.; Jung, J.Y.; Suh, D.; Choi, J.Y.; Lee, S.U.; Choi, Y.J.; Kwak, Y.H.; Kim, D.K. Impact of the COVID-19 outbreak on trends in emergency department utilization in children: A multicenter retrospective observational study in Seoul metropolitan area, Korea. *J. Korean Med. Sci.* **2021**, *36*, e44. [CrossRef]
16. Chen, J.Y.H.; Chang, F.Y.; Lin, C.S.; Wang, C.H.; Tsai, S.H.; Lee, C.C.; Chen, S.J. Impact of the COVID-19 pandemic on the loading and quality of an emergency department in Taiwan: Enlightenment from a low-risk country in a public health crisis. *J. Clin. Med.* **2021**, *10*, 1150. [CrossRef] [PubMed]
17. Lin, C.F.; Huang, Y.H.; Cheng, C.Y.; Wu, K.H.; Tang, K.S.; Chiu, I.M. Public health interventions for the COVID-19 pandemic reduce respiratory tract infection-related visits at pediatric emergency departments in Taiwan. *Front. Public Health* **2020**, *8*, 604089. [CrossRef] [PubMed]
18. Marin, J.R.; Weaver, M.D.; Yealy, D.M.; Mannix, R.C. Trends in visits for traumatic brain injury to emergency departments in the United States. *JAMA* **2014**, *311*, 1917–1919. [CrossRef] [PubMed]
19. Pandor, A.; Harnan, S.; Goodacre, S.; Pickering, A.; Fitzgerald, P.; Rees, A. Diagnostic accuracy of clinical characteristics for identifying CT abnormality after minor brain injury: A systematic review and meta-analysis. *J. Neurotrauma* **2012**, *29*, 707–718. [CrossRef]
20. Santing, J.A.L.; van den Brand, C.L.; Jellema, K. Traumatic brain injury during the SARS-CoV-2 pandemic. *Neurotrauma Rep.* **2020**, *1*, 5–7. [CrossRef]
21. Jayakumar, N.; Kennion, O.; Villabona, A.R.; Paranathala, M.; Holliman, D. Neurosurgical referral patterns during the coronavirus disease 2019 pandemic: A United Kingdom experience. *World Neurosurg.* **2020**, *144*, e414–e420. [CrossRef]
22. Karthigeyan, M.; Dhandapani, S.; Salunke, P.; Sahoo, S.K.; Kataria, M.S.; Singh, A.; Gendle, C.; Panchal, C.; Chhabra, R.; Jain, K.; et al. The collateral fallout of COVID19 lockdown on patients with head injury from north-west India. *Acta Neurochir.* **2021**, *163*, 1053–1060. [CrossRef]

23. Horan, J.; Duddy, J.C.; Gilmartin, B.; Amoo, M.; Nolan, D.; Corr, P.; Husien, M.B.; Bolger, C. The impact of COVID-19 on trauma referrals to a National Neurosurgical Centre. *Ir. J. Med. Sci.* **2021**, *190*, 1281–1293. [CrossRef]
24. Agarwal, M.; Udare, A.; Alabousi, A.; van der Pol, C.B.; Ramonas, L.; Mascola, K.; Edmonds, B.; Ramonas, M. Impact of the COVID-19 pandemic on emergency CT head utilization in Ontario—An observational study of tertiary academic hospitals. *Emerg. Radiol.* **2020**, *27*, 791–797. [CrossRef]
25. Esteban, P.L.; Querolt Coll, J.; Xicola Martínez, M.; Camí Biayna, J.; Delgado-Flores, L. Has COVID-19 affected the number and severity of visits to a traumatology emergency department? *Bone Jt. Open* **2020**, *1*, 617–620. [CrossRef]
26. Faried, A.; Hidajat, N.N.; Harsono, A.B.; Giwangkancana, G.W.; Hartantri, Y.; Imron, A.; Arifin, M.Z. Delayed definitive treatment of life-threatening neurosurgery patient with suspected coronavirus disease 2019 infection in the midst of pandemic: Report of two cases. *Surg. Neurol. Int.* **2021**, *12*, 18. [CrossRef]
27. Servadei, F.; Cannizzaro, D. Effects on traumatic brain injured patients of COVID pandemia: Which responses from neurosurgical departments? *Acta Neurochir.* **2021**, *163*, 1051–1052. [CrossRef]
28. Al Saiegh, F.; Mouchtouris, N.; Khanna, O.; Baldassari, M.; Theofanis, T.; Ghosh, R.; Tjoumakaris, S.; Gooch, M.R.; Herial, N.; Zarzour, H.; et al. Battle-tested guidelines and operational protocols for neurosurgical practice in times of a pandemic: Lessons learned from COVID-19. *World Neurosurg.* **2021**, *146*, 20–25. [CrossRef]
29. Chen, P.; Xiong, X.H.; Chen, Y.; Wang, K.; Zhang, Q.T.; Zhou, W.; Deng, Y.B. Perioperative management strategy of severe traumatic brain injury during the outbreak of COVID-19. *Chin. J. Traumatol.* **2020**, *23*, 202–206. [CrossRef]
30. Hernigou, J.; Morel, X.; Callewier, A.; Bath, O.; Hernigou, P. Staying home during "COVID-19" decreased fractures, but trauma did not quarantine in one hundred and twelve adults and twenty eight children and the "tsunami of recommendations" could not lockdown twelve elective operations. *Int. Orthop.* **2020**, *44*, 1473–1480. [CrossRef] [PubMed]
31. Megaloikonomos, P.D.; Thaler, M.; Igoumenou, V.G.; Bonanzinga, T.; Ostojic, M.; Couto, A.F.; Diallo, J.; Khosravi, I. Impact of the COVID-19 pandemic on orthopaedic and trauma surgery training in Europe. *Int. Orthop.* **2020**, *44*, 1611–1619. [CrossRef]
32. Why Taiwan is Beating COVID-19—Again. Available online: https://thediplomat.com/2021/07/why-taiwan-is-beating-covid-19-again/ (accessed on 21 September 2021).
33. Establishment and Application of Traffic Accident Injury Data Collection System (2/2). Available online: https://www.iot.gov.tw/cp-78-12430-1759c-1.html (accessed on 16 November 2020). (In Chinese)
34. Ahmad, I.A.; Osei, E. Occupational health and safety measures in healthcare settings during COVID-19: Strategies for protecting staff, patients and visitors. *Disaster Med. Public Health Prep.* **2021**, 1–9. [CrossRef] [PubMed]
35. McCabe, R.; Schmit, N.; Christen, P.; D'Aeth, J.C.; Løchen, A.; Rizmie, D.; Nayagam, S.; Miraldo, M.; Aylin, P.; Bottle, A.; et al. Adapting hospital capacity to meet changing demands during the COVID-19 pandemic. *BMC Med.* **2020**, *18*, 329. [CrossRef] [PubMed]

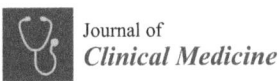

Article

Suppression of Electrographic Seizures Is Associated with Amelioration of QTc Interval Prolongation in Patients with Traumatic Brain Injury

Wojciech Dabrowski [1,*], Dorota Siwicka-Gieroba [1], Todd T. Schlegel [2,3], Chiara Robba [4], Sami Zaid [5], Magdalena Bielacz [6], Andrzej Jaroszyński [7] and Rafael Badenes [8]

1. Department of Anaesthesiology and Intensive Therapy, Medical University of Lublin, 20-954 Lublin, Poland; dsiw@wp.pl
2. Department of Molecular Medicine and Surgery, Karolinska Institute, SE-171 76 Stockholm, Sweden; ttschlegel@gmail.com
3. Nicollier-Schlegel SARL, 1270 Trélex, Switzerland
4. Department of Anaesthesia and Intensive Care, Policlinico San Martino, 16100 Genova, Italy; kiarobba@gmail.com
5. Department of Anaesthesia, Al-Emadi-Hospital, Al HilalWest, D Ring Road, Doha P.O. Box 50000, Qatar; sami1zaid@gmail.com
6. Institute of Tourism and Recreation, State Vocational College of Szymon Szymonowicz, 22-400 Zamosc, Poland; magda.bielacz@gmail.com
7. Department of Nephrology, Institute of Medical Science, Jan Kochanowski University of Kielce, 25-736 Kielce, Poland; jaroszynskiaj@interia.pl
8. Department of Anaesthesiology and Intensive Care, Hospital Clinico Universitario de Valencia, University of Valencia, 46010 Valencia, Spain; rafaelbadenes@gmail.com
* Correspondence: w.dabrowski5@yahoo.com

Abstract: Introduction: Disorders in electroencephalography (EEG) are commonly noted in patients with traumatic brain injury (TBI) and may be associated with electrocardiographic disturbances. Electrographic seizures (ESz) are the most common features in these patients. This study aimed to explore the relationship between ESz and possible changes in QTc interval and spatial QRS-T angle both during ESz and after ESz resolution. Methods: Adult patients with TBI were studied. Surface 12-lead ECGs were recorded using a Cardiax device during ESz events and 15 min after their effective suppression using barbiturate infusion. The ESz events were diagnosed using Masimo Root or bispectral index (BIS) devices. Results: Of the 348 patients considered for possible inclusion, ESz were noted in 72, with ECG being recorded in 21. Prolonged QTc was noted during ESz but significantly ameliorated after ESz suppression (540.19 ± 60.68 ms vs. 478.67 ± 38.52 ms, $p < 0.001$). The spatial QRS-T angle was comparable during ESz and after treatment. Regional cerebral oximetry increased following ESz suppression (from 58.4% ± 6.2 to 60.5% ± 4.2 ($p < 0.01$) and from 58.2% ± 7.2 to 60.8% ± 4.8 ($p < 0.05$) in the left and right hemispheres, respectively). Conclusion: QTc interval prolongation occurs during ESz events in TBI patients but both it and regional cerebral oximetry are improved after suppression of seizures.

Keywords: seizure; traumatic brain injury; QTc interval; spatial QTS-T angle; brain–heart interaction

1. Introduction

Electrocardiographic disorders are frequently associated with seizures, which are often observed in patients with traumatic brain injury (TBI). Post-traumatic seizures occur in 21–27% of patients and are generally associated with hemorrhagic lesions of the temporal lobe [1–3]. The first event of recorded seizures mostly occurs in the first 24 h after TBI, with over one-third being electrographic seizures (ESz—electrographic seizures) [1]. TBI-related seizures can also be induced by increased intracranial pressure (ICP), cerebral metabolic crises connected with disturbances in oxidative metabolism and glucose consumption, and impaired redox status of the brain [3]. On the other hand, seizures impair cerebral metabolism and may induce systemic disorders in the extra-cerebral organs, including cardiac injury [4].

Cerebral-related cardiac disorders commonly result from activation of the brain–heart axis, with electrocardiographic disorders being frequent derangements observed in patients with acute brain damage [5–8]. Recently, significant prolongation in the QTc interval and increased spatial QRS-T angles in a cohort of TBI patients with a Glasgow Coma Score (GCS) below eight were documented [6]. Some studies reported a strict relationship between prolonged QTc interval and seizures based on standard full electroencephalography (EEG) measurement [7,8]. However, no study so far has explored the relationship between TBI-related ESz and changes in the QTc interval or spatial QRS-T angle. The aim of this study was to analyze changes in the spatial QRS-T angle and QTc interval during ESz and after ESz resolution by EEG in a cohort of TBI patients.

2. Methods

We used Strengthening the Reporting of Observational Studies in Epidemiology (STROBE) guidelines [9]. This study is part of a larger prospective observational study performed at the First Clinic of Intensive Care at the Medical University of Lublin, Poland. The study was conducted in accordance with the intensive care unit (ICU) protocol for the monitoring of patients with TBI and the Declaration of Helsinki; the protocol was approved by the Institutional Review Board and the Bioethics Committee of the Medical University at Lublin, Poland (KE-0254/136/2018). Informed consent was obtained from the legal representatives of patients as all included patients were sedated and mechanically ventilated.

Inclusion criteria were adult patients with TBI and GCS below 8 and the presence of ESz. The main exclusion criterion was a history of epilepsy. Additionally, patients below 18 years old, pregnant, or with the presence of thoracic injury, drug overdoses, or a history of neoplastic, cardiac, or acute or chronic hepatic or renal diseases were excluded. Heart rate (HR), continuous mean arterial pressure (MAP), regional cerebral oximetry (SrO_2), and peripheral saturation (SpO_2) were monitored in all patients; hemodynamic variables were obtained using an EV 1000 platform (Edwards Lifescience, Irvine, CA, USA). Immediately after admission to the ICU, EEG electrodes were placed on the forehead and temporal hairline skin for EEG monitoring using Masimo Root with a SEDLine monitor (Irvine, CA, USA) or a bispectral complete 4-channel monitor (BIS, Medtronic, MN, USA).

All patients were sedated with propofol (AstraZeneca, Macclesfield, UK) and fentanyl (Polfa, Warsaw, Poland) and mechanically ventilated; the inspired fraction of oxygen (FiO_2) was adjusted to maintain oxygen saturation (SpO_2) between 92 and 98% and SrO_2 higher than 50%. Immediately after admission to the ICU, patients received hyperosmotic therapy with 15% mannitol at 1.5 g/kg body weight to reduce ICP, if required. The hyperosmotic therapy was discontinued in patients with plasma osmolality higher than 310 mOsm/kg H_2O. All patients received continuous infusion of potassium to maintain blood concentration between 4.5 and 5 mmol/L. Blood potassium, sodium, glucose, and lactate levels were measured 5 times per day. Continuous norepinephrine infusion and balanced crystalloids (Sterofundin ISO, Melsungen, Germany) were used to maintain MAP above 80 mmHg. According to the Fourth Edition of Brain Trauma Foundation Guidelines, the infusion of barbiturates is considered an option for second-tier therapy to control refractory elevated intracranial hypertension (ICH) [10].

2.1. ECG, Derived Vectorcardiogram (VCG), EEG, and Study Protocol

Surface 12-lead ECGs were recorded using a Cardiax PC-ECG® (MESA Medizintechnic GmbH Benediktbeuern, Germany). The recorded ECG was converted to a single median beat and transformed into three orthogonal leads—X, Y, and Z—using the inverse Dower method [11]. The value for the spatial QRS-T angle was then automatically calculated by the Cardiax software from the maximum spatial QRS and T vectors. The QT and corrected QT (QTc) intervals utilizing the Bazett, Fridericia, and Framingham corrections were also obtained directly from the Cardiax commercial software, which utilizes a median beat-related "global QT interval" algorithm similar to that described by Xue et al. [12]. The QT and QTc intervals were also assessed manually via electronic calipers by two of the co-authors independently to further validate the automatically assessed values. The ECG and derived VCG measurements were performed during ESz events and 15 min after effective suppression of seizures with barbiturate infusion (thiopental, Rotexmadica, Trittau, G) at the dose of 50 µg·kg^{-1}·min^{-1}.

EEG disorders were analyzed based on frontopolar (forehead hairline montage) EEG recorded with a Masimo Root monitor or a bispectral complete 4-channel (BIS-4) monitor. Both of these technologies are commonly used at our institution to measure the level of sedation. The capacity of the Masimo device for EEG recording has been previously established [13–15]. In all patients, changes in EEG were observed within the first 7 days of treatment. Electrographic seizures were defined as electrographic discharges with a frequency higher than 2.5 Hz and lasting longer than 10 s. Seizure morphology was categorized as epileptiform if it induced spikes or sharp waves or rhythmic evolving or if it induced evolving rhythmic patterns [15–17]. Electrographic status epilepticus was defined as an ESz for more than 10 continuous minutes or for a total duration of more than 20 min in any 60-minute period of recording [16]. These criteria were adapted for disorders in EEG observed in the BIS or Masimo device. Additionally, changes in EEG were recorded as the color density spectral array (DSA), with upward arches on the y-axis (increased frequency and amplitude in EEG) reflected in warmer colors (larger red area in DSA) [18–20].

2.2. Statistical Analysis

The Shapiro–Wilk test was used to test the normality of the distribution of the results. Means and standard deviations (SDs) were calculated for all variables. Student's unpaired *t*-test was used, and analysis was performed using Statistica 13.1 (StatSoft, Tulsa, OK, USA). For variables with non-normal distribution, the Wilcoxon signed-rank, Mann–Whitney U, Kruskal–Wallis ANOVA, and post hoc Dunnett's multiple comparison tests were used. The power of the statistical tests was assessed by the G*Power test. A *p*-value < 0.05 was considered significant.

3. Results

In total, 348 patients (134 female and 214 male) aged 18–90 years and treated for TBI with ICH were initially considered for inclusion. Among these, 115 patients were excluded as they presented with thoracic injury, a history of severe cardiac diseases (N = 111), or pacemaker implantation (N = 4). Finally, 233 patients treated for isolated TBI (iTBI, N = 124) and polytrauma with TBI (pTBI, N = 109) were included to the present study. Eighty-two patients (35.19%) died at day 28, following foraminal herniation (N = 54; 65.85%) or post-traumatic multiorgan failure (N = 28; 33.14%).

Immediately after admission into the ICU, all patients achieved an appropriate level of sedation with continuous propofol and fentanyl infusion, and the depth of sedation ranged between 10 and 20 on the bispectral index (BIS) and 5 and 17 on the Patient State Index (PSI). Any EEG abnormalities were monitored in all patients immediately after admission to the ICU. Episodes of ESz were noted in 72 patients (30.9%) between 12 h and the fifth day after admission in the ICU. In 54 cases, the episodes of ESz were documented on the screenshots in Masimo or BIS-4, and subsequently, ESz was successfully treated; however, changes in ECG during ESz were documented in only 21 patients (7 female and 14 male) aged 19–58 years (mean 39 ± 13). The mean GCS at hospital admission was 4.86 ± 1.6. In all cases, ESz status lasted for more than 15 min before treatment. Of the 21 patients included in the analysis, 11 were treated for cerebral edema (with or without intracerebral hemorrhage), 8 for subarachnoid hemorrhage, and 2 for epidural hematoma. Continuous infusion of thiopental at the dose of 50 µg·kg^{-1}·min^{-1} successfully suppressed ESz in all patients, and any EEG abnormalities were observed during and immediately after thiopental administration with a slight decrease in BIS or PSI values. This treatment was continued for a minimum of 12 h. Nine patients died within 28 days of treatment—three due to foraminal herniation within 7 days of treatment and six after 7 but before 28 days due to foraminal herniation. Twelve patients were discharged from the ICU; however, all remained bedridden with neurological conditions.

During ESz, the QTc interval was pathologically prolonged, and the prolongation was significantly ameliorated 15 min after ESz suppression independently of the method (automated or manual) or correction formula used in all patients (Table 1). Examples of changes in EEG monitored by BIS-4 are presented in Figure 1, and the ESz and ECG monitored by Masimo Root are presented in Figures 2 and 3. Spatial QRS-T angle was comparable during ESz and 15 min after ESz suppression (61.29 ± 46.51 and 60.41 ± 39.73, respectively).

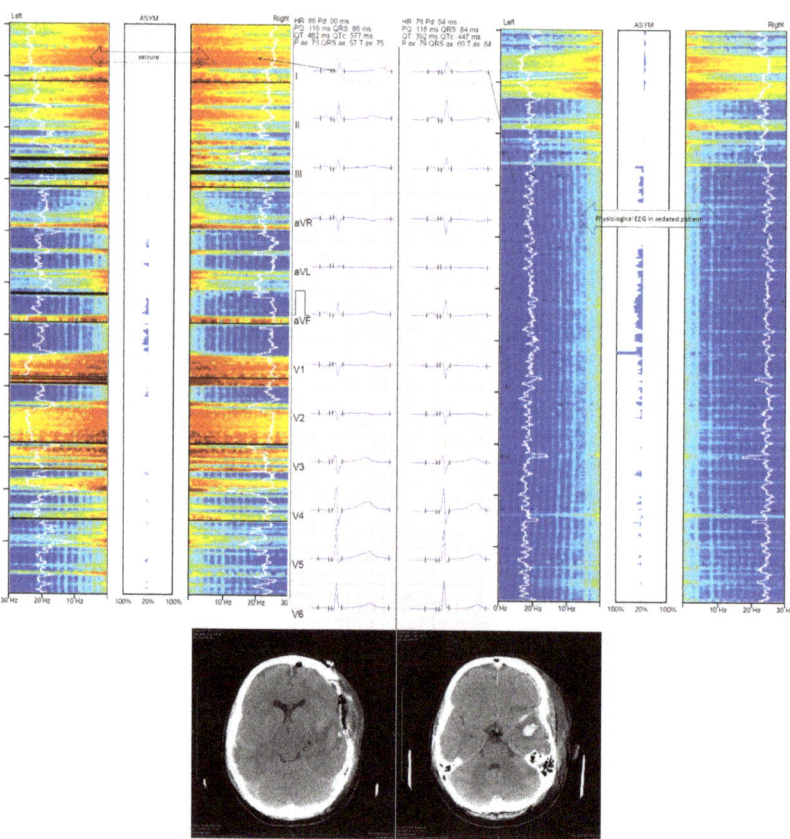

Figure 1. Changes in frontopolar electroencephalography monitored with Medtronic BIS ™ device and corrected QT (QTc) interval. The left part of the figure presents an electrographic seizure and ECG with prolonged QTc (577 ms, calculated with Bazett's formula). The right part of the figure presents ESz suppression following thiopental administration with reduction in the QTc interval (447 ms, calculated with Bazett's formula). The case shown is a 22 year-old woman who was admitted to the intensive care unit (ICU) for severe TBI. Her Glasgow Coma Score was 6. Computed tomography (CT) showed acute epidural hematoma with intracerebral hemorrhage. Immediately after CT, craniectomy was performed. According to the local ICU protocol, frontopolar electroencephalography (EEG) was used. Controlled CT was performed 24 h after surgery and showed slight cerebral edema with cerebral lesion and intracerebral hematoma in the temporal region. Despite depth sedation (BIS ranged between 10 and 20), EEG showed alternate polyspike and slow wave without clinical symptoms 24 h after the admission to the ICU. The ESz recurred for 2 h. Hence, status epilepticus was diagnosed and continuous thiopental infusion at the dose of 50 µg·kg^{-1}·min^{-1} was used to suppress ESz. Such disorders were not observed during treatment in the ICU. Patient was discharged from the ICU 32 days after trauma.

Table 1. Changes in QT and QTc intervals during electrographic seizures and 15 min after their effective suppression with barbiturate infusion. * $p < 0.05$, ** $p < 0.01$, *** $p < 0.001$—difference between QT and QTc before and after suppression of seizure (Student's *t*-test). Manual measurements comprise the averaged values from two independent co-authors.

	Manual Measurements		Automatic Measurements	
	During ESz	After ESz	During ESz	After ESz
QT	453.5 ± 66.3	416.3 ± 55.44	450.71 ± 68.9	410.14 ± 53.95 *
QTc, Bazett	544.24 ± 57.67	487.61 ± 40.37 ***	540.19 ± 60.68	478.67 ± 38.52 ***
QTc, Fridericia	511.71 ± 55.96	462.16 ± 41.95 **	507.9 ± 59	455.2 ± 39.8 **
QTc, Framingham	499.67 ± 51.91	457.19 ± 40.47 *	496.54 ± 54.6	451 ± 38.7 **

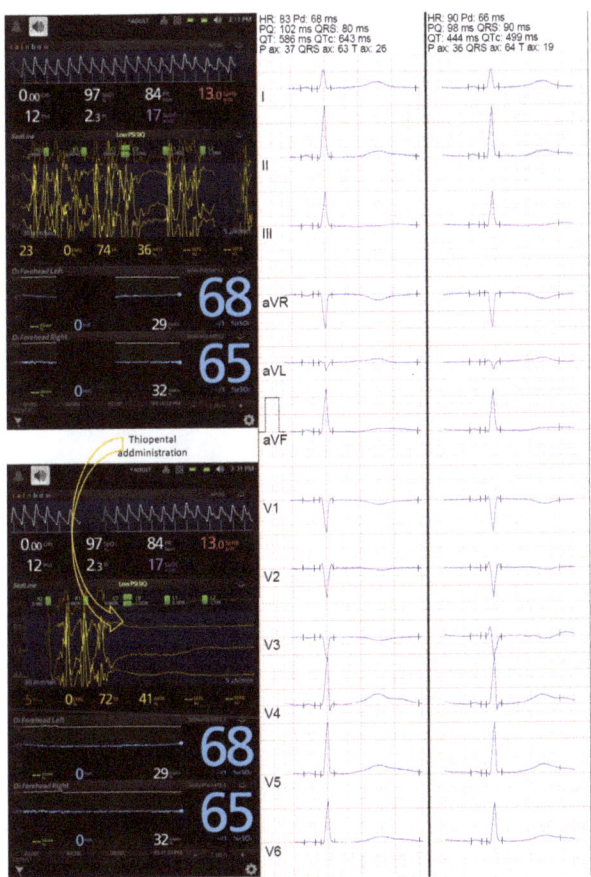

Figure 2. Changes in frontopolar electroencephalography monitored with Masimo Root device and corrected QT (QTc) interval. Prolonged QTc interval was noted during ESz, and use of thiopental suppressed the seizure successfully, which was associated with a reduction in the automated QTc (from 643 to 499 ms, calculated with Bazett's formula, and from 610 to 475 ms and 591 to 471 ms, calculated with Fridericia's formula and Framingham's formula, respectively). However, the ECG showed bifid T waves in V_4, V_5, and V_6 leads before suppression and in II, III, aVF, V_3, V_4, V_5, and V_6 15 min after ESz suppression, leading to partially spurious automated QTc results. Frontopolar EEG monitoring with the Masimo device showed seizures (upper screenshot) and their spectacular suppression following barbiturate infusion (lower screenshots).

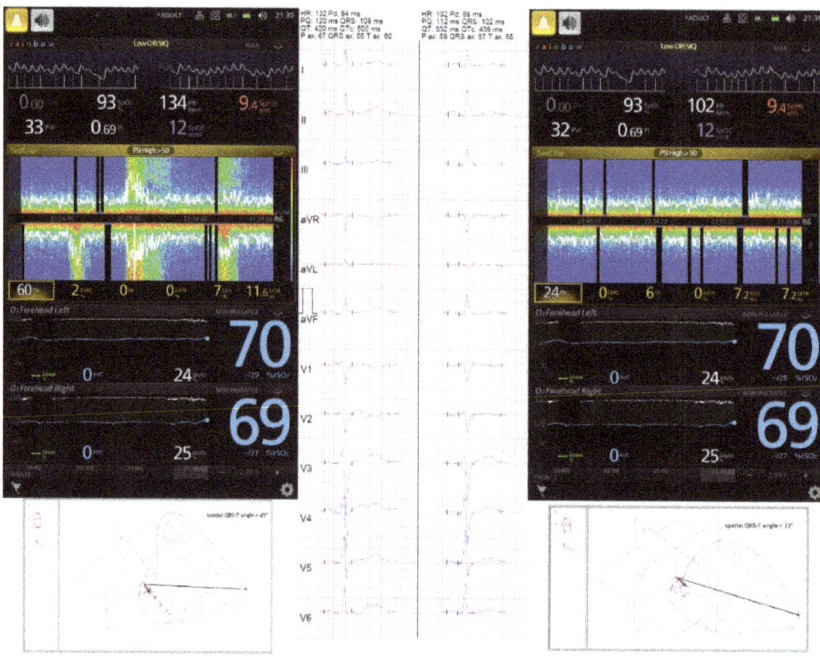

Figure 3. A 54-year-old male admitted to the intensive care unit (ICU) for severe TBI. His Glasgow Coma Score was 4. Computed tomography (CT) showed cerebral edema with reduced size of both lateral ventricles. Patient was sedated with continuous infusion of propofol and fentanyl, and hyperosmotic therapy with 15% mannitol was administered. According to the local ICU protocol, non-invasive monitoring including near-infrared spectroscopy (NIRS) and frontopolar electroencephalography (EEG) was applied. Frontopolar EEG and seizures were monitored by the Masimo Root SEDLine device. Despite deep sedation (Patient State Index was 7), the DSA image showed upward y-axis arcs in warmer colors, and the recorded EEG confirmed a polyspike and slow wave. Continuous thiopental infusion at the dose of 50 $\mu g \cdot kg^{-1} \cdot min^{-1}$ was used to suppress ESz, after which a serial 12-lead ECG showed a notably reduced QTc interval. The patient was discharged from the ICU 14 days after trauma.

The mean values of cardiac index (CI), extravascular lung water index (ELWI), pulmonary vascular permeability index (PVPI), global ejection fraction (GEF), and intrathoracic blood volume were comparable before and after ESz suppression, whereas the mean values of SrO_2 significantly increased 15 min after treatment of ESz (Table 2).

Table 2. Changes in cardiac index (CI), extravascular lung water index (ELWI), pulmonary vascular permeability index (PVPI), global ejection fraction (GEF), intrathoracic blood volume (iTBI), and regional cerebral oxygenation (SrO_2) in the right and left hemispheres during ESz and 15 min after their suppression with continuous thiopental infusion at the dose of 50 $\mu g \cdot kg^{-1} \cdot min^{-1}$. * $p < 0.05$, ** $p < 0.01$—differences in SrO_2 noted before and after suppression of ESz.

Parameter	During ESz	15 min after Thiopental Administration
CI (L/min/m^2)	3.4 ± 0.8	3.7 ± 0.9
ELWI (mL/kg)	8.2 ± 1.8	7.6 ± 2
PVPI	2.1 ± 0.5	1.9 ± 0.5
GEF (%)	27.2 ± 6.8	28.9 ± 6.4
iTBI (mL/m^2)	781.4 ± 250.4	804.4 ± 236.2
Left SrO_2 (%)	58.4 ± 6.2	60.5 ± 4.2 **
Right SrO_2 (%)	58.2 ± 7.2	60.8 ± 4.8 *

4. Discussion

The present study showed that observed electrographic abnormalities which may meet the criteria for diagnosis of ESz were associated with T wave abnormalities and prolonged QTc interval in propofol-sedated TBI patients, and that the successful treatment of ESz ameliorated the T wave abnormalities and shortened the QTc interval. Neither ESz nor successful ESz treatment appeared to modify the spatial QRS-T angle. Additionally, treatment of ESz improved SrO_2 in the left and right hemispheres. Secondarily, this study also demonstrated the potential usefulness of the Masimo and BIS technology for innovative cerebral monitoring in critically ill patients with TBI. Despite all the patients being deeply sedated, the Masimo device enabled identification of general electrographic abnormalities.

TBI-related cerebral hypoxia and ischemia can disrupt autonomic self-regulation and serve as a trigger for seizure development [21]. A rapid change in EEG oscillation may also correspond with changes in cardiac activity and different types of arrhythmias [22,23]. Seizures might affect cardiac function by impairing the repolarization phase, particularly in patients treated for refractory epilepsy [24,25]. Various types of cardiac arrhythmias have been observed in more than 90% of patients with seizures, with atrial fibrillation (AF) being the most frequent form of dysrhythmia [25]. Interestingly, the administration of anticonvulsive drugs significantly reduces ECG disorders and improves cardiac morphology in experimental models of seizures [26]. Seizure-related ventricular arrhythmias are also commonly associated with prolonged QTc interval, possibly due to hypoxemia following seizure-related respiratory dysfunction [8]. Indeed, intermittent hypoxia has been shown to be a major risk factor for life-threatening cardiac arrhythmias and sudden cardiac death [7]. Our results did not explore hypoxia-related QTc interval prolongation as the patients included in our study were mechanically ventilated and cerebral oxygenation was monitored using SrO_2, without showing any episodes of desaturation. However, significantly lower SrO_2 levels were noted during ESz compared to post-seizure. Based on these results, we speculate that suppression of electrographic seizures can improve cerebral oxygenation, but this effect requires further confirmation in larger studies.

Continuous monitoring of electrophysiological function in critically ill patients has been extensively studied in the last decade [15,18,19]. In the present study we utilized a new and convenient method for assessing cerebral EEG in critically ill patients treated for TBI. Continuous monitoring of EEG, particularly with DSA that is displayed on processed EEG, shows the power spectrum of EEG, which may be useful for detecting even short episodes of ESz. Detection of ESz in deeply sedated patients is difficult and requires continuous EEG monitoring. To facilitate the interpretation of EEG, several quantitative EEG display tools have been developed to diagnose EEG disorders, and DSA is one of them [15,20,27]. It has been documented that even non-physician personnel can identify ESz in DSA [18,19,27]. Additionally, such qualitative techniques show a high sensitivity, specificity, and accuracy for seizure detection in those personnel who have no experience in critical care EEG and seizure detection [18,19]. Compared to the gold standard of raw data read by experienced epileptologists, Dericioglu and colleagues documented an overall sensitivity of 93%, specificity of 91–95%, and accuracy of 0.93 of DSA in the detection of ESz [18]. Similarly high sensitivity and specificity in the detection of seizures using color DSA were described by Steward and colleagues [28]. Seizure evolution may be accompanied by increases in the frequency and amplitude of frontotemporal EEG signals that appear in DSA images, showing upward y-axis arcs in warmer colors [20,26]. In our cases, we observed that the color spectrum ranged from blue to dark red (from minimum to maximum power), which could document seizure events [15]. Continuous monitoring of EEG waves also enabled the detection of polyspike waves associated with ESz in deeply sedated patients [15,18]. We noted ESz in 30.9% of patients; however, we were able to document changes in ECG during ESz only in one-third of the studied patients because the seizure resolved spontaneously or the doctor on duty documented the seizure episode in the screenshot and implemented continuous thiopental infusion before ECG examination. Based on our experience, we can strongly recommend the use of continuous EEG monitoring in critically ill, unconscious TBI patients.

Other potential mechanisms underlying seizure-induced QTc interval prolongation include the stimulation of the intrinsic adrenergic pathway, leading to disorders in cardiac repolarization, also previously described in ESz [29]. Autonomic dysregulation following TBI might also contribute to QTc interval prolongation [5]. Finally, moderate–severe TBI with hemorrhagic contusions in the temporal lobe increases the risk of early seizure and post-traumatic epilepsy [2]. In the present study, we did not analyze the relationships between episodes of ESz and regions of brain injury; however, we can speculate that a prolonged QTc interval is directly associated with abnormal electroencephalographic brain activity, which could suggest brain–heart interaction [30].

Several medications may also prolong the QTc interval [31,32]. The included patients were sedated using continuous propofol and fentanyl infusion, and both drugs may affect the QTc interval. Propofol is well known to increase the risk of Torsades de Pointes dysrhythmia, which can frequently induce sudden cardiac death [33,34]. Additionally, propofol may cause prolongation of the QTc interval and result in a higher incidence of bradycardia and junctional rhythm than barbiturates can [31]. In the present study, some patients received furosemide to force diuresis, a loop diuretic that could also prolong the QTc interval [29,32]. Notably, furosemide and fentanyl only rarely prolong the QTc interval in critically ill patients, especially in association with electrolyte disturbances [33]. Interestingly, we noted a significant reduction in the QTc interval after ESz suppression with thiopental, a drug known to induce QTc interval prolongation [32]. Therefore, we can speculate that changes in QTc interval may depend more on the seizures induced by the primary cerebral pathology than on the medications administered.

Limitations

The first major limitation of the present study is that EEG was limited to the frontopolar region because both the Masimo and BIS-4 monitors only allow EEG monitoring in the frontal and temporal lobes. It should also be stressed that EEG abnormalities occurring in the other regions of the brain may also affect ECG as well as stimulate the frontal and temporal lobes to pathological activities. Additionally, changes in the color spectrum may reflect changes in EEG and ICP-related changes but also rhythmic/periodic artefacts, thus reducing the accuracy of quantitative EEG measurement. The second major limitation was that the EEG signal was evaluated by physicians without formal training in neurophysiology but with a lot of experience in the use of quantitative EEG and DSA. Thirdly, all EEG abnormalities were observed in the Masimo or the BIS device and were not confirmed in a standard EEG, but only full EEG could confirm a diagnosis of every electrographic pathology. Another important limitation of the study is the low power of our statistical analysis due to the small number of patients who had both ECG recordings and well-documented ESz. The small number of patients with well-documented ECG during ESz results in part from the lack of specific alarms for EEG disorders in the Masimo technology. Had such alarms existed, they might have allowed for more prompt recognition and treatment of cerebral electrical derangements as well as a larger study group. We did not analyze the duration of ESz in relation to the ECG, and it has been documented that long-standing seizures may induce cardiac remodeling with altered intracellular Ca^{+2} homeostasis and ECG abnormalities, including QTc interval prolongation [35]. We monitored frontopolar EEG for 7 days of treatment. Although we did not observe recurrent episodes of ESz during the study period, they could have recurred after the studied period. Finally, we noted a significant improvement of SrO_2 following ESz suppression; however, the increase in SrO_2 in the left and right hemispheres may also have resulted from a decrease in ICP following thiopental administration. In fact, a moderate inverse relationship between ICP and SrO_2 has been documented in TBI patients [36,37]. Another important limitation of our study is the lack of a control group. We used continuous thiopental infusion to ameliorate ESz; however, many other medications are also commonly used for the treatment of such disorders (e.g., valproic acid or benzodiazepines). Noteworthily, all of these drugs may affect QTc. Therefore, changes in QTc should be compared with those observed in patients with spontaneous ESz termination, because only this analysis would unambiguously confirm the relationships between brain pathology and cardiac dysfunction, which is known as brain–heart interaction.

Our report focused in particular on automated measurements for the QT and QTc intervals. However, no automated algorithm for QTc determination produces perfect results, especially in the face of poorly defined T waves. While our manual measurements of the QTc intervals confirmed the overall QTc-related changes, they did so with less statistical significance, suggesting that methodological (i.e., automated algorithmic) factors can also falsely contribute to increases in automated QTc intervals when T waves are or become very poorly defined. Additionally, we observed significant shortening of the QTc interval following pharmacological suppression of ESz; however, we did not perform ECGs before the seizures, and prolonged QTc intervals might also result from TBI. Nonetheless, the study corroborated that the brain–heart interaction and QTc interval prolongations previously noted during/after seizure activity unrelated to TBI can also occur after TBI. Specifically, it demonstrated not only a strong relationship between TBI-induced ESz and prolonged QTc intervals but also the amelioration of prolonged QTc intervals after the treatment of ESz even in the face of QTc interval-prolonging barbiturate (thiopental) therapy in sedated TBI patients. Our findings support the concept of brain–heart cross-talk [38–45] and may pave the way to further larger observational or randomized controlled studies on this topic.

5. Conclusions

Pharmacological suppression of electrographic abnormalities which may meet the criteria to detect ESz in patients with severe TBI is associated with electrocardiographic T wave changes and shortened QTc intervals noted 15 min after seizure suppression. Additionally, treatment of electrographic seizures appears to improve SrO_2 in both the left and right cerebral hemispheres. Our findings may support that pathological brain activity affects cardiac function, which is commonly known as brain–heart cross-talk. Additionally, we suggest that continuous monitoring of EEG can be useful to detect electrographic abnormalities. However, the relationship between electrographic abnormalities and ECG requires further study in TBI patients.

Author Contributions: Conceptualization, W.D. and A.J.; data collection, D.S.-G. and W.D.; statistical analysis, W.D., S.Z., M.B. and C.R.; writing—original draft preparation, W.D., T.T.S., S.Z., M.B., C.R. and R.B. All authors have read and agreed to the published version of the manuscript.

Funding: This research received no external funding.

Institutional Review Board Statement: The study was conducted according to the guidelines of the Declaration of Helsinki, and approved by the Institutional Review Board and the Bioethics Committee of the Medical University at Lublin, Poland with the consent number KE-0254/136/2018.

Informed Consent Statement: Informed consent was obtained from all subjects involved in the study or their legal representatives while the patients were unconscious and deeply sedated.

Data Availability Statement: The data presented in this study are openly available with the author.

Acknowledgments: The authors thank the neurologists from Department of Neurology Medical University of Lublin who helped us to diagnose ESz in the Masimo device.

Conflicts of Interest: The authors declare no conflict of interest.

References

1. Sun, Y.; Yu, J.; Yuan, Q.; Wu, X.; Wu, X.; Hu, J. Early post-traumatic seizures are associated with valproic acid plasma concentrations and UGT1A6/CYP2C9 genetic polymorphisms in patients with severe traumatic brain injury. *Scand. J. Trauma Resusc. Emerg. Med.* **2017**, *25*, 85. [CrossRef]
2. Tubi, M.A.; Lutkenhoff, E.; Blanco, M.B.; McArthur, D.; Villablanca, P.; Ellingson, B.; Diaz-Arrastia, R.; Van Ness, P.; Real, C.; Shrestha, V.; et al. Early seizures and temporal lobe trauma predict post-traumatic epilepsy: A longitudinal study. *Neurobiol. Dis.* **2018**, *18*, 30152–30159. [CrossRef]
3. Zimmermann, L.L.; Diaz-Arrastia, R.; Vespa, P.M. Seizures and the role of anticonvulsant after traumatic brain injury. *Neurosurg. Clin. N. Am.* **2016**, *27*, 499–508. [CrossRef] [PubMed]
4. Mohamed, J.; Scott, B.W. Impaired cardiorespiratory function during focal limbic seizures: A role for serotonergic brainstem nuclei. *J. Neurosci.* **2016**, *36*, 8777–8779. [CrossRef]
5. Chen, Z.; Venkat, P.; Seyfried, D.; Chopp, M.; Yan, T.; Chen, J. Brain-heart interaction. Cardiac complication after stroke. *Circ. Res.* **2017**, *121*, 451–468. [CrossRef] [PubMed]
6. Dabrowski, W.; Schlegel, T.T.; Wosko, J.; Rola, R.; Rzecki, Z.; Malbrain, M.; Jaroszynki, A. Changes in spatial QRS-T angle and QTc interval in patients with traumatic brain injury with or without intra-abdominal hypertension. *J. Electrocardiol.* **2018**, *51*, 499–507. [CrossRef]
7. Moseley, B.D.; Wirrell, E.C.; Nickels, K.; Johnson, J.N.; Ackerman, M.J.; Britton, J. Electrocardiographic and oximetric changes during partial complex and generalized seizures. *Epilepsy Res.* **2011**, *95*, 237–245. [CrossRef] [PubMed]
8. Sadrnia, S.; Yousefi, P.; Jalali, L. Correlation between seizure in children and prolonged QT interval. *ARYA Atheroscler.* **2013**, *9*, 7–10.
9. Von Elm, E.; Altman, D.G.; Egger, M.; Pocock, S.J.; Gøtzsche, P.C.; Vandenbroucke, J.P. The Strengthening the Reporting of Observational Studies in Epidemiology (STROBE) Statement: Guidelines for reporting observational studies. *Int. J. Surg.* **2014**, *12*, 1495–1499. [CrossRef]
10. Carney, N.; Totten, A.M.; O'Reilly, C.; Ullman, J.S.; Hawryluk, G.W.J.; Bell, M.J.; Bratton, S.L.; Chesnut, R.; Harris, O.A.; Kissoon, N.; et al. Guidelines for the management of severe traumatic brain injury, Fourth edition. *Neurosurgery* **2017**, *80*, 6–15. [CrossRef]
11. Cortez, D.L.; Schlegel, T.T. When deriving the spatial QRS-T angle from the 12-lead electrocardiogram, which transform is more Frank: Regression or inverse dower? *J. Electrocardiol.* **2010**, *42*, 302–309. [CrossRef] [PubMed]
12. Xue, J.Q. QT interval measurement. What can we really expect? *Comput. Cardiol.* **2006**, *33*, 385–388.
13. John, E.R.; Prichep, L.S.; Fridman, J.; Easton, P. Neurometrics: Computer-assisted differential diagnosis of brain dysfunctions. *Science* **1988**, *239*, 162–169. [CrossRef]
14. Prichep, L.S.; John, E.R.; Gugino, L.D.; Kox, W.; Chabot, R.J. Quantitative EEG Assessment of Changes in the Level of Sedation/Hypnosis during Surgery Under General Anesthesia: I. The Patient State Index (PSI) II. Variable Resolution Electromagnetic Tomography (VARETA). In *Memory and Awareness in Anesthesia IV*; Jordan, C., Vaughan, D.J.A., Newton, D.E.F., Eds.; Imperial College Press: London, UK, 2000; pp. 97–107.
15. Pensirikul, A.D.; Beslow, L.A.; Kessler, S.K.; Sachez, S.M.; Topjian, A.A.; Dlugos, D.J.; Abend, N.S. Density spectral array for seizure identification in critically ill children. *J. Clin. Neurophysiol.* **2013**, *30*, 371–375. [CrossRef]
16. Hirsch, L.J.; Fong, M.W.K.; Leitinger, M.; LaRoche, S.M.; Beniczky, S.; Abend, N.S.; Lee, J.W.; Wusthoff, C.J.; Hahn, C.D.; Westover, M.B.; et al. American Clinical Neurophysiology Society's standardized critical care EEG terminology: 2021 version. *J. Clin. Neurophysiol.* **2021**, *38*, 1–29. [CrossRef] [PubMed]
17. Smith, S.J.M. EEG in the diagnosis, classification, and management of patients with epilepsy. *J. Neurol. Neurosurg. Psychiatry* **2005**, *76* (Suppl. II), ii2–ii7. [CrossRef]
18. Dericioglu, N.; Yetim, E.; Bas, D.F.; Bilgen, N.; Caglar, G.; Arsava, E.M.; Topcuoglu, M.A. Non-expert use of quantitative EEG displays for seizure identification in the adult neuro-intensive care unit. *Epilepsy Res.* **2015**, *109*, 48–56. [CrossRef]
19. Kang, J.H.; Sherill, G.C.; Sinha, S.R.; Swisher, C.B. A trial of real-time electrographic seizure detection by neuro-ICU nurses using a panel of quantitative EEG trends. *Neurocrit. Care* **2019**, *31*, 312–320. [CrossRef]
20. Hernàndez-Hernàndez, M.A.; Fernàndex-Torre, J.L. Color density spectral array of bilateral bispectral index system: Electroencephalographic correlate in comatose patients with nonconvulsive status epilepticus. *Seizure* **2016**, *34*, 18–25. [CrossRef]
21. Schueke, S.U.; Bermeo, A.C.; Alexopoulos, A.V.; Burgess, R.C. Anoxia-ischemia: A mechanism of seizure termination in ictal asystole. *Epilepsia* **2010**, *51*, 170–173.
22. Jiang, H.; He, B.; Guo, X.; Wang, X.; Guo, M.; Wang, Z.; Xue, T.; Li, H.; Xu, T.; Ye, S.; et al. Brain-Heart interactions underlying traditional Tibetan Buddhist meditation. *Cereb. Cortex* **2020**, *30*, 439–450. [CrossRef]
23. Patron, E.; Mennella, R.; MesserottiBenvenuti, S.; Thayer, J.F. The frontal cortex is a heart-brake: Reduction in delta oscillations is associated with heart rate deceleration. *Neuroimage* **2019**, *188*, 403–410. [CrossRef]
24. Dogan, E.A.; Dogan, U.; Yildiz, G.U.; Akilli, H.; Genc, E.; Genc, B.O.; Gok, H. Evaluation of cardiac repolarization indices in well-controlled partial epilepsy: 12-Lead ECG findings. *Epilepsy Res.* **2010**, *90*, 157–163. [CrossRef]
25. Hocker, S.; Prasad, A.; Rabinstein, A.A. Cardiac injury in refractory status epilepticus. *Epilepsia* **2013**, *54*, 518–522. [CrossRef]
26. Read, M.I.; Andreianova, A.A.; Harrison, J.C.; Goulton, C.S.; Sammut, I.A.; Kerr, D.S. Cardiac electrographic and morphological changes following status epilepticus: Effect of clonidine. *Seizure* **2014**, *23*, 55–61. [CrossRef] [PubMed]

27. Swisher, C.B.; White, C.R.; Mace, B.E.; Dombrowski, K.E.; Husain, A.M.; Kolls, B.J.; Radtke, R.R.; Tran, T.T.; Sinhs, S.R. Diagnostic accuracy of electrographic seizure detection by neurophysiologists and non-neurophysiologists in the adult ICU using a panel of quantitative EEG trends. *J. Clin. Neurophysiol.* **2015**, *32*, 324–330. [CrossRef] [PubMed]
28. Steward, C.P.; Otsubo, H.; Ochi, A.; Sharma, R.; Hutchison, J.S.; Hahn, C.D. Seizure identification in the ICU using quantitative EEG displays. *Neurology* **2010**, *75*, 1501–1508. [CrossRef]
29. Brotherstone, R.; Blackhall, B.; McLellan, A. Lenghening of corrected QT during epileptic seizure. *Epilepsia* **2010**, *51*, 221–232. [CrossRef] [PubMed]
30. Battaglini, D.; Robba, C.; da Silva, L.A.; Dos Santos Samary, C.; Leme Silva, P.; Dal Pizzol, F.; Pelosi, P.; Rocco, P.R.M. Brain-heart interaction after acute ischemic stroke. *Crit. Care* **2020**, *24*, 163. [CrossRef]
31. Etchegoyen, C.V.; Kelle, G.A.; Mrad, S.; Cheng, S.; Di Girolamo, G. Drug-induced QT interval prolongation in the intensive care unit. *Curr. Clin. Pharmacol.* **2017**, *12*, 210–222. [CrossRef]
32. Siniscalchi, A.; Scaglione, F.; Sanzaro, E.; Iemolo, F.; Albertini, G.; Quirino, G.; Manes, M.T.; Gratteri, S.; Mercuri, N.B.; De Sarro, G.; et al. Effects of phenobarbital and levetiracetam on PR and QTc intervals in patients with post-stroke seizure. *Clin. Drug Investig.* **2014**, *34*, 879–886. [CrossRef] [PubMed]
33. Abrich, V.A.; Ramakrishna, H.; Metha, A.; Mookadam, F.; Srivathsan, K. The possible role of propofol in drug-induced torsade's de pointes: A real-world single-center analysis. *Int. J. Cariol.* **2017**, *232*, 243–246. [CrossRef]
34. Wutzler, A.; De Asmundis, C.; Matsuda, H.; Bennehr, M.; Loehr, L.; Voelk, K.; Jungmann, J.; Humer, M.; Attanasio, P.; Parwani, A.; et al. Effects of propofol on ventricular repolarization and incidence of malignant arrhythmias in adults. *J. Electrocardiol.* **2018**, *51*, 170–174. [CrossRef] [PubMed]
35. Brewster, A.L.; Marzec, K.; Hairston, A.; Ho, M.; Anderson, A.E.; Lai, Y.C. Early cardiac electrographic and molecular remodelling in a model of status epilepticus and acquired epilepsy. *Epilepsia* **2016**, *57*, 1907–1915. [CrossRef]
36. Davie, S.; Mutch, W.A.C.; Monterola, M.; Fidler, K.; Funk, D.J. The incidence and magnitude of cerebral desaturation in traumatic brain injury: An observational cohort study. *J. Neurosurg. Anesthesiol.* **2021**, *33*, 258–262. [CrossRef]
37. Zuluaga, M.T.; Exch, M.E.; Cvijanovich, N.Z.; Gupta, N.; McQuillen, P.S. Diagnosis influences response of cerebral near infrared spectroscopy to intracranial hypertension in children. *Pediatr. Crit. Care Med.* **2010**, *11*, 514–522. [CrossRef] [PubMed]
38. Gopinath, R.; Ayya, S.S. Neurogenic stress cardiomyopathy: What do we need to know. *Ann. Card Anaesth.* **2018**, *21*, 228–234. [CrossRef]
39. Prasad Hrishi, A.; Ruby Lionel, K.; Prathapadas, U. Head rules over the heart: Cardiac manifestations of cerebral disorders. *Indian J. Crit. Care Med.* **2019**, *23*, 329–335. [PubMed]
40. Georgakopoulos, A.; Pianou, N.; Anagnostopoulos, C. Central nervous system disorders affecting the heart-insights from radionuclide imaging. *Hell. J. Nucl. Med.* **2016**, *19*, 189–192.
41. Mazzeo, A.T.; Micalizzi, A.; Mascia, L.; Scicolone, A.; Siracusano, L. Brain-heart crosstalk: The many faces of stress-related cardiomyopathy syndromes in anaesthesia and intensive care. *Br. J. Anaesth.* **2014**, *112*, 803–815. [CrossRef]
42. Simonassi, F.; Ball, L.; Badenes, R.; Millone, M.; Citerio, G.; Zona, G.; Pelosi, P.; Robba, C. Hemodynamic monitoring in patients with subarachnoid hemorrhage: A systematic review and meta-analysis. *J. Neurosurg. Anesthesiol.* **2020**, in press. [CrossRef]
43. Owusu, K.; Stredny, E.S.; Williamson, G.; Carr, Z.J.; Karamchandani, K. Cardiovascular collapse in a patient with parotid abscess: Dangerous cross talk between the brain and heart: A case report. *A&A Pract.* **2019**, *13*, 281–283.
44. Dimitri, G.M.; Agrawal, S.; Young, A.; Donnelly, J.; Liu, X.; Smielewski, P.; Hutchinson, P.; Czosnyka, M.; Lio, P.; Haubrich, C. Simultaneous transients of intracranial pressure and heart rate in traumatic brain injury: Methods of analysis. *Acta Neurochir. Suppl.* **2018**, *126*, 147–151. [PubMed]
45. Dimitri, G.M.; Agrawal, S.; Young, A.; Donnelly, J.; Liu, X.; Smielewski, P.; Hutchinson, P.; Czosnyka, M.; Lió, P.; Haubrich, C. A multiplex network approach for the analysis of intracranial pressure and heartrate data in traumatic brain injured patients. *Appl. Netw. Sci.* **2017**, *2*, 29. [CrossRef] [PubMed]

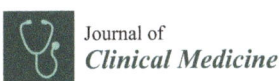

Article

Can Cranioplasty Be Considered a Tool to Improve Cognitive Recovery Following Traumatic Brain Injury? A 5-Years Retrospective Study

Francesco Corallo, Viviana Lo Buono *, Rocco Salvatore Calabrò and Maria Cristina De Cola

IRCCS Centro Neurolesi "Bonino-Pulejo", Via Palermo S.S. 113, C.da Casazza, 98124 Messina, Italy; francesco.corallo@irccsme.it (F.C.); roccos.calabro@irccsme.it (R.S.C.); mariacristina.decola@irccsme.it (M.C.D.C.)
* Correspondence: viv.lobuono@gmail.com; Tel.: +39-090-60128112

Abstract: Cranioplasty (CP) is a neurosurgical intervention of skull repairing following a decompressive craniectomy. Unfortunately, the impact of cranioplasty on cognitive and motor function is still controversial. Fifteen TBI subjects aged 26–54 years with CP after decompressive craniectomy were selected in this observational retrospective study. As per routine clinical practice, a neuropsychological evaluation carried out immediately before the cranioplasty (Pre CP) and one month after the cranioplasty (T0) was used to measure changes due to CP surgery. This assessment was performed each year for 5 years after discharge in order to investigate long-term cognitive changes (T1-T5). Before cranioplasty, about 53.3% of subjects presented a mild to severe cognitive impairment and about 40.0% a normal cognition. After CP, we found a significant improvement in all neuropsychological test scores. The more significant differences in cognitive recovery were detected after four years from CP. Notably, we found significant differences between T4 and T0-T1, as well as between T5 and T0-T1-T2 in all battery tests. This retrospective study further suggests the importance of CP in the complex management of patients with TBI showing how these patients might improve their cognitive function over a long period after the surgical procedure.

Keywords: cranioplasty; cognitive improvement; traumatic brain injury; neuropsychology

1. Introduction

Cranioplasty (CP) is a neurosurgical intervention of skull repairing and represents a second-line procedure in patients who have undergone decompressive craniectomy (DC) following a traumatic brain injury (TBI) [1], middle cerebral artery (MCA) infarction, or removal of cranial vault tumors [2]. The most appropriate time to perform cranioplasty, as well as its effect on functional outcome, remains debatable. Indeed, multiple confounding factors, including the material used, surgical technique, cognitive function, and general medical complications, seem to affect early and long-term outcomes [3–5].

In particular, the impact of cranioplasty on cognitive and motor function is also controversial. Patients with TBI show a wide range of neurocognitive and psychologic deficits after DC [6]. Although several studies have documented clinical improvements after cranioplasty in patients with severe brain injury, the reasons behind the possible mechanisms that induce such clinical improvement are not fully understood [7]. Patient improvement could be due to reduction in local cerebral compression caused by atmospheric pressure and increased cerebrospinal fluid hydrodynamics with potential improvement in local and global cerebral hemodynamics, blood flow, and metabolism [8].

A neuropsychological assessment is the best approach for understanding the nature, the severity, and the modality of cognitive complaints. This important measure of outcome is much more representative of the prognosis of neurosurgical patients than other outcome scales [9]. When cognitive complaints are reported or persist following brain injury, neuropsychological testing is useful for addressing diagnostic issues as well as treatment and rehabilitation planning [10].

This is why, beyond motor improvements, neurological rehabilitation should also be focused on cognitive functions recovery after a CP, especially during the first months after the surgery procedure [11,12]. However, only a limited number of studies on long-term neurological outcomes after a CP surgery are available, and very few concerning the cognitive recovery of these patients [13,14].

The purpose of this study was then to observe the long-term effects on cognitive recovery of patients with TBI after cranioplasty.

2. Materials and Methods

Twenty-two subjects with TBI submitted to decompressive craniectomy and attended the Neuro-rehabilitation Unit of the IRCCS Centro Neurolesi "Bonino Pulejo" of Messina between January 2015 and December 2020. However, five patients were excluded because of missing data, and two died due to unspecified causes. Therefore, fifteen subjects (five women and ten men), aged 26–54 years, were selected and included in this retrospective study. Data was extracted from the hospital database.

As per routine clinical practice, a neuropsychological evaluation carried out immediately before the cranioplasty (Pre CP) and 1 month after the cranioplasty (T0) was used to measure changes due to cranioplasty surgery. This assessment was performed each year for 5 years after discharge in order to investigate long-term cognitive changes (T1–T5).

A standardized battery of tests was used to measure in detail the main cognitive areas involved in TBI. The assessment included a test to globally evaluate cognitive functions, i.e., the Mini-Mental Status Examination (MMSE) [15], and specific scales to investigate multiple cognitive domains, such as memory (the Rey Auditory Verbal Learning Test [16] -RAVLI immediate and RAVLR recall- and Digit Span [17]), comprehension (Token Test [18]) and executive functions and attention (Trail Making Test-TMT [19]). In addition, the Hamilton Rating Scale for depression (HAM-D) and anxiety (HAM-A) [20,21] were also administered to evaluate the possible impact of mood and anxiety on cognition. For all scales and tests, the Italian language validated versions were used. A complete description of these assessments is provided in Table 1.

Table 1. The neuropsychological battery used for the assessment.

Neuropsychological Assessment
Mini Mental State Examination (MMSE)
The MMSE is a 30-point scale commonly used by healthcare providers to evaluate the global cognitive state as a screening test. The time of administration is about 10 min. Each correct answer provides 1 point. A score < 24 indicates cognitive impairment.
Rey Auditory Verbal Learning Test (RAVLT)
This test is divided into two parts: Immediate (RAVLT.I) and Delayed Recall (RAVLT.R). In the Immediate Recall, the examiner reads 15 words and asks the patient to repeat all the memorized words in the patient's preferred order. This task provides information about episodic verbal memory, encoding and learning strategies. For the evaluation of the long-term memory (RAVLT.R), the patient is asked to repeat the memorized words from the same 15-words list, after 15 min. In the meantime, between the Immediate and the Delayed Recall tests, a nonverbal and visuospatial test was administered in order to avoid any interference with the memory processes. Cut-off: 28.53 (RAVLT.I) and 4.69 (RAVLT.R)
Digit Span (DS)
The DS test is a widely used neuropsychological measure known as a test of attention and working memory. The DS consists of a forward recall part and backward recall part for digit sequences. Each part is considered to assess somewhat different cognitive processes. Cut-off: 3.75

Table 1. *Cont.*

Neuropsychological Assessment
Token
The Token test is used as a selective measure for the presence of aphasia and as an indicator for the severity of aphasia. All commands in the test consist of no redundant words, referring to circles and rectangles in different colors and sizes (large and small). To perform the requested action, every content word has to be decoded. Cut-off: 26.50
Trail Making Test (TMT)
The Trail Making Test is a widely used test to assess executive function in patients with neurological disease. Successful performance of the TMT requires a variety of mental abilities, including letter and number recognition mental flexibility, visual scanning, and motor function. The task requires connecting 25 circles distributed over a sheet of paper. In Part A, the circles are numbered 1–25, and the patient should draw lines to connect the numbers in ascending order. In Part B, the circles include both numbers and letters; here, the patient draws lines to connect the circles in an ascending pattern but alternating between the numbers and letters (i.e., 1-A-2-B-3-C, etc.). Trails are traced in the shortest time possible and without lifting the pen from the paper. Cut-off: 93 (A) and 282 (B)
Hamilton Rating Scale for Depression (HAM-D)
The HAM-D is the most widely used clinician-administered depression assessment scale. The 24-item version includes 24 items scored either on a 3-point or 5-point Likert-type scale (i.e., 10 items are defined from 0 to 2, and 14 items are defined from 0 to 4). A score $\geq$ 8 points defines depression as follows: a score ranged from 8–19 points defines a mild depression, a score ranged from 20–34 points defines a moderate depression, and a score $\geq$ 35 points defines a severe depression. Cut-off: 7
Hamilton Rating Scale for Anxiety (HAM-A)
The scale consists of 14 items, each defined by a series of symptoms, and measures both psychic anxiety (mental agitation and psychological distress) and somatic anxiety (physical complaints related to anxiety). Each item is scored on a scale of 0 (not present) to 4 (severe), with a total score ranged from 0–56, where below 17 indicates mild severity, 18–24 mild to moderate severity, and 25–30 moderate to severe. Cut-off: 17

In order to avoid the 'practice or learning effects' related to the repeated experience with the task, similar tests (but with different items for the same task) were administered, when possible.

Statistical Analysis

The Lilliefors (Kolmogorov–Smirnov) test was used to verify variables' normality, whereas the Levene test to assess the equality of variances among times. Because of reduced sample dimension, the not-normality of all variables, and the homoscedasticity of almost all of them, we chose a no-parametrical approach to perform inferential statistical analysis. Thus, the Wilcoxon signed-rank test was applied to detect significant pre-post cranioplasty changes of neuropsychological outcomes, and the Friedman test was used to compare these outcomes at different time points (T0–T5) in order to assess changes over time after the CP. On the variables in which the Friedman test detected a significance, the Conover test was applied considering the Bonferroni's correction (post-hoc analysis). All analysis was performed by using the 4.0.5 version of the open-source software R, by setting $p < 0.05$ as the significance level.

3. Results

Tables 2 and 3 report a detailed description of each subject before and after CP, respectively. Through MMSE cut-offs, we subdivided the sample in patients with nearly normal cognition, mild, and/or severe cognitive impairment. Before CP, about 53.3% of subjects presented a mild to severe cognitive impairment, about 40.0% a normal cognition, and in one subject, the MMSE was not administrable. Notably, in 2 of the 15 subjects, the tools concerning attention, executive functions, and memory before CP (Table 2), as well as at one month-follow-up, were not administrable (Table 3). However, over two years (i.e., at T2), all of our patients were able to complete the assessment. In addition, after CP, we found a significant improvement in all neuropsychological test scores (Table 3).

Table 2. Sample characteristics before reconstructive surgery.

ID	Sex	Age [1]	MMSE	TMT.A	TMT.B	RAVLT.I	RAVLT.R	TOKEN	DS	HAM.A	HAM.D
01	M	26	26	200	346	28.53	4.6	30	6	18	21
02	M	46	8	NA	NA	NA	NA	24.5	NA	16	18
03	F	41	24	280	512	31.25	3.3	33.5	5	19	21
04	M	29	NA	NA	NA	NA	NA	NA	NA	NA	NA
05	M	33	23	350	600	26.5	3.6	32.7	4	20	21
06	M	46	21	206	585	21.5	1.5	9.5	2	18	19
07	F	54	23	350	600	26.5	3.6	32.7	4	20	21
08	M	36	21	206	585	21.5	1.5	9.5	2	18	19
09	M	35	18	200	458	26	5	14.5	4	14	16
10	F	34	25	289	562	32.25	4.3	32.5	6	16	18
11	M	28	26	200	346	28.53	4.6	30	6	18	21
12	M	45	21	206	585	21.5	1.5	9.5	2	18	19
13	M	37	22	206	585	21.5	1.5	9.5	2	18	19
14	F	39	25	289	562	32.25	4.3	32.5	6	16	18
15	F	42	24	280	512	31.25	3.3	33.5	5	19	21

[1] Age is expressed in years. LEGEND: MMSE = Mini Mental State Examination; TMT = Trail Making Test; RAVL.I = Rey Auditory Verbal Learning (immediate); RAVL.R = Rey Auditory Verbal Learning (recall); HAM.D = Hamilton Rating Scale for depression; HAM.A = Hamilton Rating Scale for anxiety; DS = Digit span.

Table 3. Sample characteristics one month after reconstructive surgery.

ID	DC-CP [1]	MMSE	TMT.A	TMT.B	RAVLT.I	RAVLT.R	TOKEN	DS	HAM.A	HAM.D
01	1	28	60	100	29.53	7.6	32	7	12	10
02	9	10	NA	NA	NA	NA	26.5	NA	10	12
03	4	28	81	100	34.5	7	32.5	7	9	6
04	1	7	NA	NA	NA	NA	8.25	NA	NA	NA
05	9	28	55	120	33.5	7.6	32.7	6	10	10
06	10	26	90	240	30.5	6.5	20.4	6	10	6
07	11	28	55	120	33.5	7.6	32.7	6	10	10
08	12	26	100	240	30.5	6.5	20.4	6	10	6
09	12	24	120	300	38	9	30.25	5	10	12
10	8	26	80	180	33.5	6.7	32.5	6	10	10
11	2	28	60	100	29.53	7.6	32	7	12	10
12	11	26	90	240	30.5	6.5	20.4	6	10	6
13	12	26	100	240	30.5	6.5	20.4	6	10	6
14	9	26	80	180	33.5	6.7	32.5	6	10	10
15	6	28	81	100	34.5	7	32.5	7	9	6
Pre-Post changes p-values		0.001	0.002	0.002	0.002	0.002	0.014	0.003	<0.001	0.001

[1] The time passed between compressive craniectomy and cranioplasty (DC-CP) is expressed in months. LEGEND: MMSE = Mini Mental State Examination; TMT = Trail Making Test; RAVL.I = Rey Auditory Verbal Learning (immediate); RAVL.R = Rey Auditory Verbal Learning (recall); HAM.D = Hamilton Rating Scale for depression; HAM.A = Hamilton Rating Scale for anxiety; DS = Digit span.

Friedman's test detected significant differences in all outcomes except Digit Span, as reported in Table 4. All significant differences found by the post-hoc test are depicted in green in Figure 1.

Table 4. Subjects' scores over time, comparison analysis results by Friedman's test and Conover test.

Assessment	Scores at Each Examination (Median (First-Third Quartile))						Friedman Test	Post-Hoc Analysis	
	T0	T1	T2	T3	T4	T5	p-Value	Sign. Diff.	p-Value *
MMSE	26.0 (26.0–28.0)	28.0 (6.0–28.0)	28.0 (26.0–28.0)	28.0 (26.0–28.0)	28.0 (27.0–29.0)	28.0 (27.0–29.5)	<0.001	T4-T0 T5-T0 T5-T1	<0.001 <0.001 0.003
TMT.A TMT.B	81.0 (60.0–90.0) 180.0 (100.0–240.0)	81.0 (70.0–100.0) 180.0 (110.0–240.0)	80.0 (65.0–90.0) 170.0 (105.0–200.0)	60.0 (135.0–165.0) 160.0 (105.0–170.0)	50.0 (45.0–55.0) 100.0 (95.0–150.0)	40.0 (40.0–50.0) 90.0 (80.0–95.0)	<0.001	T4-T0 T5-T0 T4-T1 T5-T1 T5-T2	<0.001 <0.001 <0.001 <0.001 0.001
RAVLT.I RAVLT.R	33.5 (30.5–33.5) 7.0 (6.5–7.6)	33.5 (30.5–33.5) 7.0 (6.5–7.6)	34.0 (31.2–35.7) 7.0 (7.0–7.6)	35.0 (32.0–36.0) 7.0 (7.0–7.6)	35.0 (32.5–36.5) 8.0 (8.0–8.0)	36.0 (34.0–39.0) 8.0 (8.0–8.0)	<0.001	T4-T0 T5-T0 T4-T1 T5-T1 T5-T2	<0.001 <0.001 <0.001 <0.001 0.002
DIGIT SPAN	6.0 (6.0–7.0)	6.0 (6.0–7.0)	6.0 (6.0–7.0)	6.0 (6.0–7.0)	6.0 (6.0–7.0)	6.0 (6.0–7.0)	0.05	-	-
TOKEN	32.0 (20.4–32.5)	32.0 (20.4–32.5)	32.0 (30.0–32.7)	32.0 (30.0–32.7)	32.0 (30.0–32.7)	32.0 (30.0—32.7)	<0.001	T3-T0 T4-T0 T5-T0 T3-T1 T4-T1 T5-T1	0.002 <0.001 <0.001 0.003 <0.001 <0.001
HAM.A	10.0 (10.0–10.0)	10.0 (5.2–10.0)	10.0 (5.5–10.0)	9.0 (5.5–9.0)	4.0 (3.5–5.0)	3.0 (2.0–3.0)	<0.001	T4-T0 T5-T0 T4-T1 T5-T1 T4-T2 T5-T2 T5-T3	<0.001 <0.001 0.003 <0.001 0.003 <0.001 0.007
HAM.D	10.0 (6.0–10.0)	8.0 (5.2–10.0)	9.0 (5.5–10.0)	9.0 (5.5–9.0)	5.0 (4.0–6.0)	3.0 (3.0–4.0)	<0.001	T4-T0 T5-T0 T5-T1 T5-T2 T5-T3	<0.001 <0.001 <0.001 <0.001 0.001

LEGEND: MMSE = Mini Mental State Examination; TMT = Trail Making Test; RAVL.I = Rey Auditory Verbal Learning (immediate); RAVL.R = Rey Auditory Verbal Learning (recall); HAM.D = Hamilton Rating Scale for depression; HAM.A = Hamilton Rating Scale for anxiety. * with the Bonferroni's correction for six comparisons, the corrected level of significance was 0.008.

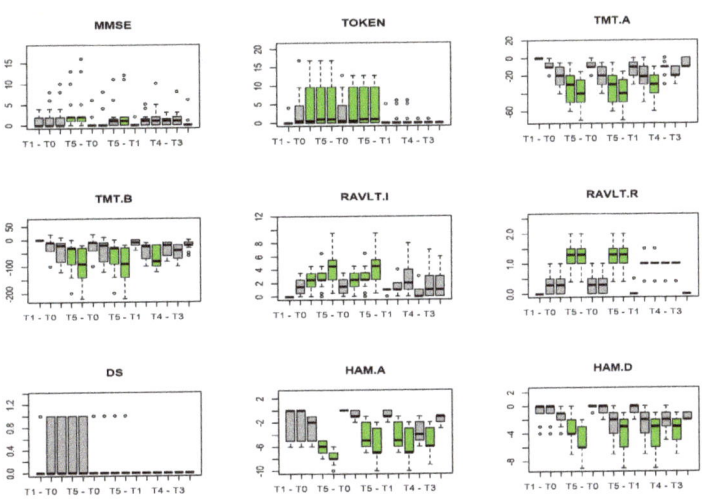

Figure 1. Boxplot of differences between times (T) for each neurophysiological test. T indicates the different time points.

Despite the absence of significant changes in Digit Span scores, the RAVLT test scores showed a gradual improvement in memory occurring over the years. The more significant differences in cognitive recovery have been detected after four years from cranioplasty. Indeed, no significant changes between T0 and T1, as well as between T1 and T2 emerged. On the contrary, we found significant differences between T4 and T0-T1, as well as between T5 and T0-T1-T2 in all battery tests. In addition, significant differences between T3 and T1 also emerged in TOKEN scores ($p = 0.003$).

4. Discussion

Cranioplasty following brain surgery is still a thorny debate. Several studies focusing on the materials used, surgical techniques, and timing to perform CP are present in the literature. However, a recent retrospective study [22] on a cohort of 40 patients with DC following severe TBI, compared with a reference population of 115 patients with DC due to other conditions, reports that a successful cranioplasty predicts a favorable outcome after 1 year, whereas patient outcome as assessed before cranioplasty does not predict cranioplasty success or failure.

To the best of our knowledge, this is the first study dealing with long-term cognitive and emotional outcomes of patients with TBI who underwent decompressive craniectomy. The findings of this retrospective study showed that cognitive performance may continue to improve over the years after cranioplasty, and in some cases, until a nearly complete neurological recovery. Overall, the more significant differences in cognitive recovery in our sample have been detected after four years from CP, given that no significant changes between T0 and T1, as well as between T1 and T2 emerged.

The improvement in neurological status after CP was not so surprising for different reasons. First, we must consider that our patients were young, hence with a higher "cognitive reserve" due to a better neuronal plasticity; and that patients following TBI usually present a better recovery, even after months/years from the acute event [23]. The mechanisms subtending these improvements after CP could be the increase of cerebral blood flow and neural metabolism, as well as changes in cerebrospinal fluid hydrodynamic. In order to repair structural defects caused by DC, cranioplasty seems to be the best way to balance the atmospheric pressure on the cranial defects. Increasing the overall intracranial compliance, cerebrospinal fluid velocity, and the flow in the craniospinal junction may promote better blood flow circulation, especially at the cerebral cortex level, also the modifying metabolic gap. Therefore, the increase in cerebral blood flow could be the key component to boost neuralplasticity and then motor and cognitive functioning [5,12]. After all, cranioplasty can remarkably improve cerebrospinal fluid (CSF) dynamics and provide cortical perfusion for both the ipsilateral and contralateral hemispheres. In their study, Shahid et al. [24] reported an improvement in cerebral perfusion in different lobes in around 94% of patients. Sarubbo et al. [25] observed a progressive decline of cortical perfusion in the injured hemisphere and a stable perfusion in the contralateral hemisphere after surgery, hypothesizing a possible role of cranioplasty in restoring flow to meet the prevailing metabolic demand. An increase in CSF flow and CBF with a potentially related improvement in cognitive function was also observed by other authors. The causative impact of CSF on neurological function, however, requires further study.

Second, patients performed neuropsychological rehabilitation during the hospitalization, which promoted an improvement in cognitive function [26–28]. Therefore, part of the recovery could be due to such specific training. Previous studies have shown that if an intensive and multidisciplinary rehabilitation program starts early, then the cognitive and motor recovery will be better. Therefore, it is possible to attribute part of the recovery occurring immediately after the CP to this surgical procedure, while the gradual improvement of cognitive and functional outcomes is probably due to a competitive effect between the surgical procedure and rehabilitation [29–31].

Third, most of the subjects did not have a severe cognitive impairment before CP. It is well-known that the severity of the brain injury and the degree of pre-cranioplasty deficits may influence the degree of cerebral blood flow improvement after CP and the patient's subsequent neurological recovery [22]. However, in our study, in three subjects with a severe deficit in attention, executive functions, and memory before CP, and/or at one-month follow-up, the improvement was so high over three to four years after the injury that they were eventually able to complete the assessment with satisfactory scores.

Only a few studies have strictly focused on cognitive recovery after this surgical procedure, and the assessment was often performed with different tools [4–8]. On the contrary, many studies have aimed to understand the right timing to perform cranioplasty after DC. Thus, most studies report about functional and cognitive improvements in patients with severe TBI, especially when the surgical procedure has been performed within three to twelve months after the event [23]. Indeed, early CP was found to improve cognitive function by restoring CSF hydrodynamics, intracranial compliance, and cerebral blood flow when neurocognitive changes are at their peak [26]. However, when is the right timing to perform CP is still controversial because it variably affects functional recovery and is also a risk factor for infections and other complications [32,33]. Archavlis et al. [34], in a 10-year retrospective study on a cohort of 200 patients, observed that patients who performed CP within 7 weeks from the decompressive craniectomy had an improvement of 78% (measured by the GCS) versus the 46% observed in patients who underwent cranioplasty after 7–12 weeks and only 12% after 12 weeks. Di Stefano et al. [35] found a low probability of complications when CP was performed within 3 months from the decompressive craniectomy, whereas the work by Corallo et al. [36] sustains that the timing of cranioplasty is independent of neurologic outcomes. However, the recent review by De Cola et al. [12] concluded that CP performed within 3 months from DC may lead to greater effects on motor functions, whereas for the cognitive domain, the best choice seems to be performing CP from 3 to 6 months, especially if the patient has received neuropsychological rehabilitation.

The novelty of this study is the long-term observation of cognitive and emotional outcomes in the TBI population after cranioplasty. In our opinion, long-term cognitive follow-ups of patients are fundamental to understand if there was a complete recovery, as the significantly improvement over the years highlighted by our findings. Beyond the recovery immediately observed after cranioplasty, this study reports a clear improvement even in patients who initially had a minor and slow recovery. In this prospective, the timing of cranioplasty could become less important, since the effects can distribute over time, and patients continued to improve.

Last but not least, our findings also report a significant improvement in mood, most likely concurring with long-term acceptance of the traumatic event and the return to a normal life.

The main limitation of the study consists in the small sample size, and therefore our results, though promising, needs to be interpreted with caution. Larger and multicenter studies should be fostered to confirm these promising findings. Moreover, the retrospective nature of the study may cause some information bias since we used existing records, as well as a bias due to the lack of a control group. However, we did not assess CP effects on recovery, but we only observed the recovery over time. In fact, the long-term follow-ups and the complete neuropsychological battery represent the main strength of the study.

5. Conclusions

This retrospective study further suggests the importance of CP in the complex management of patients with TBI showing that patients might continue to improve their cognitive function over a long period after the surgical procedure. Further larger sample prospective studies with longer follow-up period are needed to confirm these findings and better clarify the role of CP and neuropsychological rehabilitation in the functional recovery of these frail patients.

Author Contributions: Conceptualization, F.C., R.S.C. and M.C.D.C.; methodology, R.S.C. and M.C.D.C.; validation, V.L.B.; formal analysis, M.C.D.C.; investigation, F.C. and V.L.B.; data curation, F.C.; writing—original draft preparation, F.C. and M.C.D.C.; writing—review and editing, R.S.C. and V.L.B.; supervision, R.S.C. and M.C.D.C. All authors have read and agreed to the published version of the manuscript.

Funding: This research received no external funding.

Institutional Review Board Statement: The ethics committee was not necessary because the clinical data were not beyond the scope of normal clinical practice.

Informed Consent Statement: Informed consent was obtained from all subjects involved in the study.

Data Availability Statement: The data presented in this study are available on request from the corresponding author. The data are not publicly available due to Hospital policy.

Conflicts of Interest: The authors declare no conflict of interest.

References

1. Rossini, Z.; Nicolosi, F.; Kolias, A.; Hutchinson, P.J.; De Sanctis, P.; Servadei, F. The History of Decompressive Craniectomy in Traumatic Brain Injury. *Front. Neurol.* **2019**, *10*, 458. [CrossRef]
2. Brown, D.; Wijdicks, E. Decompressive craniectomy in acute brain injury. *Cerebellum Embryol. Diagn. Investig.* **2017**, *140*, 299–318. [CrossRef]
3. Champeaux, C.; Weller, J. Long-Term Survival After Decompressive Craniectomy for Malignant Brain Infarction: A 10-Year Nationwide Study. *Neurocritical Care* **2019**, *32*, 522–531. [CrossRef] [PubMed]
4. Barthélemy, E.J.; Melis, M.; Gordon, E.; Ullman, J.S.; Germano, I.M. Decompressive Craniectomy for Severe Traumatic Brain Injury: A Systematic Review. *World Neurosurg.* **2016**, *88*, 411–420. [CrossRef]
5. Corallo, F.; De Cola, M.C.; Lo Buono, V.; Marra, A.; De Luca, R.; Trinchera, A.; Bramanti, P.; Calabrò, R.S. Early vs late cranioplasty: What is better? *Int. J. Neurosci.* **2017**, *127*, 688–693. [CrossRef] [PubMed]
6. Sveikata, L.; Vasung, L.; El Rahal, A.; Bartoli, A.; Bretzner, M.; Schaller, K.; Schnider, A.; Leemann, B. Syndrome of the trephined: Clinical spectrum, risk factors, and impact of cranioplasty on neurologic recovery in a prospective cohort. *Neurosurg. Rev.* **2021**, 1–13. [CrossRef]
7. Agner, C.; Dujovny, M.; Gaviria, M. Neurocognitive assessment before and after cranioplasty. *Acta Neurochir.* **2002**, *144*, 1033–1040. [CrossRef]
8. Juul, N.; Morris, G.F.; Marshall, S.B.; Marshall, L.F. Intracranial hypertension and cerebral perfusion pressure: Influence on neurological deterioration and outcome in severe head injury. *J. Neurosurg.* **2000**, *92*, 1–6. [CrossRef]
9. Mokri, B. Orthostatic Headaches in the Syndrome of the Trephined: Resolution Following Cranioplasty. *Headache J. Head Face Pain* **2010**, *50*, 1206–1211. [CrossRef]
10. Corallo, F.; Marra, A.; Bramanti, P.; Calabrò, R.S. Effect of cranioplasty on functional and neuro-psychological recovery after severe acquired brain injury: Fact or fake? Considerations on a single case. *Funct. Neurol.* **2014**, *29*, 273–275. [CrossRef]
11. Malcolm, J.G.; Rindler, R.S.; Chu, J.K.; Chokshi, F.; Grossberg, J.A.; Pradilla, G.; Ahmad, F.U. Early Cranioplasty is Associated with Greater Neurological Improvement: A Systematic Review and Meta-Analysis. *Neurosurgery* **2018**, *82*, 278–288. [CrossRef] [PubMed]
12. De Cola, M.C.; Corallo, F.; Pria, D.; Buono, V.L.; Calabrò, R.S. Timing for cranioplasty to improve neurological outcome: A systematic review. *Brain Behav.* **2018**, *8*, e01106. [CrossRef] [PubMed]
13. Wachter, D.; Reineke, K.; Behm, T.; Rohde, V. Cranioplasty after decompressive hemicraniectomy: Underestimated surgery-associated complications? *Clin. Neurol. Neurosurg.* **2013**, *115*, 1293–1297. [CrossRef] [PubMed]
14. Morton, R.P.; Abecassis, I.J.; Hanson, J.F.; Barber, J.K.; Chen, M.; Kelly, C.M.; Nerva, J.D.; Emerson, S.N.; Ene, C.I.; Levitt, M.R.; et al. Timing of cranioplasty: A 10.75-year single-center analysis of 754 patients. *J. Neurosurg.* **2018**, *128*, 1648–1652. [CrossRef]
15. Magni, E.; Binetti, G.; Bianchetti, A.; Rozzini, R.; Trabucchi, M. Mini-Mental State Examination: A normative study in Italian elderly population. *Eur. J. Neurol.* **1996**, *3*, 198–202. [CrossRef]
16. McMINN, M.R.; Wiens, A.N.; Crossen, J.R. Rey auditory-verbal learning test: Development of norms for healthy young adults. *Clin. Neuropsychol.* **1988**, *2*, 67–87. [CrossRef]
17. Orsini, A.; Grossi, D.; Capitani, E.; Laiacona, M.; Papagno, C.; Vallar, G. Verbal and spatial immediate memory span: Norma-tive data from 1355 adults and 1112 children. *Ital. J. Neurol. Sci.* **1987**, *8*, 539–548. [CrossRef]
18. De Renzi, E.; Faglioni, P. Normative data and screening power of a shortened version of the Token Test. *Cortex* **1978**, *14*, 41–49. [CrossRef]
19. Gaudino, E.A.; Geisler, M.W.; Squires, N.K. Construct validity in the trail making test: What makes part B harder? *J. Clin. Exp. Neuropsychol.* **1995**, *17*, 529–535. [CrossRef]
20. Hamilton, M. The assessment of anxiety states by rating. *Br. J. Med. Psychol.* **1959**, *32*, 50–55. [CrossRef]
21. Hamilton, M. A rating scale for depression. *J. Neurol. Neurosurg. Psychiatr.* **1960**, *23*, 56. [CrossRef] [PubMed]

22. Posti, J.P.; Yli-Olli, M.; Heiskanen, L.; Aitasalo, K.M.J.; Rinne, J.; Vuorinen, V.; Serlo, W.; Tenovuo, O.; Vallittu, P.K.; Piitulainen, J.M. Cranioplasty After Severe Traumatic Brain Injury: Effects of Trauma and Patient Recovery on Cranioplasty Outcome. *Front. Neurol.* **2018**, *9*, 223. [CrossRef]
23. Halani, S.H.; Chu, J.K.; Malcolm, J.G.; Rindler, R.S.; Allen, J.W.; Grossberg, J.A.; Pradilla, G.; Ahmad, F.U. Effects of Cranio-plasty on Cerebral Blood Flow Following Decompressive Craniectomy: A Systematic Review of the Literature. *Neurosurgery* **2017**, *81*, 204–216. [CrossRef] [PubMed]
24. Shahid, A.H.; Mohanty, M.; Singla, N.; Mittal, B.R.; Gupta, S.K. The effect of cranioplasty following decompressive craniec-tomy on cerebral blood perfusion, neurological, and cognitive outcome. *J. Neurosurg.* **2018**, *128*, 229–235. [CrossRef] [PubMed]
25. Sarubbo, S.; Latini, F.; Ceruti, S.; Chieregato, A.; D'Esterre, C.; Lee, T.-Y.; Cavallo, M.; Fainardi, E. Temporal changes in CT perfusion values before and after cranioplasty in patients without symptoms related to external decompression: A pilot study. *Neurosurger* **2014**, *56*, 237–243. [CrossRef]
26. Erdogan, E.; Düz, B.; Kocaoglu, M.; Izci, Y.; Sirin, S.; Timurkaynak, E. The effect of cranioplasty on cerebral hemodynamics: Evaluation with transcranial Doppler sonography. *Neurol. India* **2003**, *51*, 479–481.
27. Panwar, N.; Agrawal, M.; Sinha, V.D. Postcranioplasty Quantitative Assessment of Intracranial Fluid Dynamics and Its Im-pact on Neurocognition Cranioplasty Effect: A Pilot Study. *World Neurosurg.* **2019**, *122*, e96–e107. [CrossRef]
28. Su, J.-H.; Wu, Y.-H.; Guo, N.-W.; Huang, C.-F.; Li, C.-F.; Chen, C.-H.; Huang, M.-H. The effect of cranioplasty in cognitive and functional improvement: Experience of post traumatic brain injury inpatient rehabilitation. *Kaohsiung J. Med. Sci.* **2017**, *33*, 344–350. [CrossRef]
29. Rynkowski, C.B.; Robba, C.; Loreto, M.; Theisen, A.C.W.; Kolias, A.G.; Finger, G.; Czosnyka, M.; Bianchin, M.M. Effects of Cranioplasty After Decompressive Craniectomy on Neurological Function and Cerebral Hemodynamics in Traumatic Versus Nontraumatic Brain Injury. *How Improv. Results Peripher. Nerve Surg.* **2021**, *131*, 79–82. [CrossRef]
30. Naro, A.; Billeri, L.; Manuli, A.; Balletta, T.; Cannavò, A.; Portaro, S.; Lauria, P.; Ciappina, F.; Calabrò, R.S. Breaking the ice to improve motor outcomes in patients with chronic stroke: A retrospective clinical study on neuromodulation plus robotics. *Neurol. Sci.* **2020**, *42*, 2785–2793. [CrossRef]
31. Keute, M.; Gharabaghi, A. Brain plasticity and vagus nerve stimulation. *Auton. Neurosci.* **2021**, *236*, 102876. [CrossRef] [PubMed]
32. Dang, Y.; Ping, J.; Guo, Y.; Yang, J.; Xia, X.; Huang, R.; Zhang, J.; He, J. Cranioplasty for patients with disorders of con-sciousness. *Ann. Palliat. Med.* **2021**, *10*, 8889–8899. [CrossRef]
33. Alkhaibary, A.; Alharbi, A.; Alnefaie, N.; Almubarak, A.O.; Aloraidi, A.; Khairy, S. Cranioplasty: A Comprehensive Review of the History, Materials, Surgical Aspects, and Complications. *World Neurosurg.* **2020**, *139*, 445–452. [CrossRef] [PubMed]
34. Archavlis, E.; Nievas, M.C.Y. The impact of timing of cranioplasty in patients with large cranial defects after decompressive hemi-craniectomy. *Actaneurochir* **2012**, *154*, 1055–1062.
35. Di Stefano, C.; Sturiale, C.; Trentini, P.; Bonora, R.; Rossi, D.; Cervigni, G.; Piperno, R. Unexpected neuropsychological improve-ment after cranioplasty: A case series study. *Br. J. Neurosurg.* **2012**, *26*, 827–831. [CrossRef]
36. Corallo, F.; De Cola, M.C.; Buono, V.L.; Cammaroto, S.; Marra, A.; Manuli, A.; Calabrò, R.S. Recovery of Severe Aphasia After Cranioplasty: Considerations on a Case Study. *Rehabil. Nurs.* **2020**, *45*, 238–242. [CrossRef]

MDPI
St. Alban-Anlage 66
4052 Basel
Switzerland
Tel. +41 61 683 77 34
Fax +41 61 302 89 18
www.mdpi.com

Journal of Clinical Medicine Editorial Office
E-mail: jcm@mdpi.com
www.mdpi.com/journal/jcm

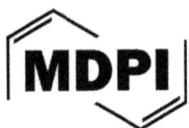

www.ingramcontent.com/pod-product-compliance
Lightning Source LLC
LaVergne TN
LVHW070644100526
838202LV00013B/877